2004

W9-BCE-424

MINORITY POPULATIONS AND HEALTH

MINORITY POPULATIONS AND HEALTH

An Introduction to Health Disparities in the United States

Thomas A. LaVeist

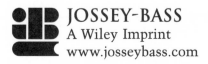

JOSSEY-BASS
A Wiley Imprint
www.josseybass.com

Published by Jossey-Bass
A Wiley Imprint
989 Market Street, San Francisco, CA 94103-1741   www.josseybass.com

Jossey-Bass books and products are available through most bookstores. To contact Jossey-Bass directly call our Customer Care Department within the U.S. at 800-956-7739, outside the U.S. at 317-572-399386 or fax 317-572-4002.

Jossey-Bass also publishes its books in a variety of electronic formats. Some content that appears in print may not be available in electronic books.

Library of Congress Cataloging-in-Publication Data

LaVeist, Thomas Alexis.
  Minority populations and health : introduction to health disparities in the United States / Thomas A. LaVeist.— 1st ed.
    p. ; cm.
  Includes bibliographical references and index.
  ISBN 0-7879-6413-1 (alk. paper)
  1. Minorities—Health and hygiene—United States. 2. Minorities—Medical care—United States. 3. Ethnic groups—Health and hygiene—United States. 4. Ethnic groups—Medical care—United States. 5. Health services accessibility—United States. 6. Discrimination in medical care—United States. 7. Equality—Health aspects—United States. 8. Health status indicators—United States. 9. Health and race—United States. 10. Health behavior—United States.
  [DNLM: 1. Health Status—United States. 2. Minority Groups—United States. 3. Delivery of Health Care—United States. 4. Health Behavior—ethnology—United States. 5. Health Services Accessibility—United States. 6. Socioeconomic Factors—United States.] I. Title.
  RA448.4.L38 2005
  362.1'089'00973—dc22

                                                                          2004030570

Printed in the United States of America
FIRST EDITION
HB Printing   10 9 8 7 6 5 4 3 2 1

CONTENTS

PART THREE: ETIOLOGY OF RACIAL/ETHNIC DIFFERENCES IN HEALTH 131

PART FOUR: RACIAL/ETHNIC GROUP–SPECIFIC HEALTH ISSUES 203

PART FIVE: CONCLUSIONS 281

TABLES AND FIGURES

Tables

Figures

PREFACE

For fifteen years I have been teaching courses on health inequality at both the undergraduate and graduate level at Johns Hopkins. I have long bemoaned the fact that nobody had written a textbook I would use in the class. I made do with article reprints and my own notes. As I compared experiences with colleagues who teach similar classes at other universities, it became clear that a textbook needed to be written.

The field has evolved and the number of people interested in health disparities and heath inequalities has grown. And there is every reason to believe that it will continue to grow for the foreseeable future. Now we need the curricula to support the expanding interest. I hope this book is a step toward creating those curricula.

Completing a book of this scope largely depends on how well you can convince others to help. Naturally, I did not possess all of the necessary knowledge to write this book alone. My learning curve was *very* steep for some of the chapters. In those cases I benefited greatly from consultations with colleagues and friends who helped me to make sense of what I was reading and writing.

At the risk of missing someone important, I would like to acknowledge each of the people who helped me along the way. Without their help I certainly could not have completed this project. It is also important that I be clear that I am listing them in alphabetical order.

I would like to thank Phillip Blanc (University of Medicine and Dentistry of New Jersey), Tamarya Carroll (Spelman College), and Paulina Lopez (Johns Hopkins University), my team of dedicated students who read drafts and ripped them apart.

Their help definitely made this a better book! I am particularly grateful to them for their input regarding what features make a textbook most usable. They helped me to view the book through the student's eye.

I am grateful for the assistance of many colleagues who graciously lent their expertise by responding to questions, sending reprints, giving me figures and charts, forwarding articles, and reading drafts of chapters. Specifically, they are Cheryl Alexander (Johns Hopkins Bloomberg School of Public Health), Lori Edwards (Shaw University), Tiffany Gary (Johns Hopkins Bloomberg School of Public Health), Darrell Gaskin (Johns Hopkins Bloomberg School of Public Health), Miryam Granthen (U.S. Department of Health and Human Services), Daniel L. Howard (Shaw University), John Lynch (University of Michigan), Katrina McDonald (Johns Hopkins University), Thomas McGuire (Harvard University), Kim Nickerson (American Psychological Association), Brian Smedley (Institute of Medicine), Sharon Smith (Johns Hopkins Bloomberg School of Public Health), David R. Williams (University of Michigan), and John M. Wallace, Jr. (University of Pittsburgh School of Social Work).

I would like to single out Dr. Duane Thomas (Johns Hopkins Bloomberg School of Public Health) for a special thank-you. Without Duane's help on the mental health chapter it might have taken me another year to complete this book. Duane was a godsend! I got a great deal of helpful advice from my fellow participants on the Spirit of 1848 (American Public Health Association Caucus) listserv. The participants on that listserv are some of the most knowledgeable and helpful people around.

The staff at Jossey-Bass were patient and understanding each time I missed deadlines (which I did often). I am grateful to them for alleviating the anxiety and helping reduce the stress associated with writing a book . They were great to work with!

I am particularly indebted to the staff of the Hopkins Center for Health Disparities Solutions for their assistance, particularly Devony Blyden, John Jackson, and Lydia Isaac. I am most indebted to Lydia Isaac for "keeping the ship afloat" during the times that I was away writing, reading drafts, and helping me to stay organized.

I would like to acknowledge my family, who are always both a help and a hindrance. My wife, Bridgette LaVeist, herself a public health professional, read drafts of several chapters while constantly asking when I would be finished. And my children: Clay, Naomi, Randall, and Carlton, your very existence drives me to work harder, while at the same time reminding me to stop and smell the roses. My first act after completing this book will be to take my four-year-old son Clay to the store to buy the model car he has been asking me about, so we can build it together.

Finally, I thank God, who continues to bless me even when I least deserve it! Thank you for the unconditional love.

T.L.

ABOUT THE AUTHOR

Thomas A. LaVeist is director of the Center for Health Disparities Solutions and professor of health policy and management at the Johns Hopkins Bloomberg School of Public Health. He teaches courses in health inequality, health disparities, and public health policy. LaVeist is a frequent visiting lecturer on minority health issues at other universities and at professional conferences and workshops. He often consults to federal agencies on minority health issues and racial disparities in health. LaVeist has conducted several important studies on related topics; his research has been funded by the National Institutes of Health, the National Center for Minority Health and Health Disparities, the Center for Disease Control, the Commonwealth Fund, the Russell Sage Foundation, the Kellogg Foundation, and the Robert Wood Johnson Foundation.

LaVeist received his bachelor of arts degree from the University of Maryland, Eastern Shore, and his doctorate in medical sociology from the University of Michigan. His dissertation was awarded the Roberta G. Simmons Outstanding Dissertation Award, for the best doctoral dissertation in medical sociology, by the American Sociological Association in 1989. He held a postdoctoral fellowship in public health at the University of Michigan, School of Public Health. LaVeist joined the Johns Hopkins faculty in 1990. He has published numerous articles in scientific journals and is author of *The DayStar Guide to Colleges for African American Students* (Kaplan Interactive, 2000), coauthor of *Eight Steps to Help Black Families Pay for College* (Princeton Review, 2003), and editor of *Race, Ethnicity, and Health: A Public Health Reader* (Jossey-Bass, 2002).

MINORITY POPULATIONS AND HEALTH

CHAPTER ONE

HISTORICAL ASPECTS OF RACE/ETHNICITY AND HEALTH

The history of the relationship between the U.S. government and racial/ethnic minorities plays an important role in understanding why health disparities exist and how they might be eliminated. In this introduction I will provide a brief overview of the history that has led to the contemporary state of health disparities. I will then discuss likely future trends and why the study of minority health is important. I will then end the chapter with a discussion of decisions made in deciding the terminology that will be used to refer to the various racial/ethnic groups to be discussed in this book.

Historical Background

Figure 1.1 summarizes the status of African Americans throughout the history of the United States. The exact date the first Africans arrived in the country is in dispute. Some historians place this as early as Columbus's first voyage, but the most commonly cited date is August 1619 (Quarles, 1987). From that point until President Lincoln issued the Emancipation Proclamation in 1863 (freeing the Africans who lived in the states that had seceded from the country, but not those in states that were not part of the confederacy), the country's African population was primarily slaves, although in every state there were some who were not slaves. The period of slavery lasted 244 years—63.4 percent of the time between 1619 and 2004.

FIGURE 1.1.   CHANGING STATUS OF AFRICAN AMERICANS IN U.S.
HISTORY, 1619–2004.

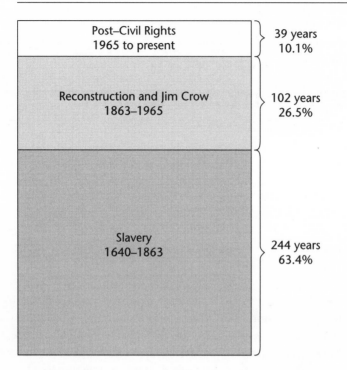

BOX 1.1.   THIRTEENTH, FOURTEENTH, AND FIFTEENTH
AMENDMENTS TO THE U.S. CONSTITUTION.

The Thirteenth Amendment, ratified in 1865, outlawed slavery in the United States and all territories.

The Fourteenth Amendment, ratified in 1868, gave citizenship to all persons born in the U.S. or naturalized.

The Fifteenth Amendment, ratified in 1870, barred states from prohibiting any male citizen from voting. All females received the right to vote with the ratification of the Nineteenth Amendment in 1920.

The end of slavery throughout the country came when the Thirteenth Amendment to the U.S. Constitution was ratified in 1865. This also began the Reconstruction era and the "Jim Crow" period, in which the black codes relegated racial and ethnic minorities to second-class citizenship. These state laws limited or even prohibited racial minorities from exercising voting rights, reducing them to receiving substandard health care and education (Quarles, 1987; Smith, 1999).

In the early twentieth century, separate health care facilities for African Americans began to be developed, mainly by churches. Medical schools for Black doctors were created because most existing medical schools would not admit African Americans. These medical schools and Black hospitals were not as well funded as their segregated counterparts. When African Americans did have interactions with the White medical system (typically in segregated wards), the discourteous nature of the interpersonal communications during these medical encounters produced inequalities in medical treatment. These factors, along with other historical events such as the Tuskegee Syphilis Study, led to racial and ethnic disparities in the access to and utilization of health services and to distrust of the medical care system among racial and ethnic minorities.

In many ways the history of African Americans parallels the history of Native Americans. The arrival of the European settlers in the New World led to the introduction of diseases not native to the continent (such as measles and yellow fever). Disease outbreaks along with war led to the decimation of the Native American population. The importation of Africans to serve as free labor introduced a new group who, along with Native Americans, were barred from access to state-of-the-art health care, clean water, and good quality housing. In 1830, thirty-three years before the Emancipation Proclamation, the United States Congress passed the Indian Removal

---

BOX 1.2.   THE FIVE CIVILIZED TRIBES.

The *Civilized Tribes* were the five American Indian tribes living in the southeastern United States before forced relocation. They were among the first tribes to encounter European settlers. Over time the settlers and tribe members intermarried. By the early 1800s, these tribes had established businesses and their own constitutions, codes of law, and judicial systems. The Civilized Tribes are

Cherokee (Muskogee Confederation): Georgia

Seminole: Florida

Creek: Alabama and Georgia

Chickisaw: Mississippi

Choctaw: Mississippi

Act, which was signed into law by President Andrew Jackson. The act ushered in a period of forcible removal of the so-called five Civilized Tribes and their relocation (referred to as the Trail of Tears) to reservations in the Oklahoma territory.

BOX 1.3.   BLACK MEDICAL SCHOOLS.

Today there are four historically Black medical schools: Howard University College of Medicine in Washington, D.C.; Meherry Medical College in Nashville, Tennessee; Charles R. Drew University of Medicine and Science in Los Angeles, California; and Morehouse School of Medicine in Atlanta, Georgia.

BOX 1.4.   THE TUSKEGEE SYPHILIS STUDY.

The Tuskegee Syphilis Study, carried out in Macon County, Alabama, from 1932 to 1972, is an example of medical research gone wrong. The United States Public Health Service, in trying to learn more about syphilis and justify treatment programs for blacks, withheld adequate treatment from a group of poor black men who had the disease, causing needless pain and suffering for the men and their loved ones. . . .

The study involved 600 black men—399 with syphilis and 201 who did not have the disease. Researchers told the men they were being treated for "bad blood," a local term used to describe several ailments, including syphilis, anemia, and fatigue. In truth, they did not receive the proper treatment needed to cure their illness. In exchange for taking part in the study, the men received free medical exams, free meals, and burial insurance. Although originally projected to last 6 months, the study actually went on for 40 years. . . .

In the summer of 1973, a class-action lawsuit filed by the National Association for the Advancement of Colored People (NAACP) ended in a settlement that gave more than $9 million to the study participants. As part of the settlement, the U.S. government promised to give free medical and burial services to all living participants. The Tuskegee Health Benefit Program was established to provide these services. It also gave health services for wives, widows, and children who had been infected because of the study.

Source: Centers for Disease Control and Prevention, "CDC Tuskegee Syphilis Study Page," http://www.cdc.gov/nchstp/od/tuskegee/index.html.

BOX 1.5.   THE CIVIL RIGHTS AND VOTING RIGHTS ACTS.

The Civil Rights Act of 1964 prohibited discrimination in public accommodations such as mass transportation, restaurants, and hotels on the basis of race, color, religion, or national origin.

The Voting Rights Act of 1965 eliminated discriminatory election practices. Specifically, it suspended literacy tests and provided for the appointment of federal examiners (with the power to register qualified citizens to vote) in those jurisdictions that were "covered," according to a formula provided in the statute. In addition, under Section 5 of the Act, covered jurisdictions were required to obtain "preclearance" for new voting practices and procedures from either the District Court for the District of Columbia or the United States Attorney General. Section 2 of the Act, which closely followed the language of the Fifteenth Amendment, applied a nationwide prohibition of denial or abridgment of the right to vote on account of race or color.

Treaties between the U.S. government and the various American Indian tribes typically promised education and health care. The responsibility for provision of health care was left to the U.S. Army, which was neither equipped nor provided the resources necessary to provide adequate care. Later the U.S. government established the Bureau of Indian Affairs (BIA), which assumed responsibility for providing health care to the American Indian population. The establishment of the Indian Health Service in 1955 led to the creation of a federal agency whose primary mission was the provision of health care to Native Americans. That same year, Rosa Parks's refusal to give up her seat on a Montgomery, Alabama, bus sparking the bus boycott that ignited the Civil Rights movement of the 1950s and 1960s (Morris, 1986).

Coming out of the civil rights movement were the Civil Rights Act of 1964 and the Voting Rights Act of 1965. These acts dismantled the most limiting components of the "Jim Crow" laws (black codes) and fulfilled the constitutional guarantees contained in the Fourteenth and Fifteenth Amendments. The Civil Rights movement shifted governmental policy away from support of racially discriminatory social norms such as racially segregated hospitals. As governmental policy shifted, the power of government shifted away from support of discrimination in favor of the enforcement of policies to dismantle discrimination in health care settings.

Today, health care facilities face the threat of government sanctions if they are found to be engaging in racially discriminatory practices. Minority health care providers can be found treating White patients, and it is not unusual to find White and non-White patients sharing hospital rooms. Yet although rigid segregation and overt discrimination are now illegal, the consequences are still with us. The health status disparities and health care disparities that have resulted are outlined in the chapters that follow.

FIGURE 1.2.   PROJECTED PERCENTAGE OF RESIDENT
U.S. POPULATION BY RACE/ETHNICITY, 2010–2070.

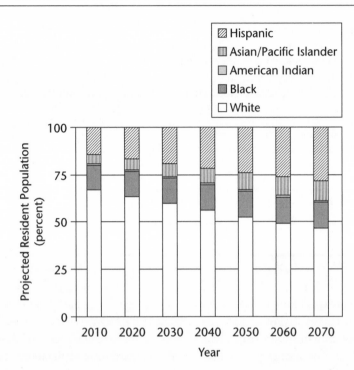

Source: U.S. Bureau of the Census, "Projections of the Resident Population by Race, Hispanic Origin, and Nativity: Middle Series, 1999 to 2100" (NP-T5).

Why Is It Important to Study Minority Health?

The last few decades of the twentieth century witnessed an explosion in the number of racial/ethnic minorities, particularly Hispanics/Latinos/Chicanos and Asians. This increase has occurred largely because of immigration, but that's not the only reason. Every major racial/ethnic group for which the U.S. government keeps records (African American-Black, Native American-American Indian-Alaska Native, Asian-Pacific Islander, and Hispanic-Latino-Chicano) has a higher fertility rate than White Americans. For this reason the U.S. Bureau of the Census projects that by the middle of the twenty-first century the United States will be a "majority-minority" country (see Figure 1.2). Whites will make up less than 50 percent of the U.S. population, and racial/ethnic groups that we now consider minorities will total more than 50 percent.

As the country undergoes this transition, health statistics for the nation as a whole will become a reflection of the health status of racial minorities. What we now call minority health will become the nation's health. And, as we will learn in the chapters that follow, racial/ethnic minorities generally have a worse health status than Whites.

At the same time, the United States is undergoing another demographic transition. The baby boomers will soon be entering their senior years—the first wave of Boomers will celebrate their sixty-fifth birthdays in 2011. As this happens, the ranks of the elderly will expand tremendously, and this will continue for several decades. These two demographic trends—an aging society combined with increasing proportions of minorities—will place increasing demands on a health care system that seems ill-prepared to handle it. Thus it's important for minority health to be a central feature of training programs in public health, medicine, nursing, social work, pharmaceutical science, and other disciplines that relate to health, such as the biological and the social sciences. We must prepare the next generation of health professionals to work with and in minority populations.

A Note on Terminology and Placing Humans in Categories

Group identity is very important to humans. It goes to the core of who we are and where we see ourselves fitting into the world. There is nothing more human than to think in terms of in-groups. At a fundamental psychological level, we think of ourselves as belonging to *this* group and *not* belonging to *that* group. And we all belong to many groups.

We know how to identify others in our in-groups. Sometimes we can identify in-group members via a secret handshake. Other times we determine membership by more subtle means, such as physical appearance. The process of identifying in-group members is easiest when there is a secret handshake, password, or similar objective process. It is easier to tell who is in the group and who is not; either they know the

---

BOX 1.6.   HISPANIC/LATINOS CROSS ALL OTHER MAJOR RACIAL/ETHNIC GROUPS.

Black Hispanic	Cuba, Dominican Republic, Puerto Rico
White Hispanic	Cuba, Dominican Republic, Puerto Rico, Argentina, Colombia
Indian Hispanic	Latin American Indians, Peru, Ecuador, Mexico
Asian Hispanic	Filipinos

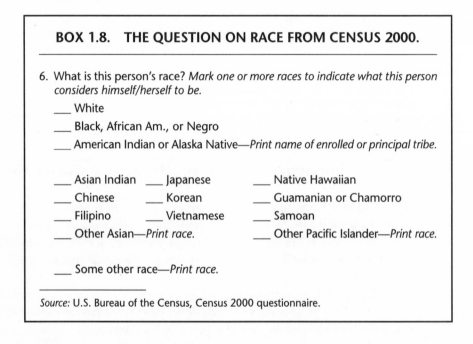

BOX 1.7. OMB DIRECTIVE 15.

The Office of Budget and Management's Directive 15 established standards for the collection of data on race and ethnicity. The original version of OMB Directive 15 was released in 1977; version 2 was issued in 1997.

BOX 1.8. THE QUESTION ON RACE FROM CENSUS 2000.

6. What is this person's race? *Mark one or more races to indicate what this person considers himself/herself to be.*
___ White
___ Black, African Am., or Negro
___ American Indian or Alaska Native—*Print name of enrolled or principal tribe.*

___ Asian Indian   ___ Japanese   ___ Native Hawaiian
___ Chinese   ___ Korean   ___ Guamanian or Chamorro
___ Filipino   ___ Vietnamese   ___ Samoan
___ Other Asian—*Print race.*   ___ Other Pacific Islander—*Print race.*

___ Some other race—*Print race.*

Source: U.S. Bureau of the Census, Census 2000 questionnaire.

handshake or they don't. But when it comes to racial or ethnic groups, there is no secret handshake. Instead, we try to identify groups by appearance, culture, nationality, and so on.

Variation in humans exists across many domains, such as skin color, hair texture, nationality, culture, shared history, language, or religion. These domains overlap. A person could be a Cuban American of African descent who has lived most of his or her life in a predominantly Chamorro community in the Marianas Islands and speaks mainly Chamoru on a daily basis. Which group does this person belong to?

An extreme example? Yes. But the point is that human variation does not conform to categories. However, categories are all we have to work with.

The United States' Office of Management and Budget (OMB) went through a multiyear process of determining how to create a set of categories that capture human variation within the United States. This process included countless hearings and studies and many hours of deliberation. It was a serious process undertaken by serious people. In the end those categories serve the purpose of being broad enough that nearly everyone can find their place in them. But the categories do not work for everyone. No set of categories can.

Often categories are too broad, combining people who really shouldn't be combined, thus obscuring the diversity of the group. For example, the Asian group includes many people from many different countries who speak very different languages. When you add Pacific Islanders (Asian/Pacific Islanders), the problem is exacerbated.

Which brings me to the question that defines my point: how do you write a book about the health of racial/ethnic minority groups in the United States while having to rely on statistics that combine individuals into categories that are less than ideal?

The second issue that one must consider is terminology. What do you call the groups?

- Black or African American?
- Hispanic or Latino or Chicano or persons of Spanish descent?
- Native American or American Indian?

The problem is a serious one because, as I have found, those who have an opinion on this issue tend to hold that opinion very strongly. That would be OK if the opinions were consistent, but they are not. I talked with many people about this issue—scholars, activists, students, cafeteria workers—even my mother. I sent out emails to people I know would have thought about these issues. I read everything I could find on the subject. I must say, nearly every one of them made a compelling argument for his or her point of view. Unfortunately, I found starkly conflicting opinions. Here is a sample of quotes from people I talked with or exchanged emails with.

- "I think I like Hispanic; Latino is for Mexicans, not us."
- "Latino is the only proper name, because Hispanic is a name created by the U.S. government."
- "We use the term American Indian—period."
- "American Indian denotes affiliation with the oppressor; you should use 'indigenous people.'"
- "Nobody uses African American in normal conversation; that's more for formal writing."
- "African American excludes native Africans living in the United States."

I could go on, but I think you see my point. No matter what terms I use, I will be making some set of readers unhappy. So as not to insult anyone, I even considered using all of the names separated by a hyphen (that is, African American-Black, Native American-American Indian-Alaska Native, Asian-Pacific Islander, and Hispanic-Latino-Chicano). Obviously that won't work for an entire book.

Census Terminology Study

In 1996 the U.S. Bureau of the Census conducted a survey to determine preferences for terms to designate racial/ethnic groups. People who identified themselves as Hispanic, White, Black, American Indian, Eskimo, Aleut, or multiracial were given a list of terms describing their respective racial or ethnic group and were asked to choose which term they preferred, or to indicate whether they preferred some other term or had no preference. Table 1.1 gives the percentage from each group preferring a particular term. These results have been collapsed across the panels.

The majority of Hispanic respondents chose *Hispanic* as the term they preferred, and about 10 percent of the Hispanics chose each of the other terms. A majority of Whites chose *White.* A large plurality of Blacks preferred the term *Black,* but almost as many chose *African American* or *Afro-American.* More than half of those identifying as American Indian or one of the classes of Alaska Native preferred either *American Indian* or *Alaska Native,* but over a third chose the more generic *Native American.* Almost 30 percent of those identifying as multiracial preferred the term *multiracial,* but about as many had no preference.

There is no consensus term that will satisfy everyone in all cases. In spite of the fact that I will be using terminology that is not favored by some set of readers, I had to make decisions that I hope will minimize the number of readers that are put off. If you are one who does not like the choices I made, I apologize. I hope you will be sympathetic to my plight and use this chapter as an opportunity to address the issue in the classroom. Ask students how they would have handled the problem. I think this will lead to a worthwhile class discussion.

I applied the following usage rules to address the various populations:

- The term *race/ethnicity* refers to the set of categories used to group individuals.
- The term *minority* refers to all of the groups generically.
- *Black* and *African American* are used interchangeably to refer to people of African descent (including African Americans, native Africans, and persons from the Caribbean and South America).
- When referring to a specific subgroup such as native Africans, I use the generic term *African* or the specific country or tribal affiliation.
- *Hispanic/Latino* is used in combination to refer to persons from Central and South America (including Mexico), the Spanish-speaking Caribbean (Puerto Rico, Cuba, and the Dominican Republic), and Brazil.
- *American Indian* refers to all indigenous Americans from what is now the continental United States.
- *Alaska Natives* refers to indigenous populations of Alaska.

TABLE 1.1.   PREFERENCE FOR RACIAL OR ETHNIC TERMINOLOGY (PERCENT DISTRIBUTION).

Preferred Terminology	Percent
Hispanic Origin	
Hispanic.	57.88
Latino	11.74
Of Spanish origin.	12.34
Some other term	7.85
No preference	10.18
White	
White	61.66
Caucasian	16.53
European American	2.35
Anglo	0.96
Some other term	1.97
No preference	16.53
Black	
Black	44.15
African American	28.07
Afro-American	12.12
Negro	3.28
Colored	1.09
Some other term	2.19
No preference	9.11
American Indian	
American Indian	49.76
Alaska Native	3.51
Native American	37.35
Some other term	3.66
No preference	5.72
Multiracial	
Multiracial	28.42
More than one race	6.03
Biracial	5.67
Mixed race	16.02
Mestizo or mestiza	2.25
Some other term	13.87
No preference	27.76

Note: Percentages may not add to 100 due to rounding.

Source: U.S. Bureau of the Census, Decennial Statistical Studies Division, "Results of the 1996 Race and Ethnic Targeted Test," Population Division Working Paper No. 18, May 1997.

- The generic terms *American Indian/Alaska Native* and *Native American* are used interchangeably.
- *Asian/Pacific Islander* refers to persons having origins in any of the original peoples of the Far East, Southeast Asia, the Indian subcontinent, or the Pacific Islands. This area includes, for example, China, India, Japan, Korea, the Philippine Islands, and Samoa.
- If the data are for Asians only, I refer to the category as *Asian* without *Pacific Islander.*
- When data on Native Hawaiians are available, I use those data. Otherwise, Native Hawaiians are combined with Pacific Islanders.
- In each case I use the lowest level of categorization available. For example, if the data allow me to talk about a specific Native American tribe, I use the tribal name. If the data are categorized only as American Indian (and specifically not Alaska Native), I use American Indian. If it is not possible to specify tribal affiliation or whether the data are for Alaska Natives or American Indians, I use the generic terms *Native American* or *American Indian/Alaska Native.*
- Finally, when referring to a specific report, study, book, or other document, I use whichever term was used in that document, even if it does not conform to the above usage rules. (See Appendix B for additional readings.)

PART ONE

CROSSCUTTING ISSUES

CHAPTER TWO

CONCEPTUAL ISSUES IN RACE/ETHNICITY AND HEALTH

Outline

Introduction
Origins of the Race Concept
Problems with the Race Concept
    Inconsistency of Race Conceptualizations
    Confounding of Race, Ethnicity, and Nationality
    Attempting to Define Race
    The Changing Measurement of Race in the U.S. Census
Office of Management and Budget Directive 15
A Conceptual Model of Race/Ethnicity and Health
Summary

Introduction

In the United States, race and ethnicity is a factor in nearly every aspect of society, including politics, economics, music, art, and literature. Race is also among the most frequently used concepts in research conducted by public health, nursing, and medical scientists. A series of studies of three leading U.S.-based scientific journals found that more than 60 percent of the studies published in these journals included race or ethnicity (Jones, LaVeist, & Lillie-Blanton, 1991; Williams, 1994). In fact, not only was race or ethnicity included in the majority of studies; the use of race/ethnicity increased during the second half of the twentieth century and is showing no sign of letting up in the twenty-first century. Because race/ethnicity is so frequently used in the health sciences, one might think that there is general agreement on the meaning of these concepts; however, this is not the case. In fact there is a great deal of disagreement among scientists about what race and ethnicity mean and what their relevance is within the realm of health care. This point will be further explained later in this chapter.

Origins of the Race Concept

The origins of the race concept are somewhat disputed. Depending on which source one uses, different scholars are credited with coining the term *race.* But while the true origin is clouded, it is clear that the term *race,* as it is used today, is a relatively recent invention. Most sources agree that it was not until the late seventeenth century that scholars set out to develop a set of categories to classify humans. However, in the early discussions of human classification, the term *race* was not used consistently or even with consistent meaning (Bernasconi, 2001). For example, Francois Bernier's 1684 essay is credited by some as the first text to specify the term, but even the title of his essay—"A New Division of the Earth, According to the Different Species or Races of Man Who Inhabit It"—implies that race is both species and subspecies.

Noted American anthropologist Ashley Montagu credited French naturalist Georges-Louis Leclerc Buffon with originating the race concept in Buffon's 1778 book (Montagu, 1964). Other scholars credit German physiologist and anthropologist Johann Friedrich Blumenbach. In 1775, Blumenbach presented a fivefold classification of the variety of man. Although he did not use the term *race* in the first or second edition of the book, he did embrace the term in the 1797 revised edition. Blumenbach classified humans into five groupings: Caucasian or White, Mongolian or Yellow, Malayan or Brown, Negro or Black, and American or Red. These classifications were made on the basis of geographic considerations and the clustering of physical features such as skin color and hair type.

Although Blumenbach's classification system was widely accepted in the eighteenth century, as it is today, his classifications are also widely disputed and rejected. With the publication of *Man's Most Dangerous Myth: The Fallacy of Race* in 1942, Montagu presented the first major attack on the scientific validity of the concept of race. Other evaluations of the validity of race began to appear in the scientific literature during the 1950s and 1960s. By the 1970s the predominant position held by most scientists was that there was no *biologic* evidence to support the existence of race groups. Some scientists—most notably anthropologists, geneticists, and evolutionary biologists—go even further and take the position that races do not exist at all. They believe that the characteristics we use to identify race (primarily skin color and hair texture) should not be viewed as any more meaningful than any other physical variation in human appearance (such as hair color, eye color, or height). That anthropologists would reject the notion of race is most interesting, because Blumenbach, one of the earliest to use the term race, is considered to be one of the founding fathers of the field of physical anthropology.

In spite of the tenuous basis upon which race stands and the growing consensus that races do not exist as a biologic concept, many have been slow to embrace the position that races do not exist. Most social scientists take the position that, while there is no biological basis for race, races are social categories that have an important impact on people's lives and on their health as well. All of this causes a great deal of confusion. For example, we know that biogenetic factors play an important role in shaping human health. And we know that there are substantial differences in the health status of various racial/ethnic groups. Therefore, isn't it obvious that race differences in health status are caused by biogenetic differences among racial/ethnic groups? This seems logical, but as this chapter will demonstrate, things are not that simple.

Problems with the Race Concept

Several studies have demonstrated problems in the use of race in health research. Some have gone so far as to recommend that we discontinue the use of race in the health sciences (Stolley, 1999; Fullilove, 1998). Although those who advocate the abolition of the use of race in the health sciences are in the minority, few would disagree that there are major problems with the term *race*. Specifically, (1) the concept has not been clearly defined nor consistently applied, (2) there is no consensus definition of race, (3) race is often confounded with other related concepts such as ethnicity and nationality, and (4) the existence of races has little support from biological or genetic research.

Inconsistency of Race Conceptualizations

Let's examine some of the problems with popular conceptualizations of race. First we will compare the race classification systems in different countries. The first three tables present the classification systems from the United States, Japan, and Brazil. Table 2.1 displays a condensed version of the pre-1989 protocol issued by the U.S. National Center for Health Statistics (NCHS), used to assign racial status on birth certificates. The table shows that a child can be assigned *White* only if both parents had been designated White. However, in every other case, the race of the father determined the race of the child. Thus, when a child is the offspring of a Japanese male and a Black female, the child is designated as Japanese, whereas the child of a Black father and a Japanese mother is designated as Black. However, the mating between a White person, regardless of their gender, and a person of any other group results in a child that is designated as a member of the non-White group. This is called the "one-drop rule," meaning that one drop of non-White blood makes a person a member of that group (Davis, 1991). In 1989 the NCHS policy was modified so that now the race of the mother determines the race of the child regardless of which combination of groups is involved.

Table 2.2 shows the classification scheme used in Japan until 1985. In that country a child was designated Japanese only if the father was Japanese. The official policy was that this scheme was to be followed without regard to the identity of the mother. In 1985, the Japanese national legislature amended the constitution so that a person would be considered Japanese if either parent was Japanese.

The Brazilian classification system is outlined in Table 2.3. In that country interracial mating is handled by assigning the offspring to a third racial category called *mulatto*. Mulatto is a classification formerly used in the United States (see Table 2.4) but long abandoned. However, with the increasing number of mixed-race persons in the United States, some have argued for the addition of a new *mixed race* category on official forms. Within the Brazilian culture, mulattos are further divided into a set of subdivisions based on the relative lightness or darkness of the person's skin.

TABLE 2.1.   U.S. POLICY FOR ASSIGNING RACIAL STATUS ON BIRTH CERTIFICATES PRIOR TO 1989.

Father	Mother	Child
White	White	White
White	Black	Black
White	Japanese	Japanese
Black	White	Black
Black	Black	Black
Black	Japanese	Black
Japanese	White	Japanese
Japanese	Black	Japanese
Japanese	Japanese	Japanese

Source: LaVeist, 1994, p. 3.

TABLE 2.2.   JAPANESE POLICY FOR ASSIGNING RACIAL/ETHNIC STATUS ON BIRTH CERTIFICATES PRIOR TO 1983.

Father	Mother	Child
White	Japanese	White
Black	Japanese	Black
Japanese	White	Japanese
Japanese	Black	Japanese

Source: LaVeist, 1994, p. 3.

TABLE 2.3. BRAZILIAN POLICY FOR ASSIGNING RACIAL/ETHNIC
STATUS ON BIRTH CERTIFICATES.

Father	Mother	Child
White	White	White
White	Black	Mulatto[a]
Black	White	Mulatto[a]
Black	Black	Black

[a]Mulatto is then broken down into fine distinctions based on physical characteristics: *Presos* (black), *Preto Retinto* (dark black), *Cabra* (slightly less black), *Cabo Verde* (slightly less black), *Escuro* (lighter still), *Mulato Esuro* (dark mulatto), *Mulato Claro* (light mulatto), *Sararas, Moreno, Blanco de terra, Blanco*.

Source: LaVeist, 1994, p. 4.

These three countries produced five different classification systems over less than a decade. Several points about this are important to highlight. First, two people with the same genetic makeup can receive a different designation depending upon which society they are born into. For example, if a black woman and her Japanese husband had a child born in the United States, that child would be designated black. If that family moved to Japan and had a second child there, that child would be considered Japanese. Second, the same person can have a different status depending upon when they are born (before or after 1985 in Japan, or before or after 1989 in the United States).

Confounding of Race, Ethnicity, and Nationality

It is common to hear people use the terms *race, ethnicity,* and *nationality* interchangeably. In fact, I intentionally did so in earlier sections of this chapter, because I wanted to illustrate a point but had not yet discussed the connections among race, ethnicity, and nationality. However, continuing to use these terms interchangeably would complicate the understanding of these concepts. Although race, ethnicity, and nationality overlap, they are not synonymous. The diagram in Figure 2.1 represents the overlap among race, ethnicity, and nationality. In the United States, the distinctions of ethnic or national variations within race groups are obscured in favor of physical appearance. For example, ethnicity refers to cultural commonality, yet in the Dominican Republic the descendants of Africans, Spaniards, and the native (or indigenous) population share a common ethnic identity. Are they all members of the same race group? Officially, in the United States these are all regarded as Hispanic (officially designated as an ethnic group; see the discussion of OMB Directive 15 in the sections that follow). However, in daily social interaction in the United States, they would be regarded as Black or White based on their appearance and their degree of acculturation into American society.

FIGURE 2.1.   RACE, ETHNICITY, AND NATIONALITY.

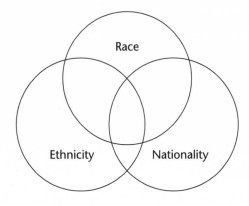

Mexican, Cuban, and El Salvadoran immigrants to America are also all categorized as Hispanic, obscuring their nationality and cultural differences. For example,
a black Cuban and a black American may share physical characteristics such as skin
color. This may result in both persons being at increased health risk—for example,
from living in poor-quality housing, due to discrimination by landlords and in the real
estate market. However, they are from distinct ethnic traditions that may result in
different dietary habits; thus they would have different dietary health risk profiles. Also,
while persons in cells A and B of Table 2.4 may both be at increased risk of exposure to housing discrimination due to their race, as measured by skin color, persons in
cells A and C may both be at increased risk of encountering barriers to accessing quality health care due to language barriers.

Here is another example: Europeans from Southern Italy, Northern Ireland, and
Southern France come from distinct cultural traditions, yet upon arrival in the United
States they are categorized as White. Rarely is this source of variation taken into account in health research. The same can be said for Native Americans and Southeast
Asians. The Yoruba of both Brazil and Nigeria share a common ethnic/cultural
heritage, yet they differ in nationality—but within the American cultural context they
both would be regarded as Black and thus be subject to the health risks associated with
being Black in America.

We often try to capture all of these concepts—ethnicity, skin color, and nationality—in one inclusive term. This results in some degree of measurement error, but
more important, the lack of conceptual clarity leaves a great deal of room for erroneous interpretations of research findings and consequently for ineffective public policy and public health programming—and possibly even ineffective medical practice.

TABLE 2.4.　THE LINK BETWEEN RACE AND HISPANIC ETHNICITY.

		Race	
		Black	**White**
Ethnicity	**Hispanic**	A Black Hispanic	C White Hispanic
	Non-Hispanic	B Black Non-Hispanic	D White Non-Hispanic

Attempting to Define Race

In examining representative medical and allied health dictionaries for definitions of race, one finds significant variation among their definitions. Some dictionaries define race in entirely biological terms; others recognize the social and political aspects of race. In *A Dictionary of Epidemiology* (Last, 1988) race is defined as "persons who are relatively homogeneous with respect to biological inheritance." This terse definition embraces the biological concept without providing guidelines for identifying individual races. Nor does this dictionary acknowledge the social or political aspects of race.

In *A Dictionary of Genetics* (King and Stansfield, 1990) race is defined as a scientific, biogenetic concept, "a phenotypically and/or geographically distinctive subspecific group, composed of individuals inhabiting a defined geographic and/or ecological region, and possessing characteristic phenotypic and gene frequencies that distinguish it from other such groups." The dictionary then adds a curious sentence that contradicts the implied scientific rigor of the first part of the definition: "The number of racial groups that one wishes to recognize within a species is usually arbitrary but suitable for the purposes under investigation."

The International Dictionary of Medicine and Biology (Becker and Landav, 1986) views race as a biological concept that defies discrete categorization: "A subspecies or other division or subdivision of a species. Human races are generally defined in terms of original geographic range and common hereditary traits which may be morphological, serological, hematological, immunological, or biochemical. The traditional division of mankind into several well recognized racial types such as Caucasoid (White), Negroid (Black), and Mongoloid (Yellow) leaves a residue of populations that are of problematical classification, and its focus on a limited range of visible characteristics tends to oversimplify and distort the picture of human variation."

Campbell's Psychiatric Dictionary (Campbell, 1981) is in fundamental agreement with the *International Dictionary of Medicine and Biology:* "The term *race* implies a blood-related group with characteristic and common hereditary traits." Likewise, this dictionary does not embrace the most commonly accepted categories of human races, stating instead: "Primary race or subspecies—the Caucasian, the Mongoloid, and the Negroid—are generalized racial types, hypothetical stocks, rather than living races." *Campbell's Psychiatric Dictionary* then goes on to advance the biological concept of "race disease" as a "group of individuals susceptible to the same disease. . . . One might conceive, therefore, as well of a gastric ulcer race, a manic depressive race, a meningococcus susceptible race, or gall-bladder race, as of the present customarily accepted Black, Yellow, or White divisions of mankind."

The Dictionary of Modern Medicine (Segen, 1992) provides the most interesting but least informative definition of race I have found among the dictionaries. This definition illustrates an attempt to incorporate the biological, political, and social conceptions of race, however unsuccessfully:

> An ethnic classification, subdivided in the U.S. into five categories, according to origin: (1) White, not Hispanic (Europe, North Africa, Middle East); (2) Black not Hispanic (Africa); (3) Hispanic; (4) American Native (Indians, Eskimos); (5) Asian and Pacific Islanders; stratification by race is of interest in several areas of medicine for a number of specific reasons. *Clinical Medicine:* Some human leukocyte antigens are more common in certain racial groups and may be associated with particular diseases, thus helping to diagnose and manage difficult cases. *Public Policy:* The Civil Rights Act of 1964 mandated equality in employment and educational policy and knowledge or race favors minority candidates. *Transfusion Medicine:* Certain red cell antigens may be relatively uncommon in a particular race and knowledge of race reduces the labor required to find a suitable unit for transfusion. *Transplantation:* Human leukocyte antigens (HLA) differ somewhat according to race and may be used to identify potential recipients for organ transplantation.

The first part of this definition is tautological in that it defines race as merely the sum of its categories as they are currently officially recognized by the United States government (see the discussion of OMB Directive 15 later in this chapter). The examples provided to demonstrate the relevance of race in medicine are also problematic. The explanations for clinical medicine, transfusion medicine, and transplantation refer to race differences in the distribution of certain HLAs (addressed in the next section of this chapter). The explanation of public policy, however, addresses a politically charged issue: affirmative action. It is not clear how this example clarifies the meaning of race at either the theoretical or the practical level. Its inclusion in the dictionary further demonstrates the lack of conceptual clarity when it comes to race. Furthermore, the description of the Civil Rights Act of 1964 is not correct. The act did not mandate equality; it made it illegal to discriminate in public accommodations (such as buses, trains, and restaurants).

Finally, *Dorland's Illustrated Medical Dictionary* (Taylor, 1988) defines race more broadly: "1. An ethnic stock, or division of mankind; in a narrower sense, a national or tribal stock; in a still narrower sense, a genealogic line of descent; a class of persons of a common lineage. In genetics, races are considered as populations having different distributions of gene frequencies. 2. A class or breed of animals; a group of individuals having certain characteristics in common, owing to a common inheritance; a subspecies." The *Dorland's* definition attempts to incorporate ethnicity, nationality, tribe, and genealogical lineage under race.

The Changing Measurement of Race in the U.S. Census

As we have seen, there is a lack of clarity regarding the definition of the term *race*. This lack of clarity has had important implications for the collection of data by race. Until the middle of the twentieth century most federal statistics (except for the census, which is a special case) were reported simply as White and non-White, combining all non-White racial/ethnic groups into one category. During the middle of the twentieth century it became standard to report data as White, Black, and Other. Even this minimal reporting was not uniformly practiced by all states. It was not until the 1980s, after the issuance of U.S. Office of Management and Budget (OMB) Directive 15, that federal statistics were routinely reported for Hispanics or Asian Americans. As such, it is sometimes difficult to compare statistics across states or across time periods.

The consequences of the lack of clarity on the definition of race can perhaps best be seen in the variety of ways in which data on race were collected in the U.S. census. Box 2.2 lists the many different ways in which race was defined and collected for every U.S. census, from the first census in 1790 through the most recent census in 2000. In the first census, data were categorized into only four groups: free White males, free White females, all other free persons, and slaves. The second census added a clarification that "Indians not taxed" were to be excluded in the tabulation of free persons. The various formats used during the remainder of the nineteenth century included years in which there was the inclusion of mulatto (mixed racial heritage), free colored persons, Chinese, and Japanese.

BOX 2.1.   OMB DIRECTIVE 15.

The Office of Budget and Management's Directive 15 established standards for the collection of data on race and ethnicity. The original version of OMB Directive 15 was released in 1977; version 2 was issued in 1997.

     The 1910 census was the first census to use the term *Other* (which was still in use as of the 2000 census). The twentieth century also saw the inclusion of additional nationalities including Filipino, Mexican, and Korean. More recent censuses, such as 1980 and 1990, expanded the Native American category to include Samoan, Eskimo, and Aleut—which disentangled these ethnic groups from the broader category of American Indian. Beginning in the 2000 census, it became permissible for individuals to select as many racial/ethnic/nationality groups as they desired.

BOX 2.2.   U.S. CENSUS RACE CATEGORIES, 1790–2000.

1790	Free White Males; Free White Females; All Other Free Persons; Slaves
1800	Free White Males; Free White Females; All Other Free Persons Except Indians Not Taxed; Slaves
1810	Free White Males; Free White Females; All Other Free Persons Except Indians Not Taxed; Slaves
1820	Free White Males; Free White Females; Free Colored Persons, All Other Persons Except Indians Not Taxed; Slaves
1830	Free White Persons; Free Colored Persons; Slaves
1840	Free White Persons; Free Colored Persons; Slaves
1850	Black; Mulatto[a]
1860	Black; Mulatto; (Indian)[b]
1880	White; Black; Mulatto; Chinese; Indian
1890	White; Black; Mulatto; Quadroon; Octoroon; Chinese; Japanese; Indian
1900	White: Black; Chinese; Japanese; Indian
1910	White; Black; Mulatto; Chinese; Japanese; Indian; Other (+ *write in*)
1920	White; Black; Mulatto; Indian; Chinese; Japanese; Filipino; Hindu; Korean; Other (+ *write in*)
1930	White; Negro; Mexican; Indian; Chinese; Japanese; Filipino; Hindu; Korean; (*other races, spell out in full*)
1940	White; Negro; Indian; Chinese; Japanese; Filipino; Hindu; Korean; (*other races, spell out in full*)
1950	White; Negro; Indian; Japanese; Chinese; Filipino; (*other race—spell out*)
1960	White; Negro; American Indian; Japanese; Chinese; Filipino; Hawaiian; Part-Hawaiian; Aleut Eskimo, and so on
1970	White; Negro or Black; American Indian; Japanese; Chinese; Filipino; Hawaiian; Korean; Other (*print race*)

1980	White; Negro or Black; Japanese; Chinese; Filipino; Korean; Vietnamese; American Indian; Asian Indian; Hawaiian; Guamanian; Samoan; Eskimo; Aleut; Other (*specify*)
1990	White; Black or Negro; American Indian; Eskimo; Aleut; Chinese; Filipino; Hawaiian; Korean; Vietnamese; Japanese; Asian Indian; Samoan; Guamanian; Other API (Asian or Pacific Islander); Other Race
2000	White; Black, African American, or Negro; American Indian or Alaska Native; Asian Indian; Chinese; Filipino; Japanese; Korean; Vietnamese; Native Hawaiian; Guamanian or Chamorro; Samoan; Other Asian (*print race*); Other Pacific Islander (*print race*); Some Other Race (*print race*)

Note: Categories are presented in the order in which they appeared on the schedules.

[a]In 1850 and 1860, free persons were enumerated on schedules for "free inhabitants"; slaves were enumerated on schedules designated for "slave inhabitants." On the free-inhabitants schedule, instructions to enumerators read, in part: "In all cases where the person is White leave the space blank in the column marked 'Color.'"

[b]Although "Indian" was not listed on the census schedule, the instructions read as follows: "'Indians'—Indians not taxed are not to be enumerated. The families of Indians who have renounced tribal rule, and who under State or Territorial laws exercise the rights of citizens, are to be enumerated. In all such cases write 'Ind.' opposite their names, in column 6, under heading 'Color.'"

Source: Nobles, 2000, pp. 1738–1745.

Office of Management and Budget Directive 15

In 1977 the Office of Management and Budget (OMB) issued Directive 15, which established standards for the collection of data on race and ethnicity. The goal of the directive was "to provide consistent and comparable data on race and ethnicity throughout the federal government for an array of statistical and administrative programs. Development of the data standards stem in large measure from new responsibilities to enforce civil rights laws. Data were needed to monitor equal access to housing, education, and employment opportunities for population groups that historically had experienced discrimination and different treatment because of their race or ethnicity."

According to the directive, "The categories that were developed represent a political-social construct designed to be used in the collection of data on the race and ethnicity of major broad population groups in this country, and are not anthropologically or scientifically based. The standards are used not only in the decennial census (which provides the 'denominator' for many measures), but also in household surveys, on administrative forms (e.g., school registration and mortgage lending applications), and in medical and other research."

The original OMB Directive 15 established four categories for data on race:

1. American Indian or Alaska Native—a person having origins in any of the original peoples of North America, and who maintains cultural identification, tribal affiliation, or community recognition.
2. Asian or Pacific Islander—a person having origins in any of the original peoples of the Far East, Southeast Asia, the Indian subcontinent, or the Pacific Islands. This area includes, for example, China, India, Japan, Korea, the Philippine Islands, and Samoa.
3. Black—a person having origins in any of the black racial groups of Africa.
4. White—a person having origins in any of the original peoples of Europe, North Africa, or the Middle East.

The standards also permit the collection of more detailed information on population groups, provided that the additional categories can be aggregated into the minimum standards established by the directive. It is also worthwhile to note that Directive 15 did not identify or designate groups as minority or disadvantaged. These designations were created by other legislation as a means of determining eligibility for participation in specific federal programs.

The directive instructs that, where possible, race/ethnicity should be captured by two separate questions. The first question asks for the individual's race (American Indian or Alaska Native, Asian or Pacific Islander, Black, or White). The second question asks for ethnicity (Hispanic origin or not of Hispanic origin). In the case of individuals with mixed racial heritage the directive offers the following: "the category which most closely reflects the individual's recognition in his community should be used for purposes of reporting on persons who are of mixed racial and/or ethnic origins."

The standards outlined by Directive 15 have been widely adopted by the federal government as well as the private sector. However, the standards have come under a great deal of criticism, particularly since the 1990 census. Most critics felt that the minimum categories set forth in Directive 15 did not reflect the increasing racial and ethnic diversity of the United States that has resulted primarily from increases in immigration and in interracial marriages. In response to the criticisms, the OMB undertook a comprehensive review of Directive 15 and in 1997 adopted three changes. First, the Asian and Pacific Islander category has been divided into two separate categories:

1. Asian—a person having origins in any of the original peoples of the Far East, Southeast Asia, or the Indian subcontinent, including, for example, Cambodia, China, India, Japan, Korea, Malaysia, Pakistan, the Philippine Islands, Thailand, and Vietnam
2. Native Hawaiian or other Pacific Islander—a person having origins in any of the original peoples of Hawaii, Guam, Samoa, or the other Pacific Islands

Second, the new standards offer the option of selecting one or more racial designations. Recommended forms for the instruction accompanying the multiple response questions are "Mark one or more" and "Select one or more." The third change adds "Latino" to "Hispanic" in the ethnicity question.

A Conceptual Model of Race/Ethnicity and Health

Up to this point the chapter has focused on the problems with the conceptualization of race. Now we will turn to a discussion of a conceptual model of how race/ethnicity influences health disparities. LaVeist (1994) developed a conceptual model of race (which has become known as the physiognomy model of race and health). The model attempts to forge a clearer interpretation of the social and behavioral factors that affect race disparities.

Figure 2.2 shows LaVeist's physiognomy model (LaVeist, 1994). The social pathway is along the left side of the model, the behavioral pathway along the right side. In the model, race is viewed as a latent factor in which skin color is the most commonly used manifest indicator. Following the left side of the model, as an individual engages the social world, others categorize that person into a race group. This process is called physiognomy, literally defined as the "art of judging human character from facial features" (*American Heritage Dictionary*, 1985). The individual, once categorized, is exposed to the social health risks associated with that group. Examples of such risks are occupational health hazards, poor-quality housing, exposure to discrimination or racism, and poorer-quality medical care. One can think of social risk factors as variables that both impact health and are generally outside of the direct control of the individual. Some examples of social risk factors are racism, sexism, socioeconomic status, social support, population density, housing quality, racial segregation, stress, or residence in a neighborhood with a high crime rate. Each of these factors has been demonstrated to be associated with health, and they all have been shown to vary by race.

The right side of Figure 2.2 recognizes that there may be characteristics of the culture of an ethnic group that influence health or illness behaviors, and thus health status. These factors may account for some degree of health disparities.

The third pathway through which racial differences in health status are produced is indicated by the arrow linking societal factors to health and illness behavior. This shows that societal factors place constraints on an individual's ability to engage in health or illness behaviors that are protective of health. For example, a person's race may lead to lower socioeconomic status, which may lead to underutilization of health services. In this example, illness behavior is directly associated not with race or ethnicity, but with social class. However, the way race is commonly analyzed, one might inaccurately ascribe such a finding to a person's race when it is really an effect of social class. Such errors lead to the assumption that there is something about a person's skin color that makes the person engage in risky behavior.

FIGURE 2.2.   CONCEPTUAL MODEL OF RACE.

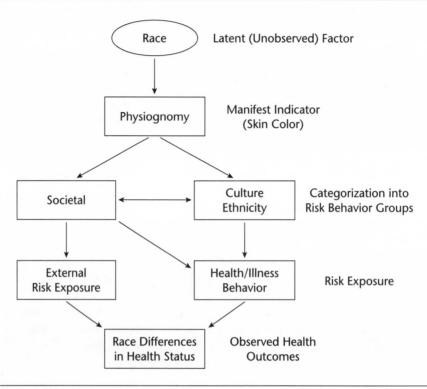

Source: LaVeist, 1994, p. 10.

Summary

This chapter outlined conceptual issues that relate to the definition of race and ethnicity. The chapter discussed the origin of the term *race* and plotted the use of the term
during the nineteenth and twentieth centuries. The public policy implications of definitions of race and ethnicity were also discussed, and the lack of a consensus definition for the term was demonstrated. Finally, the chapter discussed OMB Directive
15—which provides federal standards for the collection and reporting of data by
race—and outlined a conceptual model linking race/ethnicity to health status.

The term *race* has caused a great deal of confusion. There is no consensus definition. Often we think of human races as biologically distinct, as are different species.

However, there is no evidence of significant biological differences among racial groups. Race and ethnicity are social categories, not biological ones.

For a case study, see Appendix A. See Appendix B for additional readings.

Key Words

Race

Ethnicity

Species

Office of Management and Budget Directive 15

Physiognomy

CHAPTER THREE

THE DEMOGRAPHY OF AMERICAN RACIAL/ETHNIC MINORITIES

Outline

What Is Demography?

Demography is the science that specializes in the study of populations. Demographers focus on the size, distribution, structure, and patterns of changes of populations. Demographers approach the topic by examining the births, deaths, and migration patterns of populations within geographic areas such as nations, regions, or cities. Demographers also conduct research on other aspects of populations, such as marriage, divorce, age, sex, and race/ethnicity. This chapter will use the methods of demography to describe the population of the United States in terms of race/ethnicity, exploring historical trends as well as future projections that affect the health of populations.

The U.S. Population

Population data for the United States come from the census, which is collected every ten years by the U.S. Bureau of the Census. The census is a constitutionally mandated enumeration of the population; it is the official record of the U.S. population. Figure 3.1 depicts trends in the U.S. total and elderly populations. The figure shows a steady increase in the population between 1950 and 2000. In 1950 the total U.S. population was just over 150 million persons. By the 1970 census that number increased to more than 200 million, and by 1990 it was just over 250 million. In the year 2000 the total U.S. population was over 274.5 million. The Census Bureau projects that the total number of Americans will exceed 300 million by the year 2010 and that there will be more than 400 million Americans by 2050. There have also been increases in the number of persons over age 65: the Census Bureau projects that by the year 2020 there will be more than 50 million American seniors, more than double the 1980 number.

The increase in the number of seniors can be attributed to rising life expectancy (life expectancy will be discussed in Chapter Four) and the anticipated movement into the ranks of the elderly of the baby boom generation—the generation of Americans born during the surge of births in the twenty years immediately following the end of World War II (1946–1966). The first wave of baby boomers will reach age sixty-five in the year 2011.

FIGURE 3.1. TOTAL POPULATION AND ELDERLY POPULATION, UNITED STATES, 1950–2050.

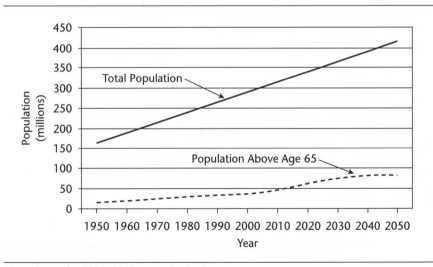

Note: Figures for 2010–2050 are projections.

Source: National Center for Health Statistics, 2003.

The Racial/Ethnic Composition of the United States

Next I will explore the racial/ethnic makeup of the United States population. Table 3.1 displays the total number and percentages for racial and ethnic groups in the United States. According to the census, in 2002 just over 75 percent of reporting U.S. residents identified themselves as White. The largest nonwhite groups were Hispanics/Latinos and African Americans. Together these groups made up slightly less than 25 percent of the total U.S. population—12.5 percent were Hispanics/Latinos and 12.3 percent were African Americans. In all, the census recorded 35.3 million Hispanics/Latinos and 34.6 million African Americans. The largest single group of Latinos came from Mexico; the next largest, from Puerto Rico. Mexican Americans accounted for over 7 percent of the U.S. population and Puerto Ricans just over 1 percent. There were about 1.2 million Cubans—less than one half of 1 percent of the total U.S. population. It is important to point out that the Hispanic/Latino and African American populations are likely

TABLE 3.1.   U.S. POPULATION BY RACE/ETHNICITY AMONG PEOPLE REPORTING ONLY ONE RACE GROUP, 2000.

Group	Number of Persons	Percentage of Total
White	211,460,626	75.1
Black	34,658,190	12.3
American Indian and Alaska Native	2,475,956	0.9
Asian	10,242,998	3.6
Asian Indian	1,678,765	0.6
Chinese	2,432,585	0.9
Filipino	1,850,314	0.7
Japanese	796,700	0.3
Korean	1,076,872	0.4
Vietnamese	1,122,528	0.4
Other Asian	1,285,234	0.5
Native Hawaiian and other Pacific Islander	398,835	0.1
Native Hawaiian	140,652	—
Guamanian or Chamorro	58,240	—
Samoan	91,029	—
Other Pacific Islander	108,914	—
Hispanic or Latino (of any race)	35,305,818	12.5
Mexican	20,640,711	7.3
Puerto Rican	3,406,178	1.2
Cuban	1,241,685	0.4
Other Hispanic	10,017,244	3.6
Total	274,595,678	100.0

Note: Percentages may not sum to 100 due to rounding.

Source: U.S. Bureau of the Census, 2001.

to be underreported because of illegal immigration and because of likely undercounts in the census (Redfern, 2001; Chao & Tsay, 1998).

The census recorded over 2.4 million American Indian and Alaska Natives (0.9 percent). Asian Americans were about 3.6 percent of the U.S. population (10.2 million persons). At 2.4 million, Chinese Americans were the largest group of Asian Americans in the country, followed by Filipino, Indian, Vietnamese, Korean, and Japanese Americans. There were 398,000 Pacific Islanders consisting of 140,000 native Hawaiians, 91,000 Samoans, and just over 58,000 Guamanians or Chamorros.

The figure shows that the U.S. population is not distributed evenly across all regions of the country (see Figure 3.2). The region with the largest population is the South; more than 35 percent of Americans live there. This contrasts with the Northeast, which has the smallest percentage of the U.S. population: just over 53 million. The Midwest and West each has slightly more than 22 percent of the population.

FIGURE 3.2.   RACIAL/ETHNIC POPULATION BY REGION.

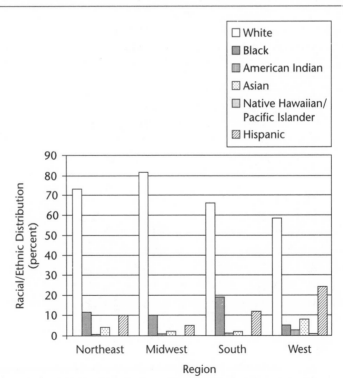

Source: U.S. Bureau of the Census, Census 2000, Redistricting Data (PL 94-171), Summary File for States and Redistricting Summary File for Puerto Rico, tabs. PL1 and PL2.

Each region varies greatly in terms of the percent of people of color, but Whites are consistently the largest group. African Americans are the largest minority group in the Northeast, Midwest, and South, and Hispanics/Latinos are the largest minority group in the West. Asians are also disproportionately represented in the West, as are American Indians, Native Hawaiians, and Pacific Islanders.

Whereas Figure 3.2 displays the percentages of each racial/ethnic group that make up each region's population, Figure 3.3 shows, for each racial/ethnic group, the distribution of its total numbers across the four regions. The figure shows that Whites are the most evenly distributed population throughout all regions of the country. As Figure 3.2 indicates, the largest proportion of whites live in the South (33.89 percent). However, no region's population is less than 18 percent Whites. The largest proportions of African Americans also live in the South (54.77 percent), but as few as 8.88 percent of African Americans live in the Western region.

Nearly 50 percent of American Indians and Asians live in the West. However, while over 20 percent of Asians live in the Northeast, fewer than 7 percent of American Indians live in the Northeast. Also, nearly 30 percent of American Indians live in the South, compared with fewer than 20 percent of Asians. The Native Hawaiian/Pacific Islander population resides almost exclusively in the West, with over 76 percent of that population living in the region. Finally, over 40 percent of Hispanics/Latinos live in the West, just over 30 percent live in the South, and nearly 15 percent live in the East. Fewer than 10 percent of Hispanics/Latinos live in the Midwest.

FIGURE 3.3.   REGIONAL DISTRIBUTION OF EACH RACIAL/ETHNIC GROUP.

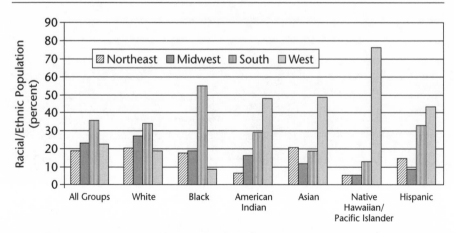

Source: U.S. Bureau of the Census, Census 2000, Redistricting Data (PL 94-171) Summary File for States and Redistricting Summary File for Puerto Rico, tabs. PL1 and PL2.

Population Projections

Between 1950 and 2000 there were significant changes in the racial composition of the United States. In 1950 nearly 85 percent of the U.S. population was White, 11 to 12 percent was African American, and American Indians and others made up roughly 5 percent. Those percentages remained constant until the 1980s, when an increase in the number of Hispanic and Asian immigrants substantially changed the demographic makeup of the country. As Figure 3.4 shows, there has been a substantial expansion of the Hispanic population. According to the 2000 census, the increase in this population has moved Hispanics past Blacks as the second largest group in the United States. Additionally, it is notable that the Asian population has also been increasing at a rapid pace. The consequence of these demographic shifts was that by the year 2000, White

FIGURE 3.4.   PERCENTAGES OF RESIDENT U.S. POPULATION BY RACE/ETHNICITY, 1950–2000.

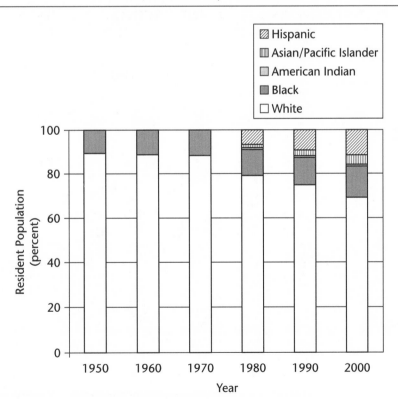

Source: National Center for Health Statistics, 2003.

Americans made up only 75 percent of the total U.S. population: a reduction of approximately 10 percentage points over fifty years.

According to projections from the U.S. Bureau of the Census, the demographic
trends depicted in Figure 3.4 are expected to continue throughout the twenty-first century. Figure 3.5 displays census projections for the years 2010 through 2070. According to these projections the expansion of the Hispanic population is expected to
comprise nearly one-fifth (20 percent) of the total U.S. population by the year 2030
and nearly a third of the population by 2070. The Asian population is also expected
to continue to expand, to nearly 10 percent of the total U.S. population by 2070. The
Census Bureau also projects that the percentage of Black Americans and American
Indians will remain relatively consistent. However, the White population is expected
to continue to decline as a percentage of the total population. By the year 2050 Whites
are projected to constitute about 50 percent of the U.S. population, and by 2060 the

FIGURE 3.5.   PROJECTED PERCENTAGES OF RESIDENT U.S. POPULATION BY RACE/ETHNICITY, 2010–2070.

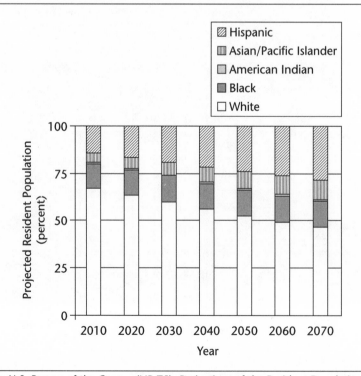

Source: U.S. Bureau of the Census (NP-T5), Projections of the Resident Population by Race,
Hispanic Origin, and Nativity: Middle Series, 1999 to 2100.

majority of Americans are projected to be from racial/ethnic groups that are now considered to be numerical minorities.

These projections are driven by several demographic trends: migration, birth rates, death rates, and differences in the age distribution of the racial/ethnic groups. Each of these demographic factors will be discussed in this chapter.

The Age Distribution of the U.S. Population

Figure 3.6 displays the age distribution of the resident U.S. population by race/ethnicity for the year 2000. For every group except Whites the proportion of the population decreases as the population ages, so that the smallest proportion of the population is the age group greater than sixty-four years old. This pattern is related to patterns of mortality rates by age (as people age the death rate increases, so their numbers are reduced).

FIGURE 3.6.   AGE DISTRIBUTION OF THE U.S. POPULATION, 2000.

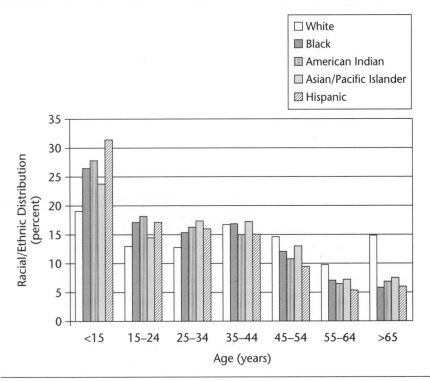

Source: National Center for Health Statistics, 2003.

Figure 3.6 also presents a partial explanation for the projections of a declining percentage of Whites and an increasing non-White percentage of the U.S. population by the middle of the twenty-first century. Figure 3.4 shows that not only does the White population have a much smaller proportion of children than other racial/ethnic groups, but Whites also have a smaller proportion of persons in the prime childbearing age range (roughly ages fifteen to forty-four). While only about 12 percent of Whites are between ages fifteen and twenty-four, more than 15 percent of Blacks, American Indians, and Hispanics are in that age group. A similar pattern can be seen for the age group twenty-five to thirty-four. Additionally, nearly 15 percent of the White population is above age sixty-four; no other racial/ethnic group has more than about 7 percent of their population in this age range.

It is also instructive to observe the pattern of age distribution of the Hispanic population. Nearly one third of the Hispanic population is below age fifteen. By the year 2020 these persons will all be within the prime childbearing age range. The same can be said for Blacks and American Indians; in these groups, more than 25 percent of the population are below age fifteen and just over 5 percent are above age sixty-four.

Fertility

Fertility (also referred to as natality) is also one of the key components of demographic change. Fertility refers to the number of offspring produced by a population. Fertility is typically expressed as a rate, either fertility rate or natality rate. The fertility rate is the number of births per 1,000 females of childbearing age. The equation to compute fertility rate is provided in Box 3.1.

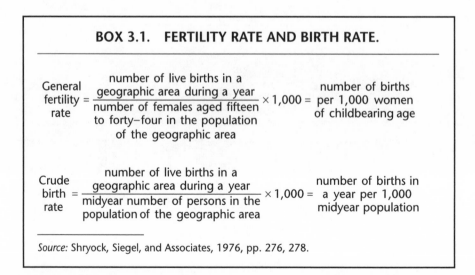

BOX 3.1.   FERTILITY RATE AND BIRTH RATE.

$$\text{General fertility rate} = \frac{\text{number of live births in a geographic area during a year}}{\text{number of females aged fifteen to forty–four in the population of the geographic area}} \times 1{,}000 = \begin{array}{l}\text{number of births} \\ \text{per 1,000 women} \\ \text{of childbearing age}\end{array}$$

$$\text{Crude birth rate} = \frac{\text{number of live births in a geographic area during a year}}{\text{midyear number of persons in the population of the geographic area}} \times 1{,}000 = \begin{array}{l}\text{number of births in} \\ \text{a year per 1,000} \\ \text{midyear population}\end{array}$$

Source: Shryock, Siegel, and Associates, 1976, pp. 276, 278.

Figure 3.7 displays the fertility rate for the United States population for the years 1950 to 2000. The figure shows a significant decline in the U.S. fertility rate for the years 1950 to 1970. After 1970, the rate of decline slowed substantially and has remained consistently around 70 births per 1,000 females between ages fifteen and forty-four.

There are differences in fertility rates by race/ethnicity, as displayed in Figure 3.8. The chart shows that Whites and American Indians have the lowest fertility rate of all racial/ethnic groups in the United States. In 2000 both of these groups had fertility rates below 60 births per 1,000 childbearing-age women. Fertility rates for Blacks and Asian/Pacific Islanders were between 65 and 70 births. Hispanics had the highest fertility rate, with a rate of nearly 100 births per 1,000 childbearing-age women in the year 2000. It is also instructive to note a nationwide pattern of declining fertility rates over the twenty-year period displayed in Figure 3.8. The single exception to this pattern is the rate of the Hispanic population, which increased, and then returned to the previous level.

Figure 3.9 shows the age distribution of mothers for the year 2000. This figure shows birth rates as opposed to fertility rates. Birth rates differ from fertility rates. Whereas fertility rates are the total number of live births per 1,000 women of childbearing age (number of live births per woman aged fifteen to forty-four times 1,000), birth rates are computed as the total number of births within a given age group over the total number of women in that age group.

FIGURE 3.7.   U.S. FERTILITY RATE, 1950–2000.

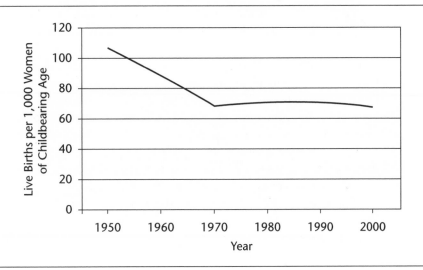

Source: National Center for Health Statistics, 2003.

FIGURE 3.8. FERTILITY RATES BY RACE/ETHNICITY, 1980–2000.

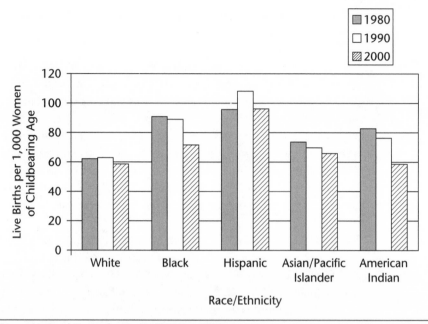

Source: National Center for Health Statistics, 2003.

Figure 3.9 shows a general pattern in which birth rates increase with age between ages twenty and thirty; after thirty there is a decline in birth rates. Although each racial/ethnic group displays this general pattern, there are differences among the groups. For Hispanic/Latinos, Native Americans, and African Americans the age group with the highest birth rate is twenty to twenty-four, and the second highest birth rates are found in the age group twenty-five to twenty-nine. This contrasts with Whites and Asian/Pacific Islanders, who have the highest birth rates in the age group twenty-five to twenty-nine, followed by the age group thirty to thirty-four. Asian/Pacific Islanders have the highest birth rates of all racial/ethnic groups for ages thirty to thirty-four, thirty-five to thirty-nine, and forty to forty-four. Conversely, the Asian/Pacific Islander population has a very low birth rate below age twenty.

In the age range twenty to twenty-four, Hispanics have a birth rate in excess of 180 births per 1,000 women; this contrasts with the Black rate of approximately 147 births, the American Indian rate of approximately 135 births, the White rate of approximately 90 births, and the Asian Pacific Islander rate of about 72 births.

FIGURE 3.9.   AGE OF MOTHER AT BIRTH BY RACE/ETHNICITY, 2000.

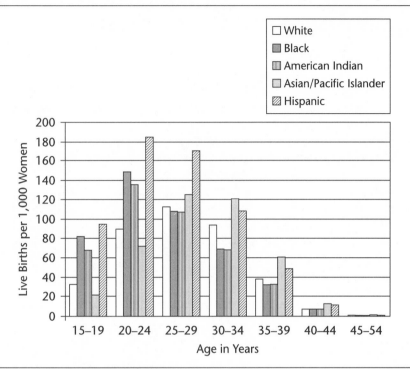

Source: National Center for Health Statistics, 2003.

Teen Childbearing

Figure 3.10 presents the percentage of live births to teen mothers for the year 2000. Note that this statistic is different from fertility rates and birth rates. The data presented in Figure 3.10 represent the percentage for a given racial/ethnic group of live births to teen mothers (number of teen births divided by all births times 100). The figure shows substantial variation across the racial/ethnic groups in teenage childbearing. Puerto Ricans have the highest percentage of births to teen mothers, followed by Blacks and American Indians, then Other Hispanic, Hawaiians, Mexicans, and Hispanics. For each of these groups, between 15 and 20 percent of the live births in the year 2000 were to mothers below age twenty. For Central Americans, Cubans, Filipinos, and Whites, the percentage of live births to teen mothers was between 5 and 10 percent. Fewer than 5 percent of births to Japanese, Chinese, and Asian/Pacific Islander women were to mothers below age twenty.

FIGURE 3.10.   TEENAGED CHILDBEARING BY
RACE/ETHNICITY, 2000.

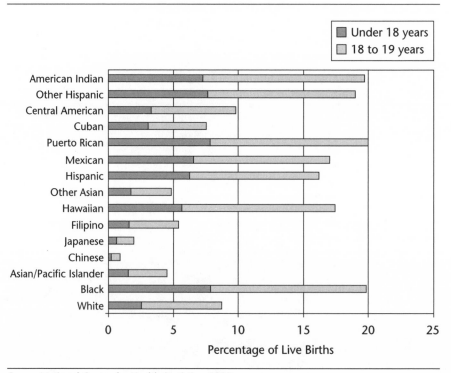

Source: National Center for Health Statistics, 2003.

Possible explanations for such large racial/ethnic variation in teen birth rates include high rates of joblessness and low rates of college attendance among African
Americans and Hispanics/Latinos, leading to lower rates of marriage (Caldas, 1994);
also, there are lower rates of contraception use among African American teens
(Besharov & Gardiner, 1997).

Nonmarital Childbearing

The pattern of births to unmarried women is similar to the pattern for teen births. As
one might expect, most teenagers who give birth are unmarried. However, while the
patterns for nonmarital childbearing and teen childbearing are similar, they are not
precisely the same. Figure 3.11 displays nonmarital childbearing for racial and ethnic
groups for the year 2000. More than 68 percent of Black births were to unmarried

FIGURE 3.11. NONMARITAL CHILDBEARING BY RACE/ETHNICITY, 2000.

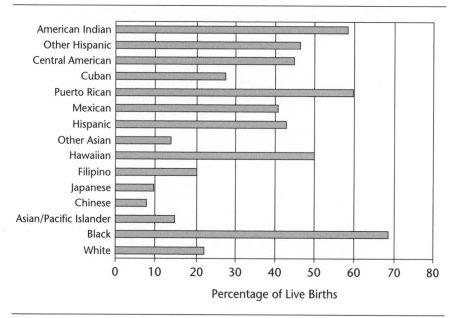

Percentage of Live Births

Source: National Center for Health Statistics, 2003.

women. This is ten percentage points higher than the births to Puerto Rican and American Indian women. Overall, Asian/Pacific Islanders have a relatively low rate of nonmarital childbearing; however, about 50 percent of all births to native Hawaiians occurred among unmarried women.

Other Hispanic groups, such as Central Americans and Mexicans, also had relatively high rates of nonmarital childbearing—between 40 and 50 percent. However, among the Hispanic groups there is fairly wide variation in rates of nonmarital childbearing. For example, the rate for Cubans was less than 30 percent, whereas the rate for Puerto Ricans was almost double that rate.

Family Formation

Patterns of nonmarital childbearing can be clearly observed by examining the data in Figure 3.12, which shows marital status of persons aged eighteen or older in the U.S. population. The figure shows that more than 50 percent of adult Whites, Hispanics, and Asian/Pacific Islanders are married. This is in stark contrast to the African American population, of which only about 35 percent of adults are married. The substantially lower rates of marriage among African Americans do not appear to be a function of high rates of divorce. The divorce rates for Black and White Americans are relatively similar, and Black rates of marital separation are relatively similar to those of Hispanics/Latinos. However, the low rate of marriage among African Americans appears to result from failing to get married in the first place, rather than high divorce rates. In fact, African Americans are the only group with a higher percentage of adults who have never married (39 percent) compared with the percentage that are married (35 percent).

As a consequence of low rates of marriage and high rates of nonmarital childbearing, Black families are often configured differently from families of other

FIGURE 3.12.   MARITAL STATUS OF PERSONS AGED 18 OR OLDER BY RACE/ETHNICITY.

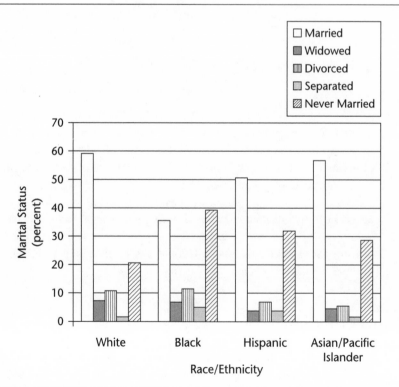

Source: U.S. Bureau of the Census, Census 2000.

racial/ethnic groups. As Figure 3.13 shows, the largest proportion of African American children under age eighteen—48.3 percent—are living in households headed only by their mother. The proportion of children living in female-headed households for Hispanics is 25 percent, nearly double the percentage of Asian/Pacific Islander children (13 percent). Only 16.1 percent of White children live in female-headed households. The percentage of Black children living in households with both of their parents is substantially lower than for the other racial/ethnic groups for which data were available (Hispanics/Latinos 65 percent, Whites 76.9 percent, and Asian/Pacific Islanders 81.2 percent).

Many studies have been conducted—mainly by social scientists such as sociologists, economists, psychologists, and anthropologists—to determine the reasons for racial/ethnic differences in marriage. It is beyond the scope of this book to fully discuss these reasons. However, the general consensus among scholars who study family

FIGURE 3.13.   CHILDREN UNDER AGE 18 LIVING WITH BOTH PARENTS OR WITH MOTHER ONLY, BY RACE/ETHNICITY.

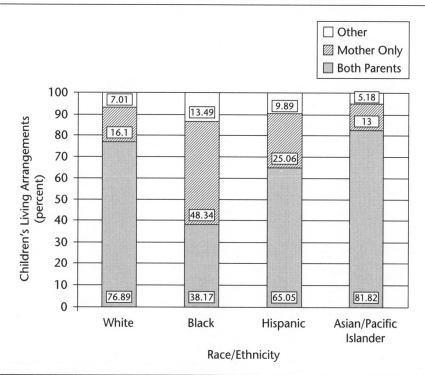

Source: U.S. Bureau of the Census, Census 2000.

issues is that the variation in marriage rates (particularly the low rate of marriage among African Americans) is caused by economic factors. These economic factors include high rates of unemployment, lower wages for similar work, and lower levels of education stemming from lower-quality schools in minority communities.

Mortality

The distribution of mortality rates by race/ethnicity will be discussed in depth in Chapter Four. However, it is important to discuss mortality within the context of demographic trends because mortality is one of the key components of demographic analysis, as mortality rates play an important role in population change. Figure 3.14 displays age-adjusted mortality rates per 100,000 persons by race/ethnicity. The figure shows that Blacks have the highest death rate among the racial/ethnic groups for which data are available. The Black mortality rate of 1,147 deaths per 100,000 persons is more than 33 percent higher than the mortality rate for Whites, who have the second highest mortality rate (860.7 deaths per 100,000 persons). The third-highest rate can be found among American Indians, who have an age-adjusted mortality rate of 716 deaths per 100,000 persons. The Hispanic age-adjusted mortality rate of 601 deaths per 100,000 persons is just over half the rate for Blacks. Asian/Pacific Islanders are the ethnic group with the lowest age-adjusted mortality rate: 517.5 deaths.

BOX 3.2. MORTALITY RATES.

$$\text{Crude mortality rate} = \frac{\text{number of deaths in a given year}}{\text{midyear number of persons in the population of the age group}} \times 1{,}000 = \text{number of deaths in a year per 1,000 of the midyear population}$$

$$\text{Age–specific mortality rate} = \frac{\text{number of deaths among persons of a given age during a year}}{\text{midyear number persons in the population of the age group}} \times 1{,}000 = \text{number of deaths of persons of a given age during a year per 1,000 of the midyear population at that age}$$

Source: Shryock, Siegel, and Associates, 1976, pp. 224, 227.

FIGURE 3.14. AGE-ADJUSTED MORTALITY RATE BY RACE/ETHNICITY, 1999.

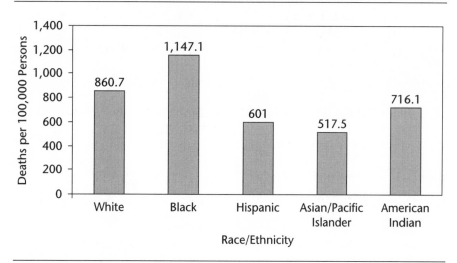

Source: National Center for Health Statistics, 2003.

Migration

Patterns in migration are perhaps the primary reason for the transition in the racial distribution of the majority of the U.S. population and the projections that the United States will become a non-White majority country by the middle of the twenty-first century. During the second half of the twentieth century the United States experienced increased in-migration. Most of that migration was among people coming from Asia or Latin America. Figure 3.15 shows the percentage of each racial group that was foreign-born for the years 1960 to 1990. The figure demonstrates a slight decline in the percentage of Whites that are foreign-born; however, during this same time

period there was a rapid increase in the percentage of foreign-born Asian/Pacific
Islanders and Hispanics. Blacks also demonstrated an upward trend in the percentage
of foreign-born, coming primarily from the Caribbean and to some extent Africa.
However, the rate of foreign-born Blacks is increasing at a much slower rate than
the rate for Asian/Pacific Islanders or Hispanics.

In 1960 just over 30 percent of Asian/Pacific Islanders were foreign-born. This
percentage had doubled by 1990, when more than 60 percent of Asian/Pacific Islanders were foreign-born. Data for the year 1960 were not available for Hispanics;
however, between 1970 and 1990 the percentage of Hispanics that were foreign-born
increased from just below 20 percent to about 35 percent.

Figure 3.16 examines migration from a different perspective: this time we look at
the actual number of foreign-born individuals immigrating into the country. By examining numbers rather than percentages, it is easier to get a sense of the magnitude of immigration and how it impacts the racial distribution of the population.

**FIGURE 3.15.   PERCENTAGE OF FOREIGN-BORN INDIVIDUALS IN
EACH RACIAL/ETHNIC GROUP, 1960–1990.**

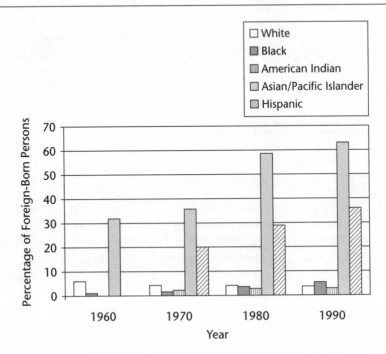

Source: U.S. Bureau of the Census, Census 2000.

Figure 3.16 shows the country of birth of the foreign-born U.S. population for each racial/ethnic group with a population of at least 500,000 persons in 1990 and 1997. In 1990 the country with the largest number of immigrants into the United States was Mexico. In that year almost 430,000 Mexicans immigrated to the United States. That number increased by more than 63 percent over the following seven years. The country with the next largest number of immigrants was the Philippines, followed by China. No other country had more than 100,000 immigrants in 1997.

It is also useful to note the rate of change in the number of immigrants from each country between 1990 and 1997. The country with the highest rate of change was the Soviet Union, with an increase of almost 120 percent. Other countries with very high rates of increase were the Dominican Republic (81 percent), India (66 percent), China (65 percent), Mexico (63 percent), and El Salvador (30 percent). Note that immigrants from these countries are classified as either Asian/Pacific Islander or Hispanic. Only two countries experienced a decline in immigration during this time span: Germany (down

FIGURE 3.16.   COUNTRY OF BIRTH OF THE FOREIGN-BORN U.S. POPULATION FOR EACH RACIAL/ETHNIC GROUP OF 500,000 OR MORE, 1990 AND 1997.

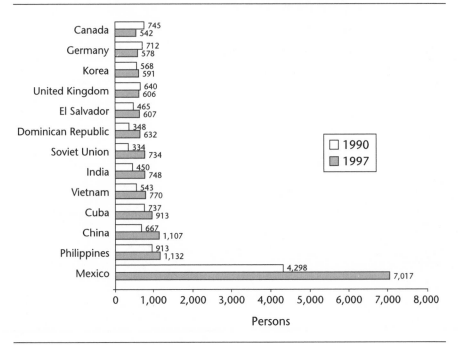

Source: U.S. Bureau of the Census, Census 2000.

18.8 percent) and the United Kingdom (down 5.3 percent). Both of these countries had been among the leading sources of immigrants to the United States in the past.

Summary

This chapter used the tools of demography to explore the degree of racial/ethnic diversity in the United States. The chapter also examined the geographic variations among the different racial and ethnic groups and assessed long-term projections for changes in the racial makeup of the U.S. population. The Census Bureau estimates that by around the middle of the twenty-first century Whites will no longer be a majority population. Reasons for these projections include immigration among Hispanics and Asians, a younger population among racial and ethnic minority groups, and higher birth rates among racial/ethnic minorities. (See Appendix B for additional readings.)

Key Words

Fertility

Crude mortality rate

Age-specific mortality rate

Age-adjustment (age-standardization)

PART TWO

MORBIDITY, MORTALITY, AND RACIAL/ETHNIC DISPARITIES IN HEALTH

CHAPTER FOUR

THE EPIDEMIOLOGICAL PROFILE OF RACIAL/ETHNIC MINORITIES

Outline

Introduction

This chapter explores the health status of the various racial/ethnic groups that make up the U.S. population. In general, the distribution of ill health is such that racial/ethnic minorities have worse health status than Whites; such differences in health status are called health disparities. The National Institutes of Health (2004) defines health disparities as "differences in the incidence, prevalence, mortality, and burden of disease and other adverse health conditions that exist among specific population groups in the United States. Research on health disparities related to socioeconomic status is also encompassed in the definition."

Health disparities must be distinguished from health care disparities. Health disparities refer to differences across racial and ethnic groups in health conditions, risks, and prognoses, whereas health care disparities refer to differences in access, utilization, quality of care, or outcomes from use of health care services. Health care disparities will be addressed in Chapter Six.

What Is Epidemiology?

Epidemiology is the study of the distribution and determinants of mortality (death) and morbidity (illness) in human populations. It is one of the fundamental sciences that support the work of public health, nursing, and medicine. Statistics are the primary tool of the epidemiologist. Statistics can be used to demonstrate how the distribution of a given disease or cause of death may be different among subpopulations such as racial/ethnic groups. This chapter will introduce several epidemiological methods and apply them to minority health to demonstrate the nature of racial and ethnic variation in mortality and morbidity within the United States. Specifically, we will examine racial/ethnic differences in mortality and morbidity. To examine mortality we will use the following indicator statistics: crude death rate, age-adjusted death rate, infant mortality rate, low birth weight, maternal mortality rate, life expectancy, and years of potential life lost. To examine morbidity we will use prevalence rates.

Comparative Mortality

Reliable data on the health status of Americans have been available since early in the twentieth century. However, until the 1940s data were very limited for African Americans. Furthermore, national health data for other ethnic groups were not available until the 1980s (in response to changes in policy related to OMB Directive 15). This makes it difficult to conduct research on minority populations and limits one's

BOX 4.1.   SOME KEY TERMS USED IN EPIDEMIOLOGY.

Term	Definition
Rate	$\dfrac{\text{Number of events in specified period}}{\text{Average population during specified time period}} \times 10^n$
Life expectancy	Number of years a given individual can expect to live, assuming that mortality conditions at the person's birth remain the same
Prevalence	The number of occurrences of a given disease or condition within a given population at a given point in time. Prevalence is typically expressed as a rate (prevalence rate). The prevalence rate is "the number of instances of a given disease or other condition in a given population at a designated time" (Last, 1988).
Incidence	The number of new cases of a given disease or condition within a given population of persons who are at risk of getting the disease at a given point in time. Incidence is typically expressed as a rate (incidence rate). Incidence rate is the number of new cases of the disease or condition divided by the number of persons exposed to risk during the time period being examined.

BOX 4.2.   OMB DIRECTIVE 15.

The Office of Budget and Management's Directive 15 established standards for the collection of data on race and ethnicity. See Chapter Two for a full discussion of Directive 15.

ability to compare present conditions to the past. However, these are the best available data. Accordingly, in this chapter we will use the available data to describe the health status of racial/ethnic groups in the United States.

Historical Trends in Mortality Rates

Figure 4.1 shows trends in age-adjusted mortality rates for the overall U.S. population, and Figure 4.2 shows similar data for U.S. racial and ethnic groups. When comparing populations it is important to refer to the relative size of the population. For example,

FIGURE 4.1.   AGE-ADJUSTED MORTALITY RATES BY SEX, 1940–2000.

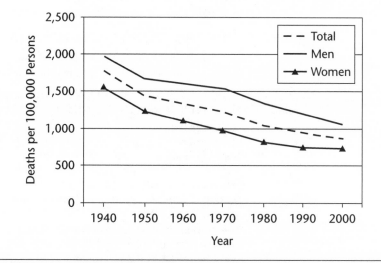

Source: National Center for Health Statistics, *National Vital Statistics Reports,* Vol. 52, No. 3,
September 18, 2003, tab. 1.

it would be misleading to compare the total number of White patients with cancer
to the total number of Asian patients with cancer, because the White U.S.-based
population is so much larger than the Asian population. To compare cancer in the
two populations it would be necessary to compute rates. Rates are typically displayed
per 100, per 1,000, per 10,000, or per 100,000.

Second, it is important that rates be adjusted for age (also referred to as age
standardization). Age-adjusting allows us to estimate the differences in mortality rates
that would exist between the two states if each state had the same age distribution.
Unadjusted (or crude) rates are limited because they do not account for differences in
the age distribution of the comparison populations (for example, crude rate equals death
divided by population times 10,000). Suppose we wanted to compare cancer death rates
between State A and State B. In State A the average age of the population is sixty years,
but in State B the average age is only forty. The crude death rate for State A would
naturally be higher. But does State A have a higher cancer mortality rate because there
are more cancer risks in the environment in State A, or is the higher rate merely a
reflection of the older age of the population in State A? Without adjusting the cancer
death rates for age analysis, it would be impossible to know.

FIGURE 4.2. AGE-ADJUSTED MORTALITY RATES BY RACE/ETHNICITY, 1940–2000.

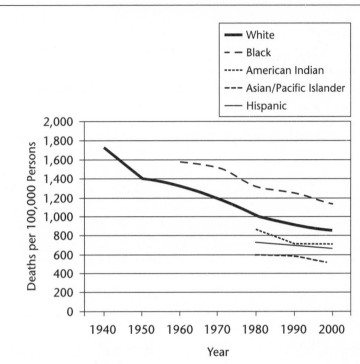

Note: Data for Hispanics are based on estimates.

Source: National Center for Health Statistics, *National Vital Statistics Reports,* Vol. 52, No. 3, September 18, 2003.

BOX 4.3. AGE ADJUSTMENT.

Age-adjustment, also called *age-standardization,* is a procedure for adjusting various rates, such as birth and death rates, to minimize the effects of differing age distributions when comparing different populations.

Racial/Ethnic Variation in Mortality Rates

Examination of Figures 4.1 and 4.2 reveals two general long-term trends. First, there has been a steady decline in age-adjusted mortality for all racial/ethnic groups throughout the twentieth century. Second, there have been persistent disparities among the sexes and the various racial/ethnic groups. In Figure 4.1 women have a lower mortality rate than men. Figure 4.2 suggests that Whites have a lower mortality rate than African Americans, Native Americans, and Hispanics/Latinos; conversely, Asian Americans have a better health profile than Whites.

These figures show deaths per 100,000 persons adjusted for the age distribution of each racial/ethnic group. In the mid-twentieth century the annual mortality rate for the United States was more than 1,700 deaths per 100,000 persons (in a given year, 1,700 out of every 100,000 persons would be expected to die). The age-adjusted mortality rate steadily declined, reaching 869 deaths per 100,000 persons by century's end. Women consistently display a lower mortality rate than men, and although death rates for both groups have experienced major declines, the gender gap has remained persistent throughout the time period displayed in the figures. In Figure 4.2 we see that the age-adjusted mortality rate for African Americans is consistently higher than the age-adjusted mortality rates for all other racial and ethnic groups. In 1960 the Black age-adjusted mortality rate was nearly 1,600 deaths per 100,000 Blacks, similar to the White rate around 1940. This disparity persisted throughout the century. By the year 2000 the Black age-adjusted mortality rate was nearly 1,200 deaths per 100,000, comparable to the White rate during the 1970s (more than twenty years earlier).

With only twenty years' worth of data for American Indians/Alaska Natives (AIAN), Asian/Pacific Islanders (API), and Hispanic/Latinos, it is difficult to make broad generalizations about comparisons over time. However, each group displays an age-adjusted mortality rate (that is, deaths from all causes) that is below the White rate. And the Asian/Pacific Islander population consistently had the lowest rate.

Age-adjusted mortality rates for the year 2001 are displayed in Figure 4.3. This figure demonstrates that the pattern displayed in the previous charts for the twentieth century has continued into the twenty-first century. The age-adjusted death rate for Black males—1,375.0—is similar to the rates experienced by White males in the early 1980s. The current Black male mortality rate is similar to the White female mortality rate of fifty years ago. The Black female mortality rate had not been as high as the current Black male mortality rate since 1960. Asian/Pacific Islanders continue to have the lowest age-adjusted mortality rate. The rate for API males was around 600 deaths per 100,000, and the female rate was just over 400 deaths. In addition, American Indian, API, and Hispanic/Latino women have age-adjusted death rates lower than 600 deaths per 100,000 persons.

FIGURE 4.3. AGE-ADJUSTED MORTALITY RATES BY RACE/ETHNICITY AND GENDER, 2001.

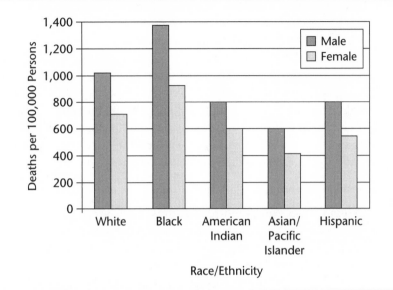

Source: National Center for Health Statistics, *National Vital Statistics Reports,* Vol. 52, No. 3, September 18, 2003, tabs. 1 and 2.

Survival Curve

Examination of the survival curve is another way in which we can compare differences in death rates across populations. The survival curve shows the proportion of a birth cohort projected to be alive as the population ages. The curve begins at 100 percent and the percent living declines as the population ages. Figure 4.4 displays the survival curve for Blacks and Whites for the year 2000. The figure shows that survivorship declines at a more rapid rate for Blacks compared with Whites. The difference between the groups widens as the population ages out of childhood, through adulthood, and into the senior years. For persons above age eighty the curve begins to converge and then tails off above age one hundred.

Infant Mortality

Infant mortality rates are often used as a marker of the general health status of a population, and these rates are often used to conduct analysis comparing across societies. Infant mortality is calculated as the total number of infant deaths divided by the total number of live births times 1,000. This statistic is interpreted as infant deaths per 1,000 live births. This use of infant mortality is widely accepted for several reasons. First, because the deaths occur among infants, who were too young to have engaged in behaviors that are injurious to their health, infant mortality allows for comparisons to be made between populations and across societies without having to account for differences in health behaviors among the individuals. (Naturally, infant mortality cannot account for differences in the behavior of pregnant women. As individuals age, they may be more or less inclined to engage in such behaviors as smoking, inactivity, or drug use, all of which may contribute to infant mortality.) Second, although cultures differ in their value systems, it is generally a universal value that societies wish for infants to survive and usually will exert effort to prevent infant deaths. Thus, infant deaths can be viewed as deaths that could not be avoided.

Neonatal and Postneonatal Mortality. In Figure 4.5, trends in infant mortality rates for various U.S.-based racial/ethnic groups are examined. The figure shows that for every racial/ethnic group the mortality rate has been declining. However, although each group has experienced declines in infant mortality, there is significant variation in rates among the groups. African Americans have the highest infant mortality rate, with a rate in excess of 13 deaths per 1,000 live births in 2000. That rate is down from 18.25 deaths per 1,000 in 1985. Blacks are followed by American Indians, whose rates

FIGURE 4.4.   SURVIVORSHIP BY RACE, 2000.

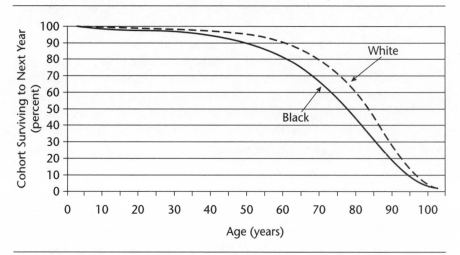

Source: National Center for Health Statistics, *National Vital Statistics Reports,* Vol. 51, No. 3, December 19, 2002, tabs. 4 and 7.

have declined from about 13 deaths per 1,000 in 1985 to just over 8 deaths in the year 2000. The lowest infant mortality rate is found among Asian/Pacific Islanders, whose rate was 4.6 deaths per 1,000 in 2000.

About two-thirds of infant deaths occur during the neonatal period, and the remaining third in the postneonatal period (see Box 4.4). Figure 4.6 compares the racial/ethnic groups' rates of infant, neonatal, and postneonatal mortality. The figure shows a pattern similar to that displayed in Figure 4.5: Blacks have the highest neonatal mortality rate and Asian/Pacific Islanders the lowest. Whites, American Indians, and Hispanics/Latinos have rates between these two groups.

FIGURE 4.5. INFANT MORTALITY RATES BY RACE/ETHNICITY, 1985–2000.

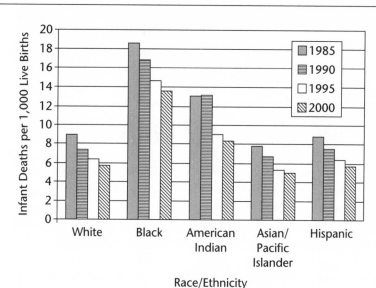

Source: National Center for Health Statistics, 2003, tab. 19.

BOX 4.4. INFANT MORTALITY, NEONATAL MORTALITY, AND POSTNEONATAL MORTALITY.

Infant mortality is typically expressed as infant deaths per 1,000 live births. Infant mortality statistics are often divided into two categories: *neonatal mortality* refers to deaths within the first twenty-eight days of birth; *postneonatal mortality* refers to deaths between twenty-nine days and one year after birth.

FIGURE 4.6.   INFANT, NEONATAL, AND POSTNEONATAL MORTALITY RATES BY RACE/ETHNICITY, 2001.

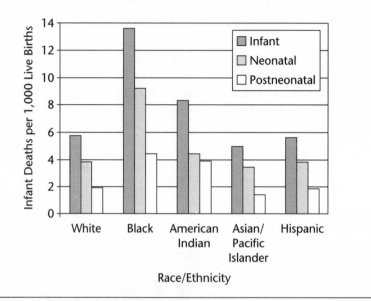

Source: National Center for Health Statistics, 2003, tab. 19.

The pattern for postneonatal mortality differs somewhat from the patterns for infants and neonatal mortality. There is far less variation among the groups in post-neonatal mortality rates. Also, the postneonatal mortality rate for Blacks is not significantly different from the rate for American Indians. It is also interesting to note that the infant, neonatal, and postneonatal mortality rates are generally similar for Whites, Asian/Pacific Islanders, and Hispanics/Latinos.

In Figure 4.7 we return to comparisons of infant mortality rates for the year 2000; however, this figure includes the more detailed classifications for ethnic groups. We first look at the subgroups comprised by the Asian/Pacific Islander population. Here we see there is significant variation in infant mortality rates of these groups. For instance, Native Hawaiians have an infant mortality rate that is exceeded only by that of Blacks. This is in contrast to the Chinese American population, which has an infant mortality rate of 3.5 deaths per 1,000 live births. No other group in this category has an infant mortality rate greater than 6 deaths per 1,000 live births.

The infant mortality rates for the Hispanic/Latino subgroups also show significant variation. Puerto Ricans have the highest infant mortality rate, a rate of more than eight deaths per thousand live births. In contrast, Cuban-Americans have the lowest rate among all Hispanic subgroups.

FIGURE 4.7.   INFANT MORTALITY RATES BY RACE/ETHNICITY, 2000.

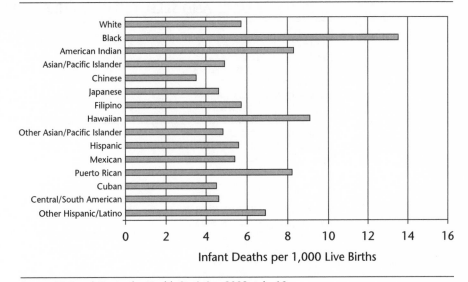

Source: National Center for Health Statistics, 2003, tab. 19.

International Comparison of Infant Mortality. By placing U.S. racial/ethnic disparities in infant mortality rates into an international context, we can get a fuller appreciation of the magnitude of the disparities among U.S.-based populations. Figure 4.8 shows infant mortality rates for selected countries compared with U.S.-based racial/ethnic groups for the year 1999. The country with the lowest infant mortality rate is Japan, with 3.4 deaths per 1,000 live births. This rate is less than half the rate for the overall U.S. population: 7 deaths per 1,000 live births. Similarly, Finland has an infant rate of less than 4 deaths per 1,000 live births. At 7 deaths per 1,000 live births, the U.S. infant mortality rate far exceeds the rates of most other industrialized countries. This is partly due to substantial variation in infant mortality rates among U.S.-based racial/ethnic groups. However, variations among minority populations do not fully explain the high U.S. infant mortality rate. The infant mortality rate for U.S. Whites—while comparable to that in the United Kingdom—is more than one infant death higher than the rates of Austria, Denmark, France, Spain, and Germany. Although it is clear that racial/ethnic disparities in infant mortality rates play some role in the relatively poor showing of the United States in international comparisons, it appears that relatively high infant mortality rates are part of a universal problem in the United States, one that affects White Americans as well.

FIGURE 4.8. INTERNATIONAL COMPARISONS OF INFANT MORTALITY RATES, UNITED STATES AND SELECTED COUNTRIES, 1999.

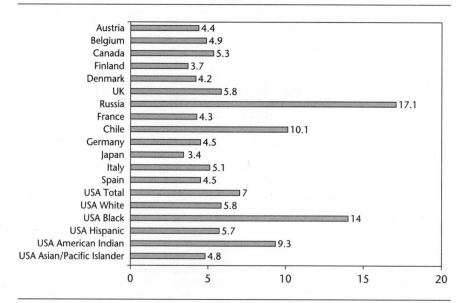

Source: National Center for Health Statistics, 2003, tabs. 19 and 25.

Low Birth Weight and Very Low Birth Weight

Low birth weight and very low birth weight are widely accepted markers of the health status of the population (see Box 4.5). Low birth weight and very low birth weight infants have a higher risk of mortality within the first year of life. In fact, birth weight is the strongest predictor of infant death. Low and very low birth weight infants are more likely to have long-term health complications and developmental difficulties. Figure 4.9 displays low birth weight and very low birth weight rates by race/ethnicity for the years 1999 through 2001.

Figure 4.9 shows that African Americans have the highest low birth weight rate among the racial/ethnic groups. About thirteen infants per thousand were considered low birth weight—double the rate for all other groups. The Black very low birth weight rate is also substantially higher than the rate for the other groups: about three per thousand births to Blacks were in the very low weight category. This rate is also double the rate for other U.S.-based racial/ethnic groups. Among the remaining groups there are only relatively modest differences in rates of the low birth weight and very low birth weight. The low birth weight rate for Asians/Pacific Islanders is slightly

---

BOX 4.5.   LOW BIRTH WEIGHT AND VERY LOW BIRTH WEIGHT

Low birth weight: Below 2,500 grams (5.5 lb)
Moderate low birth weight: Between 1,500 and 2,499 grams (3.31 to 5.4 lb.)
Very low birth weight: Below 1,500 grams (3.31 lb.)
Ultra low birth weight: Below 1,000 grams (2.2 lb.)

FIGURE 4.9.   LOW BIRTH WEIGHT AND VERY LOW BIRTH WEIGHT LIVE BIRTH RATES BY RACE/ETHNICITY, 1999–2001.

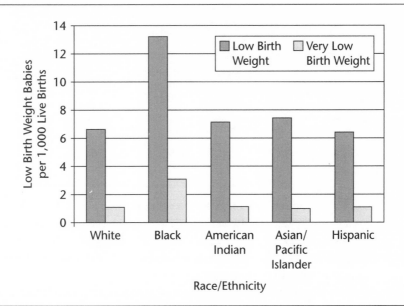

Source: National Center for Health Statistics, 2003, tabs. 14 and 15.

---

higher than the rates for American Indians and Whites, and the rate for Hispanic/
Latinos is slightly lower than for all other groups.

Maternal Mortality

Maternal mortality is still an important indicator of the health status of populations. Maternal mortality rates have experienced substantial decline during the twentieth century. Figure 4.10 shows maternal mortality rates for Whites, Blacks, and Hispanics
for the second half of the twentieth century. Please note that data for Hispanics/
Latinos were not available until the late 1980s. As the figure shows, maternal mortality

FIGURE 4.10.   MATERNAL MORTALITY RATES BY RACE/ETHNICITY, 1950–2000.

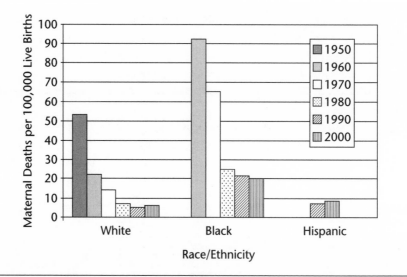

Source: National Center for Health Statistics, 2003, tab. 43.

rates for all groups have plummeted over the fifty-year period. In 1950, the White maternal mortality rate was greater than 50 deaths per 100,000 live births. By 1960 that number had dropped to just over 20 deaths. The decline in White maternal mortality continued until the end of the twentieth century—by the year 2000 the White rate was only about five deaths per 100,000 live births.

Although the pattern of infant mortality decline for African Americans is similar to that of Whites, the maternal mortality rates for African Americans remain much higher. In 1960 the African American maternal mortality rate was in excess of 90 deaths per 100,000 live births. This was more than three times the rate for Whites in 1960. Over the following decades the Black rate declined substantially; by 1990 the rate was just over 20 deaths per 100,000 live births. The Black maternal mortality rate for 1990 is equivalent to the White rate for 1960; however, the magnitude of the disparity between Blacks and Whites had widened. The Black rate of 20 deaths per 100,000 live births in the year 2000 is about four times the White rate. Finally, the available data for Hispanics shows maternal mortality rates of less than 10 deaths per 100,000 live births in both 1990 and 2000.

Life Expectancy

Life expectancy (expectation of life) is another important indicator of population health. However, unlike the other measures we have reviewed, life expectancy is hypothetical. It measures the expected number of years that the average person within a given birth cohort can expect to live if present trends in mortality rates do not change. Life expectancy can be calculated from any age; that is, one can calculate life expectancy at birth, at age one, at age forty-five, or at any other age. The most common approach is to calculate life expectancy at birth. However, it is important to note that life expectancy at birth is greatly influenced by infant mortality. In international comparisons of life expectancy this is particularly important because of tremendous disparities in infant mortality rates across countries—particularly in less economically developed countries.

Historical Trends in Life Expectancy

During the twentieth century, life expectancy in the United States increased substantially. At the beginning of the century it was relatively rare for Americans of any racial or ethnic group to live more than sixty years. By the end of the twentieth century, however, it was not unusual for Americans to exceed eighty years of life. Although life expectancy has increased for all groups, there has been a persistent disparity in life expectancy between African Americans and White Americans, as well as between males and females. Figure 4.11 shows life expectancy for male and female, African Americans and White Americans for the years 1900 to 2000.

At the beginning of the twentieth century, life expectancy for African Americans was less than thirty-five years, whereas White life expectancy was nearly fifty years. White females have consistently had the highest life expectancy throughout the century, ranging from about forty-five years to greater than eighty years by the year 2000. Early in the century White males had the second highest life expectancy; however, as the century progressed the disparity by gender overtook the racial disparity in life expectancy, and by the 1960s life expectancy for Black women equaled (and for a time exceeded) White male life expectancy. During the last three decades of the century Black women and White males had relatively equal life expectancy. Black male life expectancy has also increased substantially during the twentieth century, but it has not improved as rapidly as for Black females. Whereas life expectancy for White females reached sixty-five years in the 1940s, for White males it reached sixty-five in the 1950s and for Black females it reached sixty-five in the 1960s. It was not until late in the 1990s that Black male life expectancy reached age sixty-five.

FIGURE 4.11.   LIFE EXPECTANCY AT BIRTH BY RACE AND GENDER, UNITED STATES, 1900–2000.

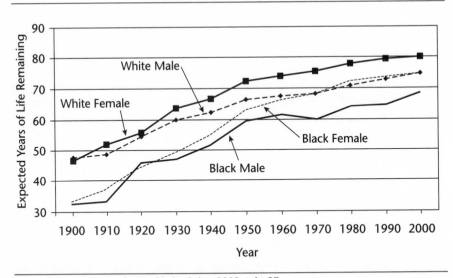

Source: National Center for Health Statistics, 2003, tab. 27.

International Comparisons in Life Expectancy

Figure 4.12 presents international comparisons of male life expectancy for the United States and selected countries for the year 1998. Similar to the findings on infant mortality, U.S. White male life expectancy is relatively consistent with that in other industrialized countries, although not as high as in such countries as Japan, Italy, the United Kingdom, and Canada. U.S. Black male life expectancy is below that in other industrialized countries.

Figure 4.13 shows that the pattern for females is similar to the male pattern; that is, White American women have life expectancy on a par with women of other industrialized nations (although not among the best) and life expectancy for Black women lags behind that for women of other industrialized nations.

Race/Ethnic Comparisons in Life Expectancy

One of the most interesting phenomena found in minority health research is the *mortality crossover.* This refers to research that shows that in old age the death rate for Black Americans is lower than the rate for White Americans (Corti et al., 1999). This reversal of mortality rates between advantaged and disadvantaged populations

FIGURE 4.12. INTERNATIONAL COMPARISONS OF MALE LIFE EXPECTANCY, UNITED STATES AND SELECTED COUNTRIES, 1998.

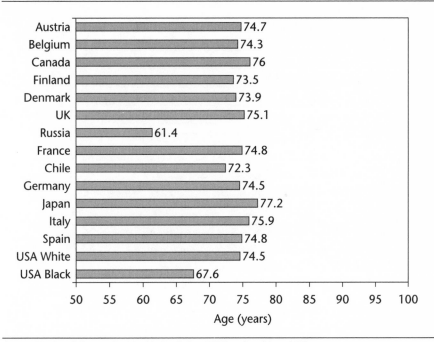

Source: National Center for Health Statistics, 2003, tabs. 26 and 27.

also occurs between Native Americans and Whites (Markides & Machalek, 1984). The crossover is illustrated in Figure 4.14, which plots life expectancy at various ages between seventy and one hundred and shows the expected number of years of life remaining for Whites and Blacks. The lines representing Black and White years of remaining life converge and then cross around age eighty. Thus, just beyond age eighty Blacks actually have a higher life expectancy than Whites.

A substantial amount of research has been devoted to the mortality crossover, and this research has created a great deal of controversy. When the mortality crossover was first discovered in the 1970s, some believed that the crossover was merely a data anomaly resulting from low-quality birth records during the early twentieth century. However, the consistency of this finding and its replication using many different research designs has led to a general consensus today that the mortality crossover is a real phenomenon and not merely a function of data anomalies.

FIGURE 4.13.   INTERNATIONAL COMPARISONS OF FEMALE LIFE EXPECTANCY, UNITED STATES AND SELECTED COUNTRIES, 1998.

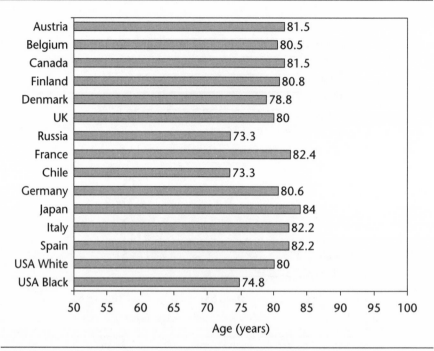

Source: National Center for Health Statistics, 2003, tabs. 26 and 27.

It is now generally accepted that the mortality crossover is caused by selective survival of the healthiest older African Americans. Below age eighty, African Americans have a high mortality rate. Those African Americans who live to age eighty are those who are particularly hearty individuals. By contrast, frail Whites are more likely to survive to age eighty. Consequently, above age eighty, the deaths of the frail Whites skew the White mortality rate to be higher, and the Black mortality rate lowers because of the relative good health of the remaining healthy African Americans.

The factors that contribute to the life span of a given individual fall into three broad categories: (1) socioenvironmental factors, (2) behavioral factors, and (3) biological inheritance. Socioenvironmental factors refer to characteristics in the physical environment that impact individuals—for example, exposure to biological,

FIGURE 4.14.   THE MORTALITY CROSSOVER.

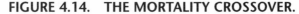

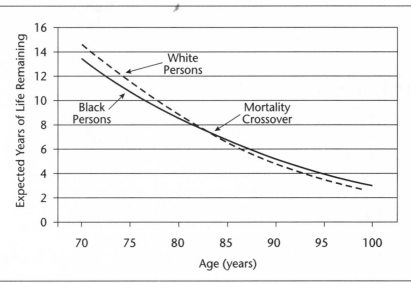

Source: National Center for Health Statistics, *National Vital Statistics Reports,* Vol. 52, No. 3, September 18, 2003, tab. 7.

chemical, or other toxic substances, or exposure to aspects of the society that are injurious to health, such as poverty, low-quality housing, stress, malnutrition, overcrowding, and the like. Behavioral factors refer to actions that an individual takes that may affect health and life span, such as smoking, lack of physical activity, underuse of available health services, and abuse of alcohol or other drugs. Biological inheritance refers to the degree to which an individual's genetic endowment predisposes that individual to long life.

One might assume that the genetic predisposition to long life is distributed within all populations in varying degrees. One can think of biological inheritance as a constant among all individuals who reached age eighty. However, given the known differences in socioenvironmental exposures and behavior, African Americans that live to be age eighty are particularly hardy individuals with an exceedingly strong biological predisposition to long life. This contrasts with Whites, who have less exposure to negative socioenvironmental exposures and health behaviors. Therefore, Blacks who reached age eighty are a unique subset of the population with a particularly strong biological inheritance, whereas Whites who reach age eighty are more representative of the general White population (not having had to endure as many social or behavioral health risks). Thus, more frail Whites reach old age than Blacks. As a result, Black and White eighty-year-olds form different subsets of their respective populations.

Leading Causes of Death

In the United States, as in other industrialized countries, the leading causes of death are chronic conditions such as heart disease, cancer, and stroke. A *chronic condition* is a health condition with a long duration, in contrast to an *acute condition*—a condition of short duration. (The term *acute* is often inaccurately used to indicate a severe condition.) Although chronic diseases are the leading causes of death in the United States as a whole, there are major differences in the leading causes of death for different racial/ethnic groups and age groups. Table 4.1 shows the leading causes of death by race/ethnicity for the United States.

The five leading causes of death for Whites, in descending order, are heart disease, cancer, stroke, asthma, and injuries. The leading causes for Blacks are the same, except that instead of asthma, diabetes is among the top five. American Indians and Hispanics have the same five leading causes as Blacks. Asian and Pacific Islanders have the same five leading causes as the White population; however, the order is somewhat different.

For Whites the seventh leading cause of death is diabetes. However, diabetes is the fifth leading cause of death for Blacks and Hispanics, and fourth for American Indians. It is notable that suicide is a leading cause of death among Whites (number ten), American Indians, and Asian/Pacific Islanders and Hispanics (number eight), yet it is not among the ten leading causes for Blacks. Additionally, homicide and HIV are among the ten leading causes of death for African Americans and Hispanics; these are not among the ten leading causes for other groups.

BOX 4.6.   CHRONIC AND ACUTE CONDITIONS.

According to the National Center for Health Statistics, a *chronic condition* is a condition that is not cured once acquired (such as heart disease and diabetes); an *acute condition* is a type of illness or injury that ordinarily lasts less than three months.

TABLE 4.1. TEN LEADING CAUSES OF DEATH, RANKED FOR EACH RACIAL/ETHNIC GROUP, 2000.

Cause of Death	Total	White	Black	American Indian	Asian/ Pacific Islander	Hispanic
Diseases of the heart	1	1	1	1	2	1
Cancer	2	2	2	2	1	2
Stroke	3	3	3	5	3	4
Chronic lower respiratory disease (asthma)	4	4	8	7	5	10
Unintended injuries	5	5	4	3	4	3
Diabetes	6	7	5	4	7	5
Influenza and pneumonia	7	6	10	9	6	
Alzheimer's disease	8	8				
Nephritis, nephritic syndrome, and nephrosis	9	9	9	10	9	
Septicemia	10					
Suicide		10		8	8	8
Homicide			6			6
HIV/AIDS			7			9
Chronic liver disease and cirrhosis				6		7
Certain conditions originating in the perinatal period					10	

Source: National Center for Health Statistics, 2003, tab. 31.

Years of Potential Life Lost

The impact of a cause of death can be demonstrated by computing the years of potential life lost before age seventy-five (YPLL-75), which indicates the average number of years of life lost per 100,000 persons, assuming that every person would otherwise live to age seventy-five. It is an important indicator of the effect of a cause of death on a population because it takes into account the age distribution of the cause of death. Since causes of death that primarily afflict younger people (such as homicide or HIV/AIDS) are responsible for a greater number of potential years of life lost, YPLL-75 is helpful in demonstrating the primary contributors to race differences in life expectancy and reflecting the societal impact of lost potential.

Table 4.2 displays years of potential life lost before age seventy-five for all racial/ethnic groups for the years 1980, 1990, and 2000. The overall number of years of potential life lost declined by 27 percent between 1980 and 2000. The trend of declining years of potential life lost was experienced by every racial/ethnic group. In the year 2000, African Americans had the highest number of YPLL-75, at 12,897.1 years per 100,000 persons. American Indians/Alaska Natives had the second highest number (7,758.2), followed by Whites (6,949.51) and Hispanics (6,037.6). The Asian/Pacific Islander population had the lowest YPLL-75, at 3,811.

Table 4.3 shows the YPLL-75 for the ten leading causes of death for each racial/ethnic group. For most racial/ethnic groups, cancer is the leading contributor to years of potential life lost. The sole exception was the American Indians and Alaska Natives group. For the other groups, cancer accounts for 17.8 to 24 percent of years of potential life lost. The leading contributor to death for American Indians/Alaska Natives is unintentional injuries, which account for more than a fifth of years of lost potential life (21.9 percent). Heart disease also takes a significant toll on lost potential years of life. It is the second largest contributor for every racial/ethnic group, accounting for 13.3 percent to 17.6 percent of potential life lost. Together cancer and heart disease account for more than 40 percent of all potential years of life lost among and API and White populations. These two chronic conditions account for more than 35 percent of YPLL for Blacks, 31.8 percent for Hispanics, and 23.3 percent for American Indians/Alaska Natives.

BOX 4.7.   YEARS OF POTENTIAL LIFE LOST.

An estimate of the number of years of life lost due to premature deaths, assuming that all persons should live to be at least age seventy-five.

TABLE 4.2.   YEARS OF POTENTIAL LIFE LOST BY AGE 75.

Race/Ethnic Group	1980	1990	2000
All groups	10,448.41	9,085.5	7,578.11
White	9,554.1	8,159.5	6,949.5
Black	17,873.4	16,593.0	12,897.1
American Indian or Alaska Native	13,390.9	9,506.2	7,758.2
Asian or Pacific Islander	5,378.4	4,705.2	3,811.1
Hispanic	—	7,963.3	6,037.6

Source: National Center for Health Statistics, 2003, tab. 30.

It is instructive to note the relatively high (compared to other groups) contribution of stroke to YPLL-75 among Asians/Pacific Islanders, and the impact of liver disease among American Indians/Alaska Natives. The impact of liver disease among American Indians/Alaska Natives (6.7 percent of total YPLL-75) is more than three times that of all other groups, with the exception of Hispanics (4.2 percent). HIV deaths account for nearly 6 percent of YPLL among Black Americans, which is more than fourfold the rate for all other groups except Hispanics (3.5 percent). The juxtaposition of suicide and homicide statistics is also interesting: although African Americans have a substantially lower number of years of life lost to suicide compared to all other groups, they have a much higher rate of homicide.

TABLE 4.3.   YEARS OF POTENTIAL LIFE LOST BY AGE 75 FOR SELECTED CAUSES OF DEATH, BY RACE/ETHNICITY, 2000.

Cause of Death	White	Black	American Indian and Alaska Native	Asian or Pacific Islander	Hispanic
Heart disease	1,175.1 (16.9%)	2,275.2 (17.6%)	1,030.1 (13.3%)	567.9 (14.9%)	821.3 (13.6%)
Stroke	183.0 (2.6%)	507.0 (3.9%)	198.1 (2.5%)	199.4 5.2%)	207.8 (3.4%)
Cancer	1,668.4 (24.0%)	2,294.7 17.8%)	995.7 (10.0%)	1,033.8 (27.1%)	1,098.2 (18.2%)
Asthma	193.8 (2.8%)	232.7 (1.8%)	151.8 (1.9%)	56.5 (1.5%)	68.5 (1.1%)
Influenza and pneumonia	76.4 (1.1%)	161.2 (1.2%)	124.0 (1.6%)	48.6 (1.3%)	76.0 (1.3%)
Liver disease	150.9 (2.2%)	185.6 (.4%)	519.4 (6.7%)	44.8 (1.2%)	252.1 (4.2%)
Diabetes	150.2 (2.2%)	383.4 (3.0%)	305.6 (3.9%)	77.0 (2.0%)	215.6 (3.5%)
HIV/AIDS	76.0 (1.1%)	763.3 (5.9%)	68.4 (.88%)	19.9 (.52%)	209.4 (3.5%)
Unintentional injury	1041.4 (15.0%)	1152.8 (8.9%)	1700.1 (21.9%)	425.7 (11.2)	920.1 (15.2%)
Suicide	389.2 (5.6%)	208.7 (1.6%)	403.1 (5.2%)	168.6 (4.4%)	188.5 (3.1%)
Homicide	113.2 (1.6%)	941.6 (7.3%)	278.5 (3.6%)	113.1 (3.0%)	335.1 (5.5%)
Totals	6,960.5	12,897.1	7,758.2	3,811.1	6,037.6

Source: National Center for Health Statistics, 2003, tab. 30.

Comparative Morbidity

Up to this point we have focused on ways of exploring racial/ethnic differences in health status by examining mortality rates and variations on mortality rates: crude death rate, age-adjusted death rate, infant mortality rate, low birth weight, maternal mortality rate, life expectancy, and years of potential life lost. Mortality data provide a valuable way of assessing the health of a population, because they come from a highly reliable source: death certificates. In the United States nearly all deaths are recorded and accounted for. Thus, there is nearly complete information on all deaths that occur in the United States.

However, examining mortality alone has limitations. For example, many of the most prevalent health problems and health risk factors (such as hypertension, high cholesterol, obesity, and depression) are not among the leading causes of death, yet they are major contributors to death. Hypertension, high cholesterol, and obesity are risk factors for heart disease. Depression is a risk factor for suicide. This is why it is important to monitor *morbidity* as well as mortality.

Morbidity is defined as any departure, subjective or objective, from a state of physiological or psychological well-being. It is the state of being sick or ill or having a disease, either physical or mental. According to the World Health Organization (1946), health is "a state of complete physical, mental, and social well-being; it is not merely the absence of disease or infirmity." Morbidity is a departure from good health. We monitor morbidity by examining prevalence and incidence rates (see Box 4.1 for definitions of these terms).

The most common way to obtain data on morbidity is through surveys. A number of ongoing surveys are conducted by the various federal agencies responsible for disease surveillance and health risk monitoring (see Box 4.8). It is important to point out that there are some limitations to survey data: telephone surveys both underrepresent the poor (who are more likely to lack access to a telephone) and rely on the respondent to be truthful and to recall important information.

Table 4.4 and the figures that follow present data from the National Health Interview Survey (NHIS). NHIS is the principal source of information on the health of the noninstitutionalized civilian population of the United States; it is one of the major data collection programs of the National Center for Health Statistics (NCHS), part of the Centers for Disease Control and Prevention. The main objective of the NHIS is to monitor the health of the United States population through the collection and analysis of data on a broad range of health topics. A major strength of this survey lies in the ability to display these health characteristics by many demographic and socioeconomic characteristics.

BOX 4.8.   FEDERAL HEALTH SURVEYS.

National Health Interview Survey (NHIS)

Behavioral Risk Factor Surveillance System (BRFSS)

National Health and Nutrition Examination Survey (NHANES)

Medical Expenditure Panel Survey (MEPS)

National Immunization Survey (NIS)

Medicare Current Beneficiary Survey (MCBS)

National Health Care Survey, which includes the following components:

- National Ambulatory Medical Care Survey (NAMCS)
- National Hospital Ambulatory Medical Care Survey (NHAMCS)
- National Survey of Ambulatory Surgery (NSAS)
- National Hospital Discharge Survey (NHDS)
- National Nursing Home Survey (NNHS)
- National Home and Hospice Care Survey (NHHCS)
- National Employer Health Insurance Survey (NEHIS)
- National Health Provider Inventory (NHPI)

Selected Prevalence Rates

Table 4.4 presents hypertension, diabetes, and dental pain prevalence rates by race/ethnicity. African Americans have the highest prevalence rate of hypertension and diabetes—more than one third of African Americans report having been diagnosed with hypertension. Native Americans have the second highest prevalence rate, followed by Whites, Dominicans, and Puerto Ricans. The lowest prevalence rates are found among Central Americans, who have a prevalence rate of 11.3 cases per 100 persons. Relatively low rates are also found among Chinese and Filipino Americans.

Native Americans have the highest diabetes prevalence rate, followed by Cuban Americans, African Americans, and Puerto Ricans. The lowest diabetes prevalence rates are among Central Americans and Asians. Finally, the prevalence rate of dental pain is highest among Native Americans, Puerto Ricans, and Chinese and African Americans.

TABLE 4.4.   PREVALENCE RATES FOR DIABETES, HYPERTENSION, AND DENTAL PAIN, BY RACE/ETHNICITY (CASES PER 100,000 PERSONS).

Race	Hypertension	Diabetes	Dental Pain
White	27.0	6.6	12.5
Black	33.7	9.6	13.9
Puerto Rican	21.3	9.5	16.5
Mexican American	18.1	7.8	12.9
Cuban American	24.6	10.2	7.4
Dominican	25.7	3.3	11.1
Central American	11.3	2.9	11.7
Asian	14.8	5.1	10.0
Chinese	13.6	4.4	14.7
Filipino	17.1	7.2	10.0
American Indian/Alaska Native	28.1	13.5	24.2

Source: National Health Interview Survey, 2002.

Disability

Activities of daily living (ADLs) are the basic tasks of everyday life, such as eating, bathing, dressing, toileting, and transferring—that is, getting into and out of a bed or chair (see Box 4.9). When people are unable to perform these activities, they must rely on other human beings and/or mechanical devices in order to maintain the basic activities of self-care. ADLs are an important indicator of the health status of a population. Impairment of ADLs is closely associated with several chronic health conditions, such as arthritis, osteoporosis, and stroke; however, many other conditions also lead to difficulty performing ADLs. Although ADL difficulties have been reported in persons of all ages, they are particularly prevalent among the elderly. Within the elderly population, disability rates rise steeply with advancing age and are especially high for persons age eighty-five and over. Measurement of the activities of daily living is critical because they have been found to be significant predictors of admission to a nursing home, use of home care, use of hospital services, living arrangements, overall Medicare expenditures, and mortality (Stark, Kane, Kane, & Finch, 1995).

ADLs are measured by survey. Individuals are asked if they are able to perform a series of tasks, such as eating, bathing, dressing themselves, and so on. Figure 4.15 displays limitations on activities of daily living by race/ethnicity. The figure shows the percentage of individuals who reported in the National Health Interview Survey that they have at least one ADL or instrumental activities of daily living (IADL) limitation. More than 25 percent of American Indians/Alaska Natives report having at least one IADL. This is substantially higher than the IADL prevalence rate for the other groups. African Americans have the second highest rate of IADLs, followed by

---

BOX 4.9. ACTIVITIES OF DAILY LIVING.

Activities of daily living (ADLs) are activities related to personal care and include bathing or showering, dressing, getting into or out of bed or a chair, using the toilet, and eating.

Instrumental activities of daily living (IADLs) are activities related to independent living; these include preparing meals, managing money, shopping for groceries or personal items, performing light or heavy housework, and using a telephone.

FIGURE 4.15. LIMITATIONS OF ACTIVITIES CAUSED BY CHRONIC CONDITIONS, ACCORDING TO SELECTED CHARACTERISTICS, UNITED STATES, 2001.

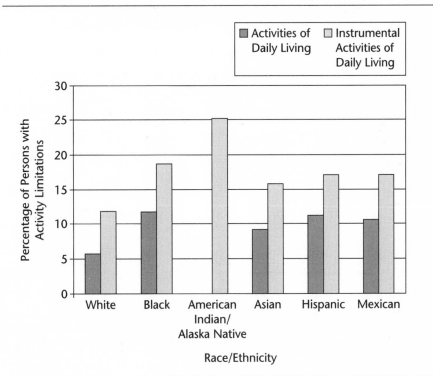

Note: Data for IADLs for American Indians/Alaska Natives are for 1999; data for ADL were not available.

Source: National Center for Health Statistics, 2003, tab. 56.

Hispanics/Latinos, Mexican Americans, and Asians. The lowest IADL prevalence rate was found among Whites, who have a rate of just below 12 percent.

The pattern for ADLs closely mirrors the rate for IADLs. Data for ADLs among American Indians were not available. African Americans have the highest ADL prevalence rate, followed by Hispanics, Mexican Americans, Asians, and Whites.

Self-Assessed Health Status

Self-assessed health status is also an important indicator of the general health of the population. It is increasingly being recognized as a valid measure for predicting future health outcomes—especially survival—among older people. It can also provide information on projected use of health services, which is useful in planning and policy development. An unfavorable assessment of overall health has been associated with increased risk of death. As with ADLs, self-assessed health is measured by survey. Survey respondents are asked the following question: "How is your health in general? Would you say it was very good, good, fair, or poor?"

Figure 4.16 reports the percentage of survey respondents who assessed their health as fair or poor. The figure shows that African Americans had the largest percentage of

FIGURE 4.16. SELF-ASSESSED HEALTH STATUS BY RACE/ETHNICITY, UNITED STATES, 2001.

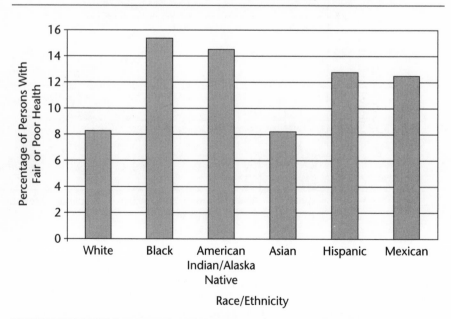

Source: National Center for Health Statistics, 2003, tab. 57.

persons indicating that they have fair or poor health (15.4 percent). They were followed closely by American Indians, who have a rate of over 14 percent. The Black rate is nearly double the rate for Asians, who have the lowest percent of persons indicating fair or poor health. About 13 percent of Hispanics and Mexican Americans reported their health as fair or poor. Slightly over 8 percent of Whites reported their health as fair or poor.

Summary

This chapter used the tools of epidemiology to explore variations in health status across a wide variety of health outcomes among U.S. racial/ethnic groups. The chapter demonstrated that there is substantial variation among the groups, with some populations consistently having better health status than others. Specifically, Asians/Pacific Islanders tend to have the best health status, followed by Whites and Hispanics/Latinos, especially Central Americans, Cuban Americans, and Mexican Americans. The African American and Native American populations and certain Hispanic/Latino populations (especially Puerto Ricans and Dominicans) tend to have worse overall health profiles. The chapter also presented the position of the United States within international comparisons of health status. We see that although the health profile of the United States ranks among those of all other industrialized nations, the United States consistently has a worse health profile than many of these nations. (See Appendix B for additional readings.)

Key Words

Health disparities

Health care disparities

Epidemiology

Age-adjusting

Survival curve

Infant mortality

Neonatal mortality

Postneonatal mortality

Low birth weight

Very low birth weight

Maternal mortality

Life expectancy

Mortality crossover

Chronic condition

Acute condition

Years of potential life lost

Activity of daily living

CHAPTER FIVE

MENTAL HEALTH

with Duane Thomas, Ph.D.

Outline

Introduction

We typically think of health and illness as polar opposites. However, as Figure 5.1 demonstrates, mental health, mental health problems, and mental illness are not precisely distinct categories; they are positions along a developmental continuum. At one end of this continuum are states of mental health: normative and expected levels of individual functioning across multiple domains of development (such as cognitive, affective, behavioral, social). At the center of the continuum are mental

FIGURE 5.1. THE MENTAL HEALTH CONTINUUM.

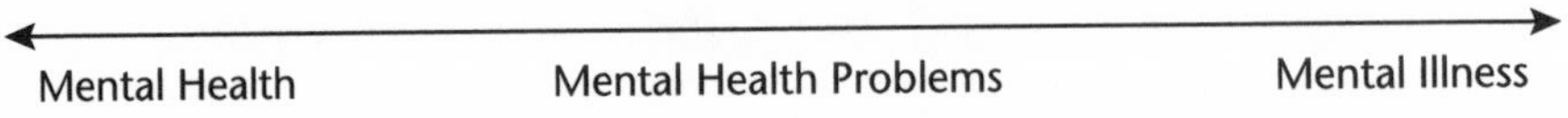

←——→

Mental Health   Mental Health Problems   Mental Illness

BOX 5.1. DEFINING COGNITIVE, AFFECTIVE, AND BEHAVIORAL FUNCTIONING.

- Cognitive functioning relates to the brain's thinking processes
- Affective functioning relates to moods, feelings, or emotions
- Behavioral functioning refers to aspects of behavior that are integrated into normative social interactions

---

health problems, which encompass emotional difficulties and predicaments that most people experience from time to time (for example, feeling sad or blue, or feeling stressed out after a trying week at work or school). At the other end are major mental illnesses, which include aberrant and disabling conditions that cause marked impairment in one's psychosocial functioning. Medically diagnosed disorders such as major depression, bipolar disorder, schizophrenia, and generalized anxiety disorder fall into this range.

In 2001 the U.S. surgeon general issued a report titled *Mental Health: Culture, Race, and Ethnicity,* (U.S. Department of Health and Human Services [DHHS], 2001), a supplement to a previously published report, *Mental Health: A Report of the Surgeon General* (U.S. DHHS, 1999). These reports offered general definitions of mental health, mental illness, and mental health problems (see Box 5.2). They described mental health as "a state of successful performance of mental function, resulting in productive activities, fulfilling relationships with other people, and the ability to adapt to change and to cope with adversity" (U.S. DHHS, 2001, p. 5). Inherent within this description is an individual's ability to successfully navigate the myriad of challenges encountered in life; this can take the form of responding in an adaptive manner to anxiety-provoking situations (such as separation from caregivers or public speaking), to daily hassles at work, to the dissolution of a romantic relationship, or to the onset of puberty or middle age. Healthy mental functioning is therefore regarded as an important factor contributing to personal well-being, to healthy interactions with others, and to successful contributions to the individual's communities and the wider society.

BOX 5.2. DEFINING MENTAL HEALTH, MENTAL ILLNESS, AND MENTAL HEALTH PROBLEMS.

- Mental health: the successful performance of mental function, resulting in productive activities, fulfilling relationships with other people, and the ability to adapt to change and to cope with adversity.
- Mental health problems: signs and symptoms of insufficient intensity or duration to meet the criteria for any mental disorder.
- Mental illness: the term that refers collectively to all mental disorders, which are health conditions characterized by alterations in thinking, mood, or behavior (or some combination thereof) associated with distress and/or impaired functioning.

Source: U.S. Department of Health and Human Services,1999, p. 7.

The surgeon general's 2001 report goes on to make the following important point: "While these elements of mental health may be identifiable, mental health itself is not easy to define more precisely because any definition is rooted in value judgments that may vary across individuals and cultures. According to a distinguished leader in the field of mental health, 'because values differ across cultures as well as among some groups (and indeed individuals) within a culture, the ideal of the uniformly acceptable definition [of mental health] is illusionary'" (Cowen, 1994).

Mental Health Problems

Mental health problems are signs or symptoms of insufficient intensity or duration to meet the criteria for any mental disorder, as outlined by statistical systems such as the tenth edition of the *International Classification of Disease* (ICD-10) and the revised fourth edition of the American Psychiatric Association's *Diagnostic and Statistical Manual of Mental Disorders* (DSM-IV-TR) (U.S. DHHS, 2001). Virtually everyone has experienced mental health problems to some degree. When under stress, anyone can exhibit behaviors that resemble some symptoms of mental disorders. For example, it is not uncommon or aberrant for children to display "symptomatology that is characteristic of separation anxiety disorder during their initial entry to preschool, or for toddlers and adolescents to go through fluctuating periods of oppositional behavior, defiance, and nonconformity" (U. S. DHHS, 2001). Furthermore, most people experience symptoms of depression after a major negative life event, such the death of a close friend or relative.

Not only can stressful life events result in mental distress, they can also have consequences for physical health. This is particularly true if one does not possess the resources to buffer the impact of the stressor (resources include coping skills, access to social support, monetary resources that can be used to purchase material needs, and so on). For example, Figure 5.2 shows the results of a study examining the effect of chronic exposure to stress on the risk of developing a rhinovirus infection (that is, the common cold). The figure shows that as the duration of exposure to stress increases, the risk of developing a cold increases (Cohen et al., 1998).

The stressful life events model (Dohrenwend & Dohrenwend, 1984; Lin & Ensel, 1989) predicts that an individual who has adaptive coping skills and/or sufficient social support from an effective support network will adapt to stressful life events, situations, experiences, frustrations, disappointments, losses, and other challenges. For individuals without such resources, stressful events and adaptational challenges can lead to a worsening of symptoms and impairment in important areas of functioning (such as work, school, or relationships). This can lead to the individual's progressing beyond experiencing behavior problems to a mental state that reaches the threshold for clinically significant mental illness.

FIGURE 5.2. CHRONIC STRESSORS AND RISK FOR THE COMMON COLD.

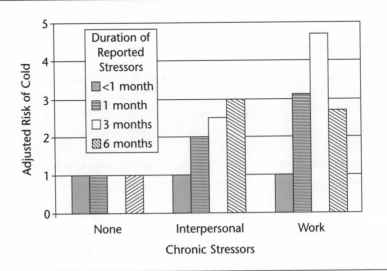

Source: Data from Cohen et al., 1998; *N* = 256.

Mental Illness

The term *mental illness* (also referred to as *psychopathology* or *abnormal behavior*) refers collectively to all diagnosed mental disorders, as identified by the DSM-IV-TR or IDC-10 classification systems (Adams & Cassidy, 1993; U.S. DHHS, 1999, 2001). Mental disorders, such as major depression, attention-deficit/hyperactivity disorder, schizophrenia, and Alzheimer's disease, are commonly found in the U.S. population. Approximately one in five adults and children has a diagnosable mental disorder (U.S. DHHS, 1999).

Mental disorders impair the individual's ability to function psychologically, socially, academically, or occupationally (American Psychiatric Association, 2000). For example, mental illness can significantly affect employee productivity and lead to a host of job-related problems. This is not surprising given that many of the symptoms typically associated with mental illness (such as fatigue, difficulty concentrating, indecision, irritability, and panic attacks) can constrain a person's ability to perform even the simplest of tasks (U.S. DHHS, 1999).

Employees who suffer from mental illness have higher absenteeism than their colleagues (Berndt et al., 1998). Mental disorders in childhood and adolescence have been linked to school avoidance, academic failure, peer rejection, high absenteeism, and poor teacher-child relations (Albano, Chorpita, & Barlow, 1996; American Psychiatric Association, 2000; Mash & Dozois, 1996).

In general, mental illness can severely lower quality of life. It can interfere with one's pursuit of educational and occupational goals, leisure activities, and personal relationships. Mental illness impairs existing relationships across settings and hinders one from coping with adversities that arise in life. Moreover, it heightens one's risk for injury, disability, and, in worst-case scenarios, premature death (for example, suicide or homicide).

Mental illness places a significant burden on health and productivity. Data collected from a large-scale study by researchers at the World Health Organization, the World Bank, and Harvard University investigated the burden of disease. The study found that mental illness ranks second in the global burden of disease (U.S. DHHS, 2001; Murray & Lopez, 1996). That is, compared to different disease conditions—including cardiovascular conditions, cancer, and other major causes of death—the burden of mental illness was identified by people around the world as a main source for loss of healthy life in terms of years lived with a disability and years of life lost to premature death.

Most Prevalent Mental Disorders in the United States

Mental disorders are common in the United States as well as other nations. According to the National Institute of Mental Health, within a given year about 22.1 percent of Americans age eighteen or older suffer from a diagnosable mental disorder. This translates into roughly forty-four million people—one-fifth of the U.S. population. Four out of the ten leading causes of disability in the United States are mental disorders—specifically, major depression, bipolar disorder, schizophrenia, and obsessive-compulsive disorder. Here we will briefly describe the most prevalent mental disorders in the United States.

Mood Disorders

Mood disorders are the most prevalent of the mental disorders. Everyone experiences changes in mood from time to time. Sometimes we feel happy, and other times we feel sad. However, when these moods go beyond the normal variation of emotions or when they start to impair our ability to function, they are considered mood disorders.

Major Depressive Disorder (MDD). A major depressive disorder is manifested by a combination of symptoms (see Box 5.3) that interfere with one's ability to work, study, sleep, eat, and enjoy once-pleasurable activities. MDD is among the leading causes of disability in the United States, affecting nearly 9.9 million Americans. The essential feature of MDD is a period of at least two weeks in which there is a depressed mood or the loss of pleasure in nearly all activities. It is important to note that in children and adolescents, MDD may manifest as an irritable or cranky mood rather than sadness and dejection. The lifetime prevalence rate for MDD is estimated to be between 10 and 25 percent for women and between 5 and 12 percent for men. As many as 15 percent of individuals with severe cases of MDD commit suicide annually.

Dysthymic Disorder. A less severe type of mood disorder, dysthymic disorder (or dysthymia) involves long-term, chronic symptoms that do not disable but keep one from peak functioning. The essential feature of the disorder is a chronically depressed mood that occurs often in an individual for at least two years. In children and adolescents, the mood may be irritable rather than depressed and occurs more often than not for at least one year. Dysthymic disorder affects approximately 6 percent of Americans. Within a given year, many people with the disorder (approximately 40 percent) will go on to experience major depressive episodes.

Bipolar Disorder. Also called *manic-depressive illness*, bipolar disorder is not as prevalent as the other mood disorders (1.2 percent of the U.S. population). It is characterized by cycling mood changes that include the presence of one or more manic episodes, or periods of abnormally and persistently elevated, expansive, or irritable mood, and one or more major depressive episodes. During the severe high periods (mania), which must last for at least one week to be considered clinically significant, individuals tend to exhibit several somatic and behavioral symptoms that include inflated self-esteem or grandiosity, decreased need for sleep, racing thoughts, increased involvement in

---

BOX 5.3.   SYMPTOMS OF DEPRESSION AND MANIA.

Depression
- Persistent sad, anxious, or "empty" mood
- Feelings of hopelessness, pessimism
- Feelings of guilt, worthlessness, helplessness
- Loss of interest or pleasure in hobbies and activities that were once enjoyed, including sex
- Decreased energy, fatigue, being "slowed down"
- Difficulty concentrating, remembering, making decisions
- Insomnia, early-morning awakening, or oversleeping
- Appetite and/or weight loss or overeating and weight gain
- Thoughts of death or suicide; suicide attempts
- Restlessness, irritability
- Persistent physical symptoms that do not respond to treatment, such as headaches, digestive disorders, and chronic pain

Mania
- Abnormal or excessive elation
- Unusual irritability
- Decreased need for sleep
- Grandiose notions
- Increased talking
- Racing thoughts
- Increased sexual desire
- Markedly increased energy
- Poor judgment
- Inappropriate social behavior

---

goal-directed activities, and excessive involvement in pleasurable but potentially harmful activities.

Suicide. Suicidal behavior is complex. Typically, the risk factors for suicide occur in combination; rarely is only one risk factor responsible. Greater than 90 percent of individuals who commit suicide had a mental disorder (most often depression) or were substance abusers (Moscicki, 2001; Conwell & Brent, 1995). Studies also show that diminished levels of neurotransmitters such as serotonin are associated with the risk for suicide (Mann, Oquendo, Underwood, & Arango, 1999). More than four times as many men as women die by suicide (Miniño, Arias, Kochanek, Murphy, & Smith, 2002), although women report *attempting* suicide during their lifetime about three times as often as men (Weissman et al., 1999). Also, as Figure 5.3 demonstrates, rates of suicide (intentional injury) vary by race/ethnicity. White men have the highest suicide rate at all ages, and black females have the lowest rates. Firearms are the most frequently used method of suicide, accounting for more than half of all suicides annually. White men account for 73 percent of all suicides (Centers for Disease Control and Prevention, 2004).

Psychotic Disorders: Schizophrenia

Schizophrenia is a severe and debilitating brain disorder that affects nearly three million (or one in every hundred) Americans. The disorder is marked by a combination of delusions (erroneous beliefs), hallucinations in any sensory modality (although auditory hallucinations are the most common), disorganized speech, grossly disorganized behavior, negative symptoms (such as flat affect), and, in some cases, catatonic motor behaviors that significantly impair social and occupational functioning. Hence, individuals with schizophrenia may hear internal voices not heard by others, or believe that other people are reading their minds, controlling their thoughts, or plotting to harm them. These symptoms may leave them fearful of and withdrawn from social situations. Schizophrenics often speak in loose associations, tangentially, and incoherently. They

FIGURE 5.3.   RACE, GENDER, AND SUICIDE, 2000.

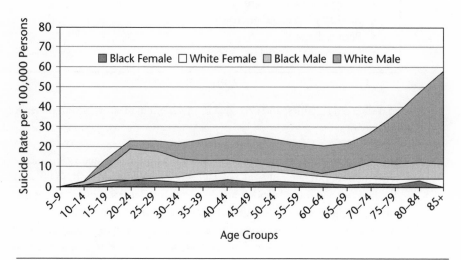

Source: National Center for Health Statistics.

may be incomprehensible to others, and their behavior may be so disorganized that it impairs their ability to perform basic self-care (such as maintaining hygiene or preparing a meal) or to conduct themselves according to norms of appropriate social behavior (for example, they may exhibit behaviors such as swearing, public masturbation, or wearing multiple overcoats on a hot day). The onset of schizophrenia typically occurs between the ages of fifteen and thirty, and affects men and women equally. Women typically develop the disease an average of five years later in life than men. Schizophrenia rarely occurs before early adolescence.

Anxiety Disorders

Anxiety disorders are serious medical illnesses that affect approximately nineteen million American adults. These disorders are also widely recognized as the most common class of psychiatric disorders affecting children and adolescents (Albano et al., 1996). The essential feature of anxiety disorders is overwhelming fear. Unlike the relatively mild, brief anxiety caused by a stressful event such as public speaking, the level of distress associated with anxiety disorders is chronic and relentless, and it can grow progressively worse if not treated. The most common forms of anxiety disorders are panic disorder, obsessive-compulsive disorder, posttraumatic stress disorder, social phobia, specific phobias, and generalized anxiety disorder.

Panic Disorder. People with panic disorder experience recurrent panic attacks, or discrete periods of intense terror or discomfort, in the absence of real threat and danger. These panic attacks can include sweating, palpitations, trembling, dizziness, shortness of breath, nausea, depersonalization, and fear of losing control or dying. The episodes can strike suddenly and unexpectedly or after exposure to or in anticipation of situational triggers or cues, either external or internal. Approximately 1.7 million Americans suffer from panic disorder.

Obsessive-Compulsive Disorder (OCD). OCD is marked by intrusive, anxious thoughts and impulses (obsessions) and engagement in ritualized, repetitive behaviors or mental acts (compulsions) to prevent or reduce anxiety or distress. Adults and some children with OCD are aware that their obsessions and compulsions are irrational, but they feel that the need to engage in behavioral or mental rituals is beyond their control. OCD affects nearly 2.3 percent of Americans annually.

Posttraumatic Stress Disorder (PTSD). PTSD is a debilitating condition characterized by intense fear, helplessness, horror, or disorganized, agitated behavior that develops following exposure to an extreme traumatic event. PTSD was first brought to public attention by war veterans, but it can result from any number of traumatic incidents, such as a mugging, rape, or torture; being kidnapped or held captive; child abuse; serious accidents, such as car or train wrecks; and natural disasters such as floods or earthquakes. Individuals with PTSD have recurrent and intrusive recollections of the traumatic events. About 5.2 million American adults (or 3.6 percent of the population) have PTSD.

Social Phobia (Social Anxiety Disorder). Social phobia involves excessive or unreasonable fear about social or performance situations. Individuals with this disorder have a persistent, intense, and chronic fear of being watched and judged by others and of being embarrassed or humiliated by their own actions. While many people with social phobia recognize that their fears may be excessive or unreasonable (this feature may be absent in children), they are unable to overcome it. They often worry for weeks in advance of a dreaded situation involving people or places. Physical symptoms often accompany the intense anxiety of social phobia and may include blushing, profuse sweating, tremors, gastrointestinal discomfort, nausea, confusion, and difficulty talking. For the estimated 5.3 million people presenting with social phobia in a given year, avoiding or anticipating feared situations can significantly interfere with normal functioning in occupational settings, social activities, and relationships.

Specific Phobias. A specific phobia is an intense and persistent fear of circumscribed objects and situations that pose little or no actual danger. Some of the more common specific phobias are centered around animals or insects, specific situations (such as escalators, tunnels, highway driving, flying, enclosed spaces), objects in the natural environment (such as heights, water, storms), injuries involving blood, invasive medical procedures, or other stimuli (such as fear of costumed characters, fear of vomiting or choking). Such phobias aren't just extreme fear; they are irrational fear of a particular object or situation; for instance, an individual with an intense, irrational fear of thunder and lightening (astraphobia) may be able to ski the world's tallest mountains with ease but be unable to refrain from panicking during a thunderstorm. Although adults with phobias realize that these fears are irrational and excessive (this may not be the case for children), they often find that confronting, or even thinking about confronting, the feared object or situation invariably brings on a panic attack or severe anxiety. About 4.4 percent of Americans in a given year suffer from some form of specific phobia.

Generalized Anxiety Disorder (GAD). GAD is much more than the normal anxiety people experience day to day. The level of anxiety associated with the disorder is chronic and consumes individuals with persistent and exaggerated worry and tension that they find difficult to control. Having this disorder means always anticipating tragedy or misfortune, often worrying excessively about health, money, family, or work. Sometimes, though, the source of the worry is hard to pinpoint. The mere thought of getting through the day may provoke anxiety. These generalized worries are accompanied by fatigue, restlessness, muscle tension, concentration difficulties, irritability, and sleep disturbances. Approximately 3 percent of Americans suffer from GAD within a given year.

Eating Disorders

Eating disorders are forms of mental illness characterized by severe disturbances in eating behavior.

Anorexia Nervosa. The primary characteristic of anorexia nervosa is the restriction of food and the refusal to maintain a minimal normal body weight. Individuals with this disorder see themselves as overweight even though they may be dangerously thin. Unusual eating habits develop, such as avoiding food and meals, picking out a few foods and eating them in small quantities, or carefully weighing and portioning food. Anorexics engage in techniques to control their weight, such as compulsive exercise, purging by means of vomiting, or abuse of laxatives, enemas, and diuretics. About 1 percent of females have anorexia nervosa. The prevalence for males is approximately one tenth that of females.

Bulimia Nervosa. Symptoms of bulimia nervosa include recurrent episodes of binge eating, characterized by eating an excessive amount of food, and purging, which involves inappropriate behavior in order to prevent weight gain, such as self-induced vomiting or misuse of laxatives, diuretics, enemas, or other medications. In lieu of purging, some people with this eating disorder may engage in inappropriate compensatory behaviors, such as fasting or excessive exercise. About 4 percent of women have bulimia nervosa. The rate of occurrence in males is approximately one tenth of that in females. Bulimia nervosa is extremely rare in children.

Childhood Disorders

Childhood disorders impair proper mental development.

Attention-Deficit/Hyperactivity Disorder (ADHD). This is a developmental disorder of self-control, marked by a persistent pattern of inattention, hyperactivity, and impulsivity. People with symptoms of inattention often fail to pay close attention to details, fail to complete tasks, have difficulties with the organization of tasks, and are easily distracted by extraneous stimuli. Hyperactivity may manifest itself by the individual's appearing to be always on the go, or driven by a motor. The individual may scurry about, talk incessantly, or find it impossible to perform a simple task like sitting still through a classroom lesson or a presentation at work. Therefore, it is common for

BOX 5.4. SUMMARY OF THE MOST PREVALENT MENTAL DISORDERS.

Mood Disorders

Major Depressive Disorder
A combination of symptoms that interfere with one's ability to work, study, sleep, eat, and enjoy pleasurable activities

Dysthymic Disorder
Long-term chronic symptoms that do not disable but keep one from functioning well or from feeling good

Bipolar Disorder
Cycling mood changes that include one or more manic episodes and one or more major depressive episodes

Suicidal Disorder
Organized attempts to harm or kill oneself

Psychotic Disorders

Schizophrenia
Brain disorder characterized by delusions, hallucinations, disorganized speech and behavior, and so on

Anxiety Disorders

Panic Disorder
Panic attacks or discrete periods of intense terror or discomfort in the absence of real threat or danger

Obsessive-Compulsive Disorder
Intrusive, anxious thoughts and impulses and engagement in ritualized or repetitive behaviors

Posttraumatic Stress Disorder
Intense fear, hopelessness, and horror following an extreme traumatic event

Social Phobia
Excessive or unreasonable fear about social or performance situations

Specific Phobias
Intense and persistent fear of objects and situations that pose little or no actual danger

Generalized Anxiety Disorder
Chronic, persistent, and exaggerated worry and tension that are difficult to control

Eating Disorders

Anorexia Nervosa
The restriction of food and the refusal to maintain a normal body weight

Bulimia Nervosa
Recurrent episodes of binge eating, excessive eating, and purging

Childhood Disorders

Attention-Deficit/Hyperactivity Disorder
Developmental disorder of self control characterized by a pattern of inattention, hyperactivity, and impulsivity

Autistic Disorder
Developmental disorder that affects a person's ability to communicate, form relationships, and respond appropriately to the environment

Cognitive Disorders

Alzheimer's Disease
Age-related irreversible brain disorder manifested by memory loss, decline in thinking, and personality changes

hyperactive children to squirm in their seats and to roam around the classroom without permission. Hyperactive teens and adults may appear to be intensely restless or fidgety. They may also try to do several things at once, bouncing around from one activity to the next. People with high levels of impulsivity are incapable of inhibiting their immediate reactions to situations or stopping to think before they act. As a result, they may blurt out inappropriate comments, interrupt or intrude on others, or find it difficult to wait for things they want or to take their turn in games. Given the nature of the disorder, individuals with ADHD experience significant problems across multiple settings and areas of functioning, particularly with respect to their general social adjustment. The prevalence of ADHD has been estimated at 3 to 7 percent in school-age children. Estimates also suggest that 30 to 80 percent of those diagnosed in childhood will continue to display evidence of some symptoms of the disorder through adolescence and adulthood.

Autistic Disorder Autism is a pervasive developmental disorder that generally affects a person's ability to communicate, form relationships, and respond appropriately to the environment. Individuals with autistic disorder have qualitative impairments in their communication, evidenced by a delay or total lack of development of spoken language, the inability to initiate or sustain a conversation with others, or the use of idiosyncratic language. The disorder also impairs one's ability to use multiple non-verbal behaviors (such as eye contact and facial expressions), to regulate social inter-action, to engage in social or emotional reciprocity, or to seek opportunities to share enjoyment, activities, and interests with other people. These social deficits make in-dividuals with autistic disorder seem oblivious to and detached from other people. Individuals with the disorder also appear locked into repetitive, stereotyped patterns of behaviors, interests, and activities, and rigid patterns of thinking. Although all in-dividuals with autism do not present exactly the same symptoms and deficits, they tend to share certain social, communication, motor, and sensory problems that affect their behavior in predictable ways. Epidemiological studies indicate that the median preva-lence rate of autistic disorder is 5 cases per 10,000 individuals (or about 0.05 percent).

Cognitive Disorders: Alzheimer's Disease (AD)

Alzheimer's disease, or dementia of the Alzheimer's type, is an age-related, irreversible brain disorder that occurs gradually and results in multiple cognitive deficits mani-fested by memory loss, decline in thinking and behavior, and personality changes. These deficits are related to the breakdown of the connections between nerve cells in the brain and the eventual death of many of these cells. About 3 percent of men and women age sixty-five to seventy-four have AD, and nearly half of those age eighty-five and older may have the disease.

Racial/Ethnic Differences in Prevalence of Mental Disorders

The prevalence rates for mental disorders in the United States are presented in Tables 5.1, 5.2, and 5.3. The tables display results from three large, well-established studies. Unfortunately, solid nationwide estimates for racial/ethnic differences in the prevalence of mental disorders are not available. The best available data come from relatively small

---

BOX 5.5.   PREVALENCE RATE.

"The number of instances of a given disease or other condition in a given pop-ulation at a designated time" (Last, 1988).

studies or larger studies that are geographically limited. Although the specific nature of racial/ethnic disparities in mental illness has not yet been definitively determined, the consensus opinion among mental health researchers is that the overall rate of mental illness among minorities is similar to the overall rate for the U.S. population, which has been estimated at over 20 percent . In short, the patterns of prevalence for specific mental disorders within the overall rate may vary somewhat, but the total prevalence appears to be similar across populations living in community settings.

Table 5.1 displays national estimates for Black and White Americans from the National Comorbidity Survey (NCS). The NCS surveyed a nationally representative sample of the U.S. population. The NCS is the best available national sample focusing on mental illness; however, it has a major limitation: it does not include individuals living in institutions such as prisons, hospitals, or nursing homes. Such individuals may likely have higher mental illness prevalence rates. Therefore, it seems likely that the estimates from such samples are conservative. The NCS included 666 Blacks and 4,498 Whites (Kessler et al., 1994). Survey respondents reported whether or not they had experienced symptoms of frequently diagnosed mental disorders in the past month, the past year, or at any time during their lives.

The NCS findings indicated that African Americans were less likely than Whites to suffer from major depression. There were also significant gender differences in rates of mental illness. Rates of depression, anxiety disorders, and phobia were higher among African American women than among African-American men. The gender pattern was similar for Whites. Overall, the NCS found that Blacks had a somewhat

TABLE 5.1.   PREVALENCE OF SELECTED MENTAL DISORDERS, NATIONAL COMORBIDITY SURVEY (PERCENTAGES).

Mental Disorder	Black (N = 666)	White (N = 4,498)	Total (N = 5,877)
	Past Twelve Months		
Major depression	8.2	9.9	10.0
Panic disorder	1.1	2.4	2.2
Phobic disorder	14.5	14.8	15.0
	Lifetime		
Major depression	11.6	17.7	16.9
Dysthymic disorder	5.4	6.7	6.5
Panic disorder	1.4	3.9	3.4
Phobic disorder	19.2	22.3	21.9

Source: U.S. Department of Health and Human Services, 2001, tab. 3-1.

TABLE 5.2.   COMPARISONS OF MENTAL DISORDERS
BETWEEN HISPANICS IN THE FRESNO STUDY
AND THE NATIONAL COMORBIDITY SURVEY
(PERCENTAGES).

	Fresno Study		*NCS*
Mental Disorder	**Immigrants**	**U.S.-Born**	**Total U.S. Population**
Mood disorder	8.0	18.7	19.5
Anxiety disorder	11.0	23.2	24.0
Any disorder	24.9	48.4	48.6

Source: U.S. Department of Health and Human Services, 2001, fig. 6-2.

lower prevalence rate for each disorder examined in the study. The pattern is similar for both twelve-month and lifetime prevalence rates (Kessler et al., 1996).

Researchers conducted a study of psychiatric disorders in a large sample of Mexican-Americans residing in Fresno County, California (Vega et al., 1998). The study found that lifetime rates of mental disorders among Mexican American immigrants were significantly lower than the rates for U.S.-born Mexican Americans. This finding is consistent with the "Hispanic epidemiologic paradox," which is discussed in greater detail in Chapter Thirteen. An additional interesting finding is that the rate of mental disorders among U.S.-born Mexican Americans closely resembles rates from the general U.S. population as reported in the NCS (see Table 5.2). By contrast, the Mexican-born Fresno residents had lower prevalence rates.

Table 5.3 compares results from the NCS with results from the Chinese American Psychiatric Epidemiological Study (CAPES), a large-scale study of the prevalence of selected disorders conducted in 1993 and 1994. The study examined rates of depression among more than 1,700 Chinese Americans in Los Angeles County, California (Takeuchi, Chung, & Shen, 1998; Sue, Sue, Sue, & Takeuchi, 1995). The study subjects were primarily Chinese immigrants; 90 percent of those sampled were born outside of the United States. The researchers conducted interviews in Cantonese, Mandarin, and English.

Results from the CAPES showed that Chinese Americans have moderate levels of depressive disorders. About 7 percent of the respondents reported experiencing depression in their lifetime, and a little over 3 percent had been depressed in the past year. These rates were lower than those found in the NCS. However, the rate of dysthymia in Chinese Americans more closely approximated findings of the NCS.

TABLE 5.3. COMPARISONS OF MENTAL DISORDERS BETWEEN CHINESE AMERICANS AND THE NATIONAL COMORBIDITY SURVEY (PERCENTAGES).

Mental Disorder	Rate in Chinese American Adults (CAPES)	Rate in National Sample of Adults (NCS)
Past Twelve Months		
Major depressive disorder	3.4	10.0
Dysthymic disorder	0.9	2.5
Lifetime		
Major depressive disorder	6.9	16.9
Dysthymic disorder	5.2	6.4

Note: CAPES = Chinese American Psychiatric Epidemiological Study.

Source: U.S. Department of Health and Human Services, 2001, tab. 5-1.

The Difficulty of Diagnosing Mental Illness

Although the available evidence suggests that the prevalence rates of mental disorders among racial/ethnic minorities are lower than or similar to those of Whites, we still cannot draw definitive conclusions. In many ways the diagnosis of mental disorders is more difficult than diagnoses in other areas of health. There are usually no laboratory tests involved in the assessment of mental disorders. Rather, a diagnosis often depends on the subjective complaints of patients, observable signs or symptoms, and behaviors associated with distress or disability. "Disability is conceptualized as impairment in one or more areas of functioning at home, work, school, or in the community" (U.S. DHHS, 2001, p. 10).

A formal diagnosis of a mental disorder is made by clinicians and hinges upon three components:

- A patient's description of the nature, intensity, frequency, patterning, and duration of symptoms
- A developmental history and signs from a mental status examination
- A clinician's observation and interpretation of the patient's behavior, including a global assessment of functional impairment

In the end, a diagnosis of a mental disorder is based on the judgment of a mental health care provider, such as a psychiatrist, a clinical or counseling psychologist, or a clinical social worker. The provider must determine whether or not the signs, symptom patterns, and impairment of functioning meet the criteria for a given diagnosis, as established by the American Psychiatric Association in its *Diagnostic and Statistical Manual of Mental Disorders* (American Psychiatric Association, 2000). This is the most widely used classification system both nationally and internationally.

Mental disorders are found worldwide (Weissman et al., 1994, 1996, 1997, 1999). Yet diagnosis is complicated because the manifestations of mental disorders vary with age, gender, race, ethnicity, and culture. Major depression provides a good example. Clinical depression for children can present as prolonged periods of irritability rather than the sadness or feelings of emptiness typical in adults. In addition, in some cultures, depression may be experienced largely in somatic terms rather than with sadness or guilt (American Psychiatric Association, 2000; Hammond & Rudolph, 1996; Tharp, 1991). Complaints of "nerves" and headaches may express depressive experiences of Latino and Mediterranean cultures; problems of the "heart," or weakness or "imbalance" may represent depressive symptoms of Middle Eastern and Asian cultures, respectively (American Psychiatric Association, 2000).

Moreover, according to a study by Manson, Shore, and Bloom (1985), words such as *depression* and *anxiety* do not exist in the languages of some American Indians and Alaska Natives. However, this of course does not preclude American Indians, Alaska Natives, and other ethnic groups who do not share a similar lexicon of symptoms of psychopathology in their respective languages from having mood or anxiety disorders. But culture can influence the communication of symptoms as well as the experience of depression and other mental illnesses. Clearly, this would complicate patient-provider communication and threaten the quality of mental health care received by patients from different ethnic and cultural groups.

Mental health care providers must determine whether a patient's signs and symptoms significantly impair functioning at home, school, work, or in other roles within the patient's community. This judgment is based, in part, on a determination of the degree to which the patient's signs and symptoms deviate from accepted social norms and standards within the patient's culture. However, if the provider is not knowledgeable about the cultural context in which the patient lives, it may be difficult to make judgments about the appropriateness of the patient's behavior or the degree to which the behavior (or signs and symptoms) will impair functioning at home, school, or work, or in the community. As such, when physician and patient are from different cultures, the interaction between them is rife with possibilities for miscommunication and misunderstanding.

Idioms of Distress and Culture-Bound Syndromes

Different cultures express, experience, and cope with feelings of distress in different ways. These differences are referred to as *idioms of distress*. One of the most common

---

BOX 5.6. SOMATIZATION.

The expression of distress through physical symptoms. Examples include stomach disturbances, excessive gas, palpitations, chest pain, dizziness, vertigo, blurred vision, burning hands and feet, or the experience of worms in the head or ants crawling under the skin. Somatization is closely related to "idioms of distress."

---

idioms of distress is *somatization*: the expression of distress through physical symptoms (Kirmayer & Young, 1998). Abdominal pain, heart palpitations, and chest pain are common forms of *somatization* (Escobar, 1987). "Some Asian groups tend to express cardiopulmonary and vestibular symptoms, such as dizziness, vertigo, and blurred vision (Hsu & Folstein, 1997). In Africa and South Asia, *somatization* sometimes takes the form of sensations of burning hands and feet or the experience of worms in the head or ants crawling under the skin" (U.S. DHHS, 2001, p. 11).

"Culture-bound syndromes are clusters of symptoms more common in some cultures than in others. For example, some Latino patients—especially women from the Caribbean—display *ataque de nervios,* a condition that includes screaming uncontrollably, attacks of crying, trembling, and verbal or physical aggression. Fainting or seizure-like episodes and suicidal gestures may sometimes accompany these symptoms (Guarnaccia, Canino, Rubio-Stipec, & Bravo, 1993). A culture-bound syndrome from Japan is *taijin kyofusho:* an intense fear that one's bodily functions give offense to others. The syndrome is listed as a diagnosis in the Japanese clinical modification of the World Health Organization (WHO) International Classification of Diseases, 10th edition" (U.S. DHHS, 2001, p. 11). Numerous other culture-bound syndromes are given in the DSM-IV-TR "Glossary of Culture-Bound Syndromes" (American Psychiatric Association, 2000).

The symptoms of mental disorders are found in all nations and in all cultures; there are similar recognizable symptoms worldwide (Weissman et al., 1994, 1996, 1997, 1999). Culture-bound syndromes are the exception. Mental health researchers have not yet determined whether culture-bound syndromes are indicative of one or more of the following possibilities:

- Culture-bound syndromes are distinct disorders that exist only in those cultures.
- Culture-bound syndromes reflect different ways in which individuals from different cultures express mental illness.
- Culture-bound syndromes reflect different ways in which the social and cultural environment interact with genes to produce disorders.
- Some combination of these.

Risk and Protective Factors for Mental Health Problems and Mental Disorders

The risk factors for mental illness are not always clear. Mental disorders are believed to have biological, psychological, social, and broader contextual origins and causes (Mash & Dozois, 1996; Sameroff, 1993). They can operate within the individual—for example, genetic susceptibility, gender, low birth weight, neurophysiological dysfunction, language disabilities, chronic physical illness, below-average intelligence, and social-cognitive deficits. Other risk factors operate through the family—for example, child abuse and neglect, maladaptive patterns of parenting, marital discord, family dysfunction, limited family resources and other poverty-related stressors, parental psychopathology, and living in foster care.

Moreover, risk factors can also be tied to the community or broader social context—for example, exposure to high levels of community violence, community disorganization, being a recent immigrant, inadequate schools, and institutional racism and discrimination. It should be noted that the risk factors associated with the development of mental health problems and mental illness are not independent of each other; they often operate in dynamic and interactive ways over time to increase risk for individual distress, functional impairment, and low quality of life. In fact, for most mental disorders, research does not support granting central etiological status to any single risk or causal factor (Mash & Dozois, 1996; Seifer, Sameroff, Baldwin, & Baldwin, 1992).

There are also several characteristics that are known to be protective against developing mental disorders. Protective factors can also be based in the individual, family, or community context. Protective factors associated with the individual include above-average intelligence, positive reference group orientation, and spirituality or religious involvement. Familial protective factors include effective parenting skills, parental employment, smaller family size, and supportive relationships with parents, siblings, or spouses. Protective factors at the community level include the availability of health and social services, presence of extended kinship networks, and strong community (and neighborhood) ties and cohesion.

Having any risk factor could increase one's risk for developing a mental disorder, but having one or more risk factors does not necessarily mean that one will develop a disorder. Having a risk factor is neither necessary nor sufficient to produce a given outcome. Each person is exposed to a unique combination of risks and protective factors that interact in complex and poorly understood ways to produce or not produce mental illness in a given individual (Institute of Medicine, 1994).

Risk and protective factors vary not only across individuals, but also across age, gender, and racial/ethnic groups. Racial/ethnic minorities are disproportionately exposed to several risk factors, such as poverty, immigration, violence, racism, and discrimination. Given this, one might expect that ethnic minorities would have a higher prevalence of mental disorders. However, as we have seen, this is not the case. One possible reason for this could be that, as research has shown, racial/ethnic minorities also have greater exposure to several important protective factors—for example, spirituality and family support.

One of the most thoroughly studied areas of mental health is the relationship between family factors and relapse of schizophrenia. Several studies have found that people with schizophrenia who returned to the community after hospitalizations to live with family members who are critical or otherwise unsupportive were more likely to relapse than those who lived with family members who were supportive (Leff & Vaughn, 1985; Kavanaugh, 1992; Bebbington & Kuipers, 1994). One study compared Mexican American and White families and found that for Mexican American families, less warm interactions were predictive of schizophrenia relapse. For Whites, the study found that the opposite was true. In other words, among Whites the warmer the family interactions with the family member with schizophrenia, the greater the likelihood that the family member would relapse (Lopez et al., 1998).

Here are a few more examples of culturally related differences in risk/protective factors. Some Asian American groups tend not to dwell upon negative thoughts because they believe that reticence is preferable to outward expression of displeasure (Hsu, 1971; Kleinman, 1977). Some also prefer to rely on themselves when coping with distress (Narikiyo & Kameoka, 1992). These strategies for coping with distress are referred to as passive coping styles. By contrast, African Americans are more likely to use more active coping styles and to rely more heavily on spirituality to help cope with adversity (Broman, 1996; Neighbors, Musick, & Williams, 1998).

Utilization of Mental Health Services

An additional issue related to racial/ethnic differences in mental health is the utilization of mental health services. In fact, more than other areas of health and medicine, the mental health field is plagued by disparities in the utilization of its services (U.S. DHHS, 2001). According to the National Comorbidity Survey (Kessler et al., 1994), African Americans with mood or anxiety disorders were less likely than Whites with similar conditions to receive care. Only 16 percent of African Americans with a diagnosable mood disorder saw a mental health specialist, and less than one-third consulted a health care provider of any type.

In addition to receiving less mental health services than Whites, African Americans tend to receive care from different types of providers as well. They are more likely to receive care from their primary care provider than from psychiatrists or psychologists, and they are more likely to seek assistance for their mental health concerns from informal sources of support such as spiritual advisers (Cooper-Patrick et al., 2002;

Cooper, Brown, Vu, Ford, & Powe, 2001; U.S. DHHS, 2001). The available studies also indicate that Latinos and Asian Americans substantially underutilize mental health services (U.S. DHHS, 2001). However, national studies of mental health services use typically do not have large enough numbers of Asian Americans to provide reliable estimates of the degree of underutilization (Takeuchi et al., 1998).

Several barriers affect the utilization of mental health care in the United States. In particular, patient, provider, and health system barriers all contribute to ethnic disparities in mental health care, including the extent to which persons from different cultural and ethnic backgrounds seek professional help for mental illness (Butcher, Narikiyo, & Vitousek, 1993; Cooper et al., 2001). Perhaps the primary reason for underutilization of mental health services is health insurance. As we will see in the Chapter Six discussion of health care services, racial/ethnic minorities (particularly Hispanics and some Asian American sub-groups) have significantly higher rates of being uninsured. Additionally, many sources of health insurance do not provide adequate coverage for mental health services. Moreover, research has documented that nonfinancial barriers, such as fragmentation of mental health services, inaccessibility of specialty treatment facilities, language barriers, cultural mistrust, and a host of therapist-related variables (for example, cultural bias or professional training) impact mental health care utilization (Butcher et al., 1993; U.S. DHHS, 2001; Hoberman, 1992).

But perhaps the biggest obstacle to the treatment and management of mental illness is the social stigma attached to it. In the United States and elsewhere, mental illness is highly stigmatized. Many cultures maintain negative attitudes and beliefs regarding mental illness. There is widespread fear and rejection of and discrimination against people with mental disorders (Corrigan & Penn, 1999). This is largely because of misunderstanding about many mental disorders. For example, many people view depression not as an illness, but rather as a character weakness.

Because of widespread social stigma, many people with mental disorders fail to seek treatment. Furthermore, people with mental disorders often do not disclose their symptoms to health care providers or researchers attempting to compile statistics on the prevalence of mental illnesses. Stigma also further degrades the quality of life and health of persons with mental disorders because of discrimination in housing, employment, and in other spheres of life, such as the development of family and other social ties. In this way, stigma can be a barrier to developing the protective factors (high socioeconomic status, family support, and so on) that can aid in lessening the severity of the mental disorder and improve the odds that treatment will be successful. The negative stigma of mental health can also affect family members of those with mental disorders. This can serve to further degrade family support, which is an important protective factor for persons with mental illness.

There have been relatively few studies of stigma and mental illness across cultures. However, the studies that have been conducted returned the following findings.

In some Asian cultures, the stigma against mental illness is so extreme that such conditions are thought to reflect poorly on family lineage and thereby diminish marriage and economic prospects for relatives of persons with mental illness—that is, even for relatives who may not personally have any symptoms of mental illness (Sue & Morishima, 1982; Ng, 1997).

One study asked Asian and White Americans in the Los Angeles area about their experiences with mental illness symptoms. Only 12 percent of Asians had mentioned mental health problems to a friend or relative, compared with about 25 percent of Whites. Only 4 percent of Asians reported that they would seek help from a psychiatrist or other mental health specialist; about 26 percent of Whites reported that they would seek such help. Also, only 3 percent of Asians reported that they would seek help from a physician; about 13 percent of Whites reported that they would (Zhang, Snowden, & Sue, 1998).

A study by Pescosolido, Monahan, Link, Stueve, and Kikuzawa (1999) presented people with a number of vignettes depicting people with mental illness, and asked respondents a series of questions regarding their attitudes toward the people in the vignettes. Study respondents generally viewed people with mental illness as dangerous and less competent to handle their own affairs; their harshest judgments were reserved for people with schizophrenia and substance use disorders. It is interesting to note, however, that neither the race/ethnicity of the individuals responding to the survey, nor the race/ethnicity of the individuals depicted in the vignettes influenced the responses given by persons responding to the survey.

Diala and his colleagues (2000) conducted a reanalysis of the National Comorbidity Survey to determine if there were racial differences in attitudes towards use of professional mental health care services. The study found that among people who have never used mental health services, African Americans tended to have more positive attitudes than Whites toward using mental health services. However, among those who had had interactions with the mental health care system, African Americans tended to have more negative attitudes towards use of mental health care services compared with Whites. Thus, the African American experiences within mental health care settings seem to have a negative effect on their attitudes regarding mental health services.

As the studies demonstrate, it is not clear whether, and to what extent, stigma regarding mental health varies by race/ethnicity. It may be that the variation that has been documented is a function of different experiences of people from different cultures as they interact with the mental health care system. There are many studies of bias and stereotyping within health care in general. Surely physicians and other health care providers are no less susceptible to general societal attitudes. Until the 1960s, most states of the United States maintained separate and segregated health care systems for Whites and non-Whites. Without question there has been substantial progress regarding race relations in health care as well as in the broader society. However, there

---

BOX 5.7. FACTORS AFFECTING BALANCED MENTAL HEALTH.

Cultural
- Language
- Idioms of distress
- Culture-bound syndromes

Health Care Utilization
- Socioeconomic status
- Insurance status
- Access to health care
- Stigma
- Negative experience

Risk
- Genetics
- Environmental characteristics
- Social context
- Individual networks
- Family networks
- Community networks

---

may still be traces of more subtle forms of discrimination within health care. Additionally, it is possible that whatever amount of discrimination remains in the health care system is more a function of social class than race/ethnicity. It is possible that biases held by health care providers may be a reflection of socioeconomic status or the culture of the medical profession (Epstein & Ayanian, 2001).

Summary

The impact of mental health on society is often overlooked. However, mental health has a tremendous impact on the economy and on quality of life for individuals and families. Often health insurance policies do not adequately cover mental health services, and a powerful stigma continues to limit utilization of services when such services are available. Racial/ethnic differences in the prevalence of mental disorders are not as pronounced as they are in the area of physical health. Yet although mental disorders are not as widespread and racial/ethnic disparities are not as common, mental health disparities do exist. In addition to racial/ethnic differences in the prevalence of mental disorders, other important aspects of mental health, such as culture-bound syndromes and idioms of distress, play an important role in our understanding of minority health. Culture-bound syndromes are mental health conditions that exist only within a specific culture. Idioms of distress are racial/ethnic differences in the presentation of disease. (See Appendix B for additional readings.)

Key Words

Mental health

Mental health problems

Mental illness

Mental disorder

Psychosocial functioning

International Classification of Diseases (ICD-10)

Diagnostic and Statistical Manual of Mental Disorders (DSM-IV-TR)

Life event

Somatization

Idioms of distress

Culture-bound syndromes

Stigma

CHAPTER SIX

HEALTH CARE SERVICES AMONG RACIAL/ETHNIC GROUPS

Outline

Introduction: Definition of Health Care

In this chapter we will explore the way in which variation in health care services can impact the health of populations. Health care disparities are to be distinguished from health status disparities. The term *health care disparities* refers to differences in the access, use, quality, or outcomes of health care services received by racial/ethnic minorities. In contrast, the term *health status disparities* refers to differences among racial/ethnic groups in health status (that is, morbidity, mortality, functional status, or disability). The National Institutes of Health (n.d.) define *health disparities* as "differences in the incidence, prevalence, mortality and burden of diseases and other adverse health conditions that exist among specific population groups in the United States.

BOX 6.1.   HEALTH STATUS AND HEALTH CARE DISPARITIES.

Health status disparities: Differences in the incidence or prevalence of disease, disability, or illness. These differences can be among racial/ethnic groups, gender groups, socioeconomic groups, or other groupings.

Health care disparities: Differences in quality of care that are not due to clinically appropriate treatment decisions or patient preferences.

Research on health disparities related to socioeconomic status is also encompassed in the definition."

This chapter will outline issues in health care disparities. Health status disparities—differences in the health profiles of various populations—were discussed in Chapter Four. The distinction between health *status* and health *care* disparities may seem like splitting hairs, but in fact this distinction is important because it is crucial to understanding the nature of the causes of health status and health care disparities. The causes of the two classes of disparity are likely different, and the methods for eliminating them are likely different as well.

Health Care Disparities

In 2002, the Institute of Medicine (IOM) issued a report titled *Unequal Treatment: Confronting Racial and Ethnic Disparities of Health Care.* The report focused on a subsection of health care disparities: racial/ethnic differences in the quality of care received. It did not address health status disparities or health care access. The IOM described the scope of the report as follows: "racial or ethnic differences in the quality of health care that are not due to access-related factors or clinical needs, preferences and appropriateness of interventions." The IOM's concept of health care disparities is depicted in Figure 6.1.

The model in Figure 6.1 shows a simulation of racial disparities in health care quality. Nonminorities receive better quality care than racial minorities. The differences between the quality of care received by minorities and nonminorities fall into two broad groupings: health care disparities and health care dissimilarities. Health care disparities are racial/ethnic differences in the outcomes or quality of care that are indicative of injustice within the health care system or in the behavior of health care providers. Health care dissimilarities refer to racial/ethnic differences that are not caused by underlying inequities; for example, differences produced by patient cultural preferences or patient choice.

FIGURE 6.1.   MODEL OF HEALTH CARE DISPARITIES.

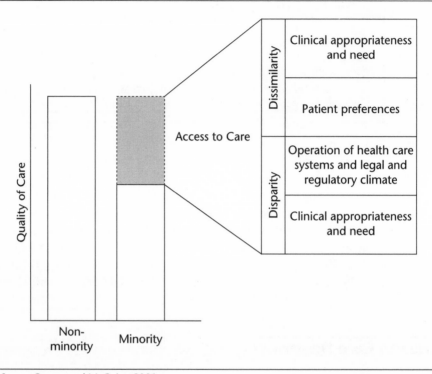

Source: Gomes and McGuire, 2001.

One might wonder where access to and use of health care fits into this model. These constitute a special case. Because health care access and use have components that are part dissimilarity and part disparity, the IOM model deals separately with access and use of health care services. We will explore access and use in the next section of this chapter.

The IOM's study and 2002 report *Unequal Treatment* was very influential. It led health care organizations and policymakers to accelerate efforts to eliminate racial and ethnic differences in care. The study reported the following conclusions:

- Racial and ethnic disparities in health care exist and, because they are associated with worse outcomes in many cases, are unacceptable.
- Racial and ethnic disparities in health care occur in the context of broader historic and contemporary social and economic inequality, and evidence of *persistent* racial and ethnic discrimination in many sectors of American life.
- Many sources—including health systems, health care providers, patients, and utilization managers—may contribute to racial and ethnic disparities in health care.

BOX 6.2.   DISTINGUISHING BETWEEN DISPARITIES
AND DISSIMILARITIES.

Disparities: Differences that are indicative of injustice or unfairness.

Dissimilarities: Differences that are not attributable to injustice or unfairness. For example, if well-informed patients choose not to accept treatment, this would lead to dissimilarities in treatment.

- Bias, stereotyping, prejudice, and clinical uncertainty on the part of health care providers may contribute to racial and ethnic disparities in health care. While indirect evidence from several lines of research supports this statement, a greater understanding of the prevalence and influence of these processes is needed and should be sought through research.
- A small number of studies suggest that racial and ethnic minority patients are more likely than white patients to refuse treatment. These studies find that differences in refusal rates are generally small and that minority patient refusal does not fully explain health care disparities.

Access to and Use of Health Care

There are differences among racial/ethnic groups in access to and use of health services. As mentioned previously, this can be viewed in part as disparity (difference caused by injustice) and in part as dissimilarity (difference not caused by injustice). Differences in access to and use of health care services are largely caused by socioeconomic inequities, such as discrimination or differences in health insurance coverage. However, differences in use of health care services are also influenced by differences in need for services and in patient preferences.

In Chapter Four it was demonstrated that there are substantial differences in health status among the racial/ethnic minority groups. This suggests that there are substantially different levels of need for heath services among the groups. Logically, if there are higher morbidity rates among racial/ethnic minorities than among nonminorities, one would suspect that racial/ethnic minorities would have a greater need for health services; this would result in higher rates of health services use among minorities.

In fact, in some cases the populations with the greatest need are also the populations with the lowest rates of health care use. Table 6.1 displays the percent of persons who reported having no health care visits—whether to a doctor's office or emergency department, or a home visit—in the past twelve months, according to

TABLE 6.1.   PERCENTAGE OF PERSONS WITH NO HEALTH CARE VISITS IN THE PAST TWELVE MONTHS, 2001.

Race/Ethnic Group	Percentage with No Visits
Total	16.5
White	14.3
Black	16.4
American Indian or Alaska Native	21.4
Asian	20.8
Hispanic	27.0
Mexican	31.4

Source: National Center for Health Statistics, 2003, tab. 70.

the National Health Interview Survey. The table shows that Mexican Americans are the group most likely to not have had any medical visits. Nearly one third of Mexican Americans had not had a single medical encounter in the preceding year. For Hispanics/Latinos as a whole, 27 percent reported having no medical encounters. They were followed by American Indians/Alaska Natives (21.4 percent) and Asians (14.3 percent).

Behavioral Model of Health Services Use

Dr. Ronald Andersen (1995) developed a model that seeks to explain patterns of use of health services. His behavioral model of health services utilization, shown in Figure 6.2, is among the most commonly used models in public health and is widely accepted among health services researchers. The model categorizes factors that contribute to use of heath services into three groups: (1) enabling factors, (2) predisposing factors, and (3) patient need for health care.

Enabling factors relate to structural or material resources that can be barriers or facilitators in seeking care. Examples of enabling factors are having health insurance; the ability to take sick time off from work; having access to transportation; or having a preexisting relationship with a health care provider. *Predisposing factors* measure the patient's inclination to use health services; this includes the patient's attitudes toward using care, which are influenced by cultural beliefs, prior experiences, and perceptions. *Need* refers to the patient's perceived need for health care services; this includes the individual's health status and the severity and duration of their symptoms. In the sections that follow, we will further explore racial/ethnic differences in enabling and predisposing factors. Racial/ethnic differences in the need for health care reflect evidence from the data described in Chapter Four.

FIGURE 6.2. BEHAVIORAL MODEL OF HEALTH SERVICES UTILIZATION.

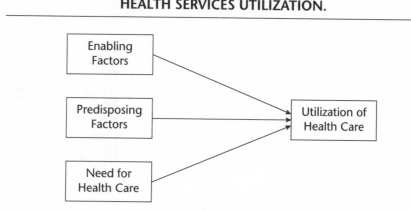

Source: Andersen, 1995.

Enabling Factors: Health Insurance

The most commonly studied enabling factor is health insurance (see Box 6.3 for a description of the major categories of health insurance). There are substantial racial/ethnic differences in sources of health insurance, as Figure 6.3 depicts.

A total of 174.1 million Americans are covered by private insurance. The next largest group of American adults—about 39.2 million in 2004—is the uninsured. About 25.2 million Americans obtain health insurance through Medicaid, and 40 million Americans are covered by Medicare.

BOX 6.3. TYPES OF HEALTH INSURANCE.

Private health insurance: The majority of Americans have private health insurance; this includes most people between the ages of eighteen and sixty-four, who obtain health insurance through their employers, and a small number of people who pay for their own health insurance.

Medicare: This is a federally run program for persons over age sixty-five. Costs are borne in part by the insured individual, who pays a monthly premium, and in part by taxpayers and corporate taxes.

Medicaid: This federally run health insurance program for low-income persons covers about 25.2 million Americans. The costs are split between the federal government and state government.

FIGURE 6.3. HEALTH INSURANCE STATUS AMONG PERSONS 18–64 YEARS OLD, 2001.

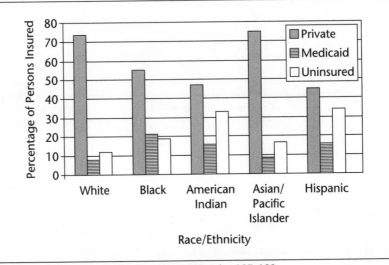

Source: National Center for Health Statistics, 2003, tabs. 127–129.

The distribution of health insurance type varies by race/ethnicity. Seventy-four percent of whites have private insurance. This contrasts with Hispanics/Latinos, of whom only 45 percent have private insurance. The racial/ethnic group with the largest percentage covered by Medicaid is African Americans: slightly more than 20 percent are covered by Medicaid, more than double the percent for Asians and Whites. More than 33 percent of Hispanic/Latinos and American Indian/Alaska Natives are uninsured, a far greater percentage than for African Americans (19.2 percent), Asians (17.1 percent), and Whites (11.9 percent).

There are several reasons for the large number of uninsured Americans. First and foremost, in the United States health insurance is linked to employment. The United States is the only industrialized nation that does not provide health care access to all citizens. Although most Americans who have health insurance obtain it through their employment, there are many jobs that do not provide health insurance. These jobs tend to be low-wage. And racial/ethnic minorities disproportionately hold these jobs; as such, racial/ethnic minorities are more likely to be uninsured compared to nonminorities.

Enabling Factors: Availability of Health Services

One consequence of the pattern of health insurance and lack thereof presented in Figure 6.3 is that there are major differences among racial/ethnic groups in having a usual source of care. Many Americans lack the continuity associated with having a health care provider who maintains a long-term relationship with the patient and is familiar with the patient's needs. The lack of this important enabling factor is believed to lead to the limited access and reduced quality of health care received by racial minorities. Figure 6.4 displays the pattern of having "no usual source of care" by race/ethnicity.

The figure shows that nearly 14 percent of White Americans do not have a usual source of care. Whites have the lowest percentage of such individuals, followed by American Indians/Alaska Natives and African Americans. About 18 percent of Asian Americans and more than 30 percent of Hispanics/Latinos do not have a usual source of care. A lack of these enabling factors is closely tied to socioeconomic status, and the inequitable distribution of health care resources within minority communities.

Predisposing Factors

Predisposing factors are often measured as a person's attitudes. Attitudes are thought to be an indicator of feelings and a predictor of actions, according to the behavioral model of health services utilization. Assuming that the enabling factors are equal, a person's decision whether or not to utilize health services is based on the patient's perception of

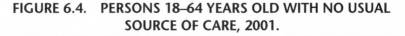

FIGURE 6.4.   PERSONS 18–64 YEARS OLD WITH NO USUAL SOURCE OF CARE, 2001.

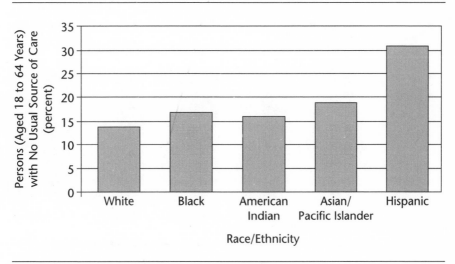

Source: National Center for Health Statistics, 2003, tab. 76.

a need for health services weighed against the perception of the possibility of having an unpleasant experience (such as discourteous treatment, pain caused by the medical treatment, general hassle associated with seeking care, and so on). If a person holds negative attitudes about the health care system, he or she may be less inclined to use health services unless the perceived need is very high. On the other hand, one would expect the threshold for use to be lower if the person holds more positive attitudes.

Satisfaction with Care   Figure 6.5 displays patients' attitudes regarding satisfaction with care. The data in the figure come from the Commonwealth Fund's Minority Health Survey (Hogue & Hargraves, 2000). The survey was designed to be a nationally representative sample of each racial/ethnic group. Patients were asked to rate their satisfaction, from "very dissatisfied" to "very satisfied." The figure shows the percentage of patients who reported being "very satisfied" in the following areas: (1) overall satisfaction, (2) satisfaction with access to their doctor, (3) how well their doctor listens to them, and (4) satisfaction regarding being treated with respect.

FIGURE 6.5.   PERCENTAGE OF PATIENTS "VERY SATISFIED" WITH THEIR HEALTH CARE, 1994.

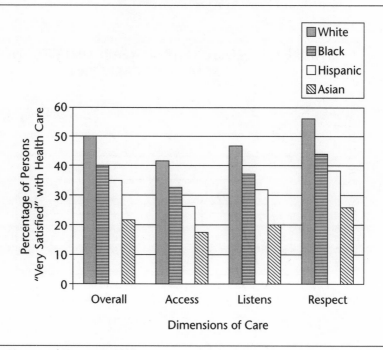

Source: Hogue and Hargraves, 2000.

There is a general pattern across all four questions: White patients were more likely to indicate they were "very satisfied" compared with patients from all other racial/ethnic groups. African Americans were the second most likely to be "very satisfied," followed by Hispanics/Latinos, then Asians.

Delving more deeply into the likely causes of lower levels of satisfaction among minorities, we come to a set of analyses conducted by researchers at the Johns Hopkins School of Public Health (LaVeist, Nickerson, & Bowie, 2000). This is a study of African American and White patients who received care for a severe heart condition at one of three hospitals in Baltimore, Maryland. Patients in this study were asked a series of questions about their feelings of trust toward health care institutions and a set of questions about their perceptions of discrimination. The results of this study are presented in Tables 6.2 and 6.3.

Mistrust of Health Care Patients were asked to react to three statements regarding mistrust of the health care system. The responses were recorded on a four-point scale (strongly disagree, disagree, agree, or strongly agree). Table 6.2 reports responses of "agree" and "strongly agree" combined. Of African American patients, 51.4 percent agreed or strongly agreed that patients have sometimes been deceived or misled in hospitals, compared with 42.4 percent of White patients. Nearly 40 percent of African American patients, compared with 24.1 percent of White patients, agreed that hospitals often want to know more about patients' personal affairs than they really need to know. And African American patients were nearly twice as likely as White patients to agree or strongly agree that hospitals have sometimes done harmful experiments on patients without their knowledge.

Perceived Discrimination Survey respondents were also read statements regarding discrimination in the health care system and asked to indicate their agreement with the statements, using the same four-point scale. Table 6.3 displays race comparisons of the percentage of survey respondents who indicated "strongly agree" or "agree," combined. The table shows a consistent racial disparity in reports of racism within health care settings. Although 67.5 percent of African American patients agreed or strongly agreed that "doctors treat African American and White people the same," nearly 87 percent of White patients felt that way. Thirty percent of African American patients endorsed the statement, "racial discrimination in a doctor's office is common," whereas only 7.3 percent of White patients endorsed that statement. African American patients were about 85 percent as likely as White patients to agree or strongly agree that African Americans and Whites receive the same kind of care at hospitals. And although 88.1 percent of White patients agreed or strongly agreed that "African Americans can receive the care they want as equally as White people can," only 61.2 percent of African American patients felt similarly.

TABLE 6.2.   RACIAL DIFFERENCES IN TRUST IN HEALTH CARE.

Statement	*Percent Agreeing*		
	Black Patients	**White Patients**	**Black-White Ratio***
Patients have sometimes been deceived or misled at hospitals.	51.4	42.4	1.21
Hospitals often want to know more about your personal affairs or business than they really need to know.	39.2	24.1	1.63
Hospitals have sometimes done harmful experiments on patients without their knowledge.	50.6	26.0	1.95

*All statistically significant at $p < .001$.

Source: LaVeist, Nickerson, & Bowie, 2000.

TABLE 6.3.   RACIAL DIFFERENCES IN PATIENTS' PERCEPTIONS OF RACISM IN HEALTH CARE SETTINGS.

Statement	*Percent Agreeing*		
	Black Patients	**White Patients**	**Black-White Ratio***
Doctors treat African American and White people the same.	67.5	86.8	0.78
Racial discrimination in a doctor's office is common.	30.0	7.3	4.11
In most hospitals, African Americans and Whites receive the same kind of care.	78.6	92.9	0.85
African Americans can receive the care they want as equally as White people can.	61.2	88.1	0.68

*All statistically significant at $p < .001$.

Source: LaVeist, Nickerson, & Bowie, 2000.

Provider Attitudes There are substantial differences by race/ethnicity in patients' perceptions of the health care system. These different perceptions are known to play a role in contributing to different rates of use of health services among racial/ethnic groups. If these perceptions are without substance, then the solution is clear: change people's perceptions. However, as we see in Table 6.4, these perceptions are based, to some extent, in objective reality.

The data presented in Table 6.4 were collected by Michelle van Ryn and Jane Burke in a study of 550 doctor-patient encounters in eleven U.S. and Canadian communities. The study included audiotapes of physician-patient interactions and self-administered questionnaires from each physician and patient. The audiotapes of the physician-patient interactions were obtained during regularly scheduled outpatient visits at academic and Veterans Administration centers, community hospitals, and private practices. Physicians were asked to complete a questionnaire for each patient immediately after the taped visit. The questionnaire included a number of questions about the patient and the physician-patient encounter. Table 6.4 summarizes the findings.

TABLE 6.4.   PHYSICIANS' RATING OF PATIENTS BY PATIENTS' RACE.

Physician Perception of Patient	*Percent Agreeing*		
	White Patient	Black Patient	Black-White Ratio*
Not at all likely to abuse alcohol or other drugs	79	67	1.18
Not at all likely to fail to comply with medical advice	57	42	1.36
Very to extremely likely to participate in the cardiac rehabilitation	47	34	1.38
Very to extremely likely to strongly desire a very physically active lifestyle	26	14	1.86
Not at all likely to lack social support	63	45	1.40
The kind of person I can see myself being friends with	34	27	1.26
Very intelligent	26	13	2.00
Very to somewhat educated	41	31	1.32
Very pleasant	53	27	1.96
Very rational	37	20	1.85

*All statistically significant at $p < .05$.

Source: van Ryn and Burke, 2002.

Physicians consistently reported more negative attitudes toward African American patients than toward White patients. The table shows that the physicians were 18 percent more likely to feel that the White patients "would not abuse alcohol or other drugs" compared with African American patients, 36 percent more likely to believe that the African American patients would be noncompliant with medical advice, and 38 percent more likely to believe that the African American patients would fail to participate in cardiac rehabilitation if it were ordered. Additionally, the physicians in the survey were 86 percent more likely to perceive White patients as "strongly desiring of a physically active lifestyle" and 40 percent more likely to feel that White patients had adequate social support. They were also 26 percent more likely to report that the patient was the "kind of person [the physician] could see [the physician] being friends with" if the patient was White.

Perhaps most telling were the results of the final four questions. Physicians were only half as likely to view African American patients as very intelligent and 32 percent less likely to view African American patients to be at least "somewhat educated." They were also 96 percent more likely to view the White patients as very pleasant and 85 percent more likely to view the White patients as very rational. It is important to note that the authors of the study also conducted more in-depth multivariate analysis to determine if these results were caused by real differences in the socioeconomic status, educational level, and so on of the White and African American patients. That analysis adjusted for patient's age, sex, health risk status, education, depressive symptoms, social assertiveness, and feelings of mastery. Van Ryn and Burke also tested for differences in the results as a function of physician characteristics such as age, race, sex, and medical specialty. Even after adjusting for these characteristics, their analysis still revealed that physicians held more negative attitudes toward African American patients than they did toward White patients.

Quality of Care

In its 2001 report, *Crossing the Quality Chasm: A New Health System for the 21st Century,* the Institute of Medicine defined *quality health care* as "providing patients with appropriate services in a technically competent manner, with good communication, shared decision-making, and cultural sensitivity." Differences in the quality of health care received among racial/ethnic groups have been noted in several dimensions of quality. Racial differences in access to surgical and medical management of heart disease are perhaps the most studied health care disparity (Sheifer, Escarce, & Schulman, 2000). Many studies have demonstrated that White patients are about twice as likely to receive cardiovascular surgical procedures (such as cardiac catheterization, percutaneous transluminal coronary angioplasty, and coronary bypass surgery) compared with African American and Hispanic/Latino patients (Ford et al., 2000).

Racial differences have been widely observed in studies of heart disease (Sheifer et al., 2000), but similar findings have been demonstrated with other conditions as well. For example, differences in screening and/or treatment have been found in cancer (McMahon et al., 1999; Mandelblatt, Yabroff, & Kerner, 1999), asthma (Ali & Osberg, 1997), participation in AIDS clinical trials (Stone, Mauch, Steger, Janas, & Craven, 1997), access to kidney transplantation (Eggers, 1995), and long-term care (Wallace, Levy-Storms, Kington, & Andersen, 1998; Mui & Burnette, 1994). Marsh, Brett, and Miller (1999) found that physicians were twice as likely to recommend hormone replacement therapy for White patients than for African Americans. Studies have demonstrated racial differences in access to care among the elderly (Buckle, Horn, Oates, & Abbey, 1992). And several studies have simultaneously examined disparities in the use of multiple procedures (Escarce, Epstein, Colby, & Schwartz, 1993; Harris, Andrews, & Elixhauser, 1997; Giacomini, 1996).

One can conclude from studies of racial and ethnic differences in access and use of health services that racial and ethnic minorities often face the prospect of seeking care in facilities with fewer resources. Also, when they obtain access to similar facilities as Whites, they often receive less optimal treatment. There are some interesting exceptions to this pattern. Studies conducted in health care systems used by active military personnel found no racial/ethnic differences in quality of care (Dominitz, Samsa, Landsman, & Provenzale, 1998). However, it should be noted that health care disparities have been documented in the Veterans Affairs Health System, which is used by retired military personnel (Whittle, Good, Conigliaro, & Lofgren, 1993).

Cultural Appropriateness of Care

Another aspect of good quality health care identified by the Institute of Medicine is cultural appropriateness, also referred to as "cultural competence." Lavizzo-Mourey and Mackenzie (1996) define cultural competence as "the demonstrated awareness and integration of three population-specific issues: health-related and cultural values, disease incidence and prevalence, and treatment efficacy." Anderson, Scrimshaw, Fullilove, Fielding, and Normand (2003) describe cultural competence as "a set of congruent behaviors, attitudes, and policies that come together in a system, agency, or among professionals and enable effective work in cross-cultural situations."

In most cases, racial/ethnic minorities are seen by health care providers who are not from the same culture. Table 6.5 presents the results of a study examining race concordance between health care providers and patients among patients who had a choice in selecting their provider (LaVeist & Nuru-Jeter, 2002). The table shows that with the exception of Asian Americans, all patients were most likely to have a White physician. Other than White physicians, the second most common configuration was for the patient to have a physician from his or her own racial/ethnic group.

**TABLE 6.5. PHYSICIAN-PATIENT RACE CONCORDANCE IN THE
1994 COMMONWEALTH MINORITY HEALTH SURVEY.**

	Patient's Race			
Physician's Race	**White** ($n = 910$)	**Black** ($n = 745$)	**Hispanic** ($n = 676$)	**Asian American** ($n = 389$)
White	779 (85.6%)	436 (58.5%)	406 (60.1%)	175 (45.0%)
Black	14 (1.5%)	162 (21.7%)	15 (2.2%)	5 (1.3%)
Hispanic	19 (2.1%)	17 (2.3%)	128 (18.9%)	2 (.5%)
Asian/Pacific Islander	68 (7.5%)	75 (10.1%)	71 (10.5%)	203 (52.2%)
Other	30 (3.3%)	55 (7.4%)	56 (8.3%)	4 (1.0%)

Source: LaVeist and Nuru-Jeter, 2002, p. 300.

Twenty-one percent of African American respondents, 18.9 percent of Hispanic/
Latino respondents, and 52.2 percent of Asian American respondents had physicians
of the same race or ethnicity. In all, 46.8 percent of respondents were race concordant with their physician.

The group that was by far the most likely to be race concordant with their physician was Whites. However, Asian Americans were more likely to be race concordant
than to have a White physician. White respondents were 3.94 times more likely than
African American respondents and 4.53 times more likely than Hispanic/Latino respondents to have a physician of the same race. However, Whites were only 1.64 times
more likely than Asian Americans to be race concordant with their physician. African
American and Hispanic/Latino respondents were also more likely than Whites to have
a physician from a minority group other than their own. Ten percent of African American and 10.5 percent of Hispanic/Latino respondents reported having an Asian
American physician, while 7.5 percent of Whites reported having an Asian American
physician. In addition, 7.4 percent of African Americans and 8.3 percent of Hispan-
ics/Latinos reported having a physician of another race, compared with only 3.3 percent of Whites. Of all groups, Asian American respondents were least likely to have a
physician who was of a non-Asian minority.

When the findings in Table 6.5 are combined with national data on racial
distribution of physicians (see Figure 6.6), an interesting picture emerges. Although minority physicians represent a small proportion of the total physicians in the country,
they provide care for a disproportionately high number of minority patients (Carlisle,
Gardner, & Liu, 1998; Libby, Zhou, & Kindig, 1997). For example, in a study of
California-based physicians, Komaromy et al. (1996) demonstrated that African
American and Hispanic/Latino physicians were more likely than their White
counterparts to care for African American, Hispanic/Latino, and low-income

FIGURE 6.6. RACIAL/ETHNIC DISTRIBUTION OF PHYSICIANS, UNITED STATES, 2000.

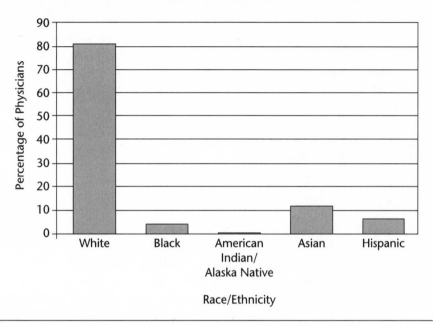

Source: U.S. Bureau of the Census, 2001.

patients. Likewise, in their national sample Moy and Bartman (1995) found that minority physicians were more likely to care for minority, medically indigent, and sicker patients.

There has been some speculation that minority patients tend to be seen by physicians of the same race because minority health care providers were the only providers available in their communities. This is a reasonable speculation, but it is not the complete explanation. It is a reasonable speculation because a study by Bertakis (1981) found that minorities do not express a preference for the race of their physician, and several studies have documented that minority physicians are more likely to practice in minority communities (Moy & Bartman, 1995). However, Saha, Taggart, Komaromy, and Bindman (2000) demonstrated that African American, White, and Hispanic/Latino patients sought care from physicians of their own race because of personal preferences and language, not because of limited options.

Only a few studies have examined whether or not patient outcomes are affected by doctor-patient race concordance. Cooper-Patrick et al. (2002) conducted a telephone survey of African American and White adults who were recent patients of a primary care practice to examine patient assessments of how well the physician incorporated patient preferences into decision-making style. Their analysis found that patients who were race concordant with their physician rated their visits as significantly more participatory than patients who were race discordant. Saha, Komaromy, Koepsell, and Bindman (1999) found that African American race-concordant patients were more likely to rate their physician as excellent and were more likely to report receiving preventive care and needed medical care. Finally, LaVeist and Nuru-Jeter (2002) found that patients of each racial and ethnic group reported the highest level of satisfaction if they were race concordant with their provider.

How Health Care Disparities Contribute to Health Status Disparities

Although health care disparities and health status disparities are distinct, they are still interrelated. Figures 6.7 through 6.9 present models that show how health care disparities can contribute to health status disparities. Figure 6.7 depicts a series of points at which race disparities are produced. The first point is the objective exposure to health risks. African Americans and other racial minorities are more likely to be exposed to socioenvironmental risks compared with Whites. For example, race disparities have been described in exposure to environmental toxins (Bullard, 2002), occupational stressors (Robinson, 1985, 1989), and residency in high-crime neighborhoods (Harburg et al., 1973).

However, while objective risk exposure is important, the health effects often are mediated by the individual's perception and/or resources to cope with them. For example, in 1994, Sherman James (2002) developed a concept he called *John Henryism*— a predisposition to cope actively with stressors believed to be a feature of African American culture. James argues that elevated blood pressure among African Americans is partly the result of the interaction of John Henryism and low social class. The interaction between objective health risk factors and a psychosocial coping style is represented in the model. The model shows that if an individual perceives that he or she is at risk, the individual will be more inclined to engage in health prevention practices and less inclined to engage in high-risk behavior. It is important to point out that even if the individual is inclined to engage in prevention behavior, he or she still might not do so. This is because individuals often encounter barriers, financial or otherwise. Thus it is possible to perceive risk and to have a proclivity to reduce the risk or increase prevention behavior, yet not follow through.

To continue the hypertension example, the objective social risk exposure of living in a high-crime area or having limited occupational opportunities is filtered through the coping mechanisms of the individual. Knowledge of increased risk for hypertension may lead an individual to want to stop living a sedentary lifestyle (inactivity being a risk

FIGURE 6.7.   SOCIAL AND BEHAVIORAL PRODUCTION OF DISPARITIES.

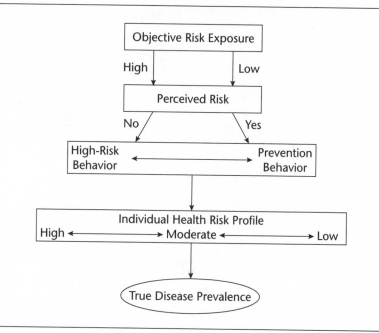

behavior for hypertension) and begin getting periodic blood-pressure checks (prevention behavior). However, suppose the individual lives in a community that is lacking in recreational options, or the individual cannot afford a gym membership. Suppose the individual does not have health insurance and cannot afford blood-pressure checks. These barriers may inhibit or even prevent the individual from making healthy lifestyle changes.

The combination of objective risk exposures, along with the individual's risk and prevention practices, influences the health risk profile of the individual. This ultimately leads to the probability of developing a disease.

Figure 6.8 shows the pathway through which individual patients go from disease recognition to accessing health care. The model seeks to highlight the many decision points that create race disparities in use of health care services. Note that in the figure each item denoted with a circle identifies a point along the pathway at which an individual is at increased risk of falling out of the care process. Underlying the use of health care services is the individual's disease or ill-health status. A *pathogen* is any disease-producing agent, such as a virus, bacteria, or other microorganism. Once a pathogen has entered the individual's body, the individual may or may not exhibit symptoms of that disease. However, even if there are symptoms, the individual may

FIGURE 6.8.   MODEL OF ACCESS TO HEALTH CARE SERVICES.

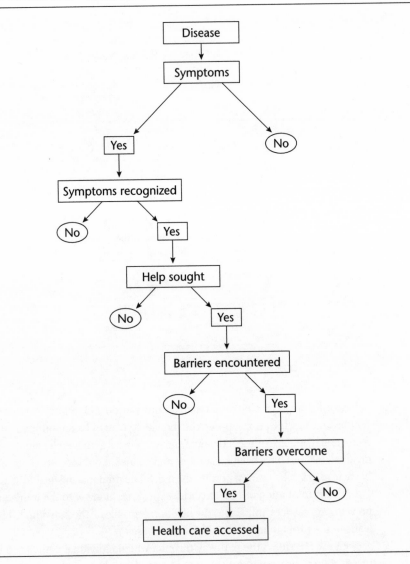

or may not recognize the symptoms as indicative of disease. This is the first decision point at which important race disparities can be produced, as significant race differences in awareness of symptoms and risk factors have been documented (Folsom, Sprafka, Luepker, & Jacobs, 1988).

Assuming that symptoms are present and the individual recognizes the symptoms, the individual then makes the determination whether or not to seek health services. That determination is influenced by a variety of predisposing characteristics (Andersen, 1995), which include the patient's attitudes, beliefs in the efficacy of health care, and previous experiences. If inclined to seek care, the individual must now assess his or her enabling factors as they relate to potential barriers to care. Does the individual have a usual source of care? Health insurance? The ability to travel to the health care provider?

Among those who seek care, there are race differences in barriers to obtaining access to care. These include financial barriers such as lack of health insurance or inability to make co-payments, but barriers to accessing care go beyond these financial barriers; they include perceived as well as realized impediments. For example, according to some studies, African American patients are more likely to express distrust of health care and more likely to perceive themselves to have been victimized by discrimination (LaVeist, Nickerson, & Bowie, 2000). These perceptions have been supported by objective findings of race differences in quality of care received (IOM, 2002), as well as studies demonstrating more negative attitudes among health care providers toward racial or ethnic minority patients (van Ryn & Burke, 2002). Although financial and nonfinancial barriers prevent many patients from accessing health care, most patients are able to overcome these barriers and access care.

Finally, as Figure 6.9 shows, even when patients are able to overcome barriers and access care, there may still be race differences in the quality of care they receive. Once in care, patients must have their symptoms correctly recognized and diagnosed. There is a large body of research literature demonstrating racial and ethnic differences in treatment decision-making (IOM, 2002). Additionally, there may be racial or ethnic disparities in access to specialty care. Thus, while patients can sometimes overcome barriers and gain access to primary care, several studies have demonstrated racial differences in referrals to specialists. Finally, assuming the correct diagnosis and treatment plan, there may be racial differences in patient compliance.

FIGURE 6.9.   HEALTH CARE QUALITY AND DISPARITIES.

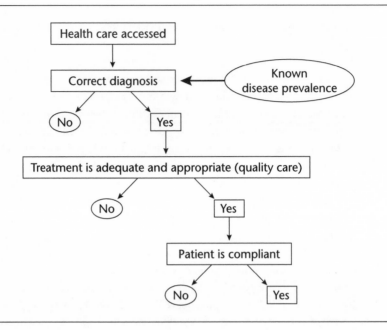

Summary

This chapter described the scientific evidence of disparities in health care and explored racial/ethnic differences in access, use, and quality of care, establishing the following points:

- Racial/ethnic minorities have significantly worse access to health care compared with nonminorities.
- Because of reduced access to care, racial/ethnic minorities have lower rates of use of health care services compared with Whites.
- There is important variation among the racial/ethnic minority groups as well; for example, Hispanic/Latinos are substantially more likely to be uninsured and to not have a usual source of care compared with other minorities.
- Even when access to care is equal, racial/ethnic minorities tend to receive lower-quality care.

For a case study, see Appendix A. See Appendix B for additional readings.

Key Words

Health care disparity

Health disparity

Health care dissimilarity

Health status disparity

Predisposing factor

Enabling factor

Cultural competence

Primary care

Access to care

Quality of care

PART THREE

ETIOLOGY OF RACIAL/ETHNIC DIFFERENCES IN HEALTH

CHAPTER SEVEN

THEORIES OF RACIAL/ETHNIC DIFFERENCES IN HEALTH

Outline

Introduction

In Chapter Four we identified substantial differences in health status across the U.S.-based racial/ethnic groups. There are no simple explanations, nor is there a consensus explanation for these health status disparities; however, a number of theories have been developed to explain them. This chapter will present each of these theories and examine the evidence that supports or refutes them. The theories have been grouped within the following three categories from the determinants of health model outlined in Figure 7.1.

- Socioenvironmental or context—causes associated with social factors or environmental exposures
- Psychosocial or behavioral—causes associated with characteristics of the individual, such as behavior or psychological factors
- Biophysiological—causes associated with genetic or biological processes

These categories are depicted in Figure 7.1 as they interrelate along a continuum to produce health status disparities.

Determinants of Health

The first category of determinants, socioenvironmental factors, includes such factors as exposure to pollution or other toxic agents, poverty, living in an urban environment, or exposure to sources of stress such as living in a high-crime environment.

Psychosocial or behavior factors refer to the person-level—factors that are mediated by individuals, such as health behavior. Examples include smoking, inactivity, and substance abuse (such as consumption of alcohol or other drugs). Psychosocial or behavior factors are more than health behaviors; they include psychological and personality characteristics of individuals, such as individual modes of coping with stress or the "human capital" at the disposal of the individual (such as financial resources, intellectual capacity, or access to information).

Biophysiological factors refer to the biological mechanisms that produce ill health. Inherited genetic predisposition to disease is one example, but this is probably a relatively small aspect of biophysiological factors. Biophysiological factors also refer to gene-environment inactions, whereby genes are modified by socioenvironmental exposures or the consequences of health behavior.

Sometimes the term *fundamental cause* is used to discuss the underlying causes of disease. However, I have intentionally avoided the use of this term because its meaning can be confusing when communicating with people who are trained in different disciplines. For example, among social scientists (such as medical sociologists, social epidemiologists, demographers, and health economists) fundamental causes of disease are those factors that emanate from the social environment (such as poverty, inequality,

FIGURE 7.1. DETERMINANTS OF HEALTH STATUS.

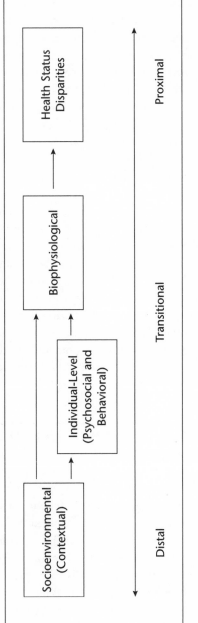

environmental exposures, and so on). However, among biological scientists fundamental causes refer to the underlying biophysiological mechanisms that lead to disease (for example, a specific gene mutation or a receptor that stops working). Instead, I will use the terms *distal, transitional,* and *proximal. Distal* causes are those further removed from disease manifestation—for example, such socioenvironmental factors as exposure to air pollution or the stress of a sudden economic downturn with massive layoffs. *Transitional* causes are factors that mediate distal causes or factors that are "closer" to disease manifestation—for example, coping with the stress of a sudden economic downturn through excessive alcohol consumption. *Proximal* causes refer to the biological factors that ultimately lead to disease.

Socioenvironmental factors (distal) often operate through psychosocial or behavioral factors (individual-level). Socioenvironmental factors help to produce the context that influences behavior or in which individual health and illness behavior occurs. For example, targeted advertising of cigarettes is part of the social context that leads to teen smoking or higher rates of smoking among minority adults.

Ultimately, all socioenvironmental and behavioral characteristics operate through biophysiological mechanisms (proximal) to produce health outcomes. Cigarette advertising (socioenvironmental factor) and the consequent act of taking up smoking (behavioral factor) will lead to death or ill health only if one is affected physiologically. The categories of determinants of disease can be viewed as a chain of relationships that link the social and physical environment to health outcomes. This view leads to the conclusion that the etiology (cause) of health disparities can occur within any of the three categories of factors.

Socioenvironmental Theories of Health Disparities

Socioenvironmental or context theories state that disparities in health status exist because of differences in race/ethnicity in the community context in which people live. The community context can lead to better or worse health outcomes depending on the nature of that community context. Thus racial/ethnic variation in exposure to health risks is greatly intensified by substantial racial and ethnic segregation within the United States. In its 1968 report to President Lyndon Johnson, the National Advisory Commission on Civil Disorders concluded, "our nation is moving toward two societies, one Black, one White—separate and unequal." More than three decades later this statement can still be supported by examining data on the level of racial segregation in the United States. Because of substantial segregation in the United States, members of different racial/ethnic groups have substantially different levels of exposure to social health risks as well as to environmental toxins.

I will outline the extent to which racial/ethnic segregation exists in the United States and then describe the context theories that relate to racial/ethnic segregation.

Racial/Ethnic Segregation

Table 7.1 displays the index of dissimilarity (IOD) for the twenty-five largest metropolitan areas in the country. The IOD is a widely used measure of racial residential segregation within geographic areas. The index is based on a scale ranging from 0 (no segregation) to 1.0 (complete segregation). The IOD can be interpreted as the percentage of a given minority group that would have to relocate to another census tract within the metropolitan area to achieve in every census tract a racial distribution equal to the distribution for the entire metropolitan area. In other words, the IOD score of 0.63 for Hispanics/Latinos living in the Los Angeles–Long Beach, California, area indicates that 63 percent of Hispanics/Latinos would have to move to a different census tract in order for the entire metropolitan area to have an even distribution of Hispanics/Latinos compared with Whites.

The table shows the IOD for African Americans, Hispanics/Latinos, Asians, and American Indians and Alaska Natives. In each case the IOD is computed with Whites as the comparison group. The table shows substantial variation across the metropolitan areas in terms of the level of segregation within each group. There is also substantial variation across the minority groups. In general, African Americans are more segregated from Whites than any other minority groups. For example, the average IOD for Blacks is 0.64, which indicates that across all twenty-five metropolitan areas about two thirds of Blacks would have to move to achieve complete racial integration with Whites. The average score for Hispanics is 0.49, and for Asian Americans, 0.41. American Indians and Alaska Natives have the lowest average IOD at 0.36.

Several studies have demonstrated a link between segregation and health disparities. These studies have found racial segregation to be correlated with mortality/morbidity rates and health-related resources for a variety of unrelated health outcomes (Acevedo-Garcia, 2002). For example, studies have found associations between segregation and

- Infant mortality (LaVeist, 1989, 1993; Yankauer, 1950)
- Adult mortality (Collins & Williams, 2002; Polednak, 1991; Fang, Madhavan, Bosworth, & Alderman, 1998; Jackson, Anderson, Johnson, & Sorlie, 2000)
- Tuberculosis (Acevedo-Garcia, 2001, 2002)
- Hospital admissions (Hart, 1997)
- The location of food stores (Morland, Poole, Roux, & Wing, 2002)

TABLE 7.1. RACIAL/ETHNIC RESIDENTIAL SEGREGATION IN THE 25 LARGEST U.S. CITIES, 2000.

Rank	MSA/ PMSA[a]	Total Population	Black/ White Dissimilarity Index	Hispanic/ White Dissimilarity Index	Asian Dissimilarity Index	American Indian/ Alaska Native Dissimilarity Index
1	Los Angeles–Long Beach, CA PMSA	9,519,338	0.664	0.631	0.479	0.474
2	New York, NY PMSA	9,314,235	0.810	0.667	0.505	0.652
3	Chicago, IL PMSA	8,272,768	0.797	0.611	0.426	0.426
4	Philadelphia, PA–NJ PMSA	5,100,931	0.720	0.601	0.437	0.426
5	Washington, DC–MD–VA–WV PMSA	4,923,153	0.625	0.480	0.385	0.336
6	Detroit, MI PMSA	4,441,551	0.846	0.456	0.460	0.329
7	Houston, TX PMSA	4,177,646	0.663	0.551	0.488	0.325
8	Atlanta, GA MSA	4,112,198	0.645	0.511	0.444	0.303
9	Dallas, TX PMSA	3,519,176	0.587	0.537	0.444	0.258
10	Boston, MA-NH PMSA	3,408,722	0.658	0.587	0.450	0.353
11	Riverside–San Bernardino, CA PMSA	3,254,821	0.449	0.425	0.371	0.267
12	Phoenix–Mesa, AZ MSA	3,251,876	0.433	0.521	0.283	0.498
13	Minneapolis–St. Paul, MN-WI MSA	2,968,806	0.576	0.465	0.427	0.403
14	Orange County, CA PMSA	2,846,289	0.371	0.551	0.398	0.344
15	San Diego, CA MSA	2,813,833	0.535	0.506	0.472	0.328
16	Nassau-Suffolk, NY PMSA	2,753,913	0.730	0.469	0.354	0.479
17	St. Louis, MO-IL MSA	2,603,607	0.731	0.273	0.413	0.254

Rank	MSA/PMSA[a]	Total Population	Black/White Dissimilarity Index	Hispanic/White Dissimilarity Index	Asian Dissimilarity Index	American Indian/Alaska Native Dissimilarity Index
18	Baltimore, MD PMSA	2,552,994	0.675	0.358	0.393	0.328
19	Seattle–Bellevue–Everett, WA PMSA	2,414,616	0.489	0.303	0.346	0.245
20	Tampa–St. Petersburg–Clearwater, FL MSA	2,395,997	0.629	0.444	0.337	0.247
21	Oakland, CA PMSA	2,392,557	0.618	0.469	0.406	0.320
22	Pittsburgh, PA MSA	2,358,695	0.671	0.290	0.486	0.351
23	Miami, FL PMSA	2,253,362	0.694	0.439	0.301	0.411
24	Cleveland–Lorain–Elyria, OH PMSA	2,250,871	0.768	0.577	0.380	0.385
25	Denver, CO PMSA	2,109,282	0.605	0.500	0.291	0.324
	Average dissimilarity		0.64	0.49	0.41	0.36

[a]PMSA = primary metropolitan statistical area; MSA = metropolitan statistical area.

Source: U.S. Bureau of the Census.

- The availability of pharmaceuticals (Morrison, Wallenstein, Natale, Senzel, & Huang, 2002)
- The availability of liquor stores (LaVeist & Wallace, 2000)

Racial segregation has been shown to be a consistent predictor of health outcomes and a partial explanation for race disparities in health. The different social and environmental contexts among minority groups that are created by racial segregation are theorized to impact health disparities through two different pathways. I will refer to these as risk exposure theory and resource deprivation theory.

Risk Exposure Theory

This theory states that a high prevalence of social or environmental health risks in predominantly minority communities leads to a higher prevalence of disease and death. Many studies have found support for the risk exposure theory. Some studies have found that environmental hazards disproportionately exist in minority communities. Other studies have focused on social risks.

The National Research Council conducted a study that observed health effects associated with living near a Superfund site or other toxic waste site. These sites contain billions of pounds of highly toxic chemicals, including mercury, dioxin, polychlorinated biphenyls, arsenic, lead, and heavy metals such as chromium. The study found a pattern of greater prevalence of health problems, such as heart disease, spontaneous abortions, congenital malformations, leukemia, learning disabilities, hyperactivity, and Hodgkin's disease near toxic sites (National Research Council, 1991). A 1987 study by the United Church of Christ's Commission for Racial Justice (1987) was the first to bring attention to the disproportionate location of toxic waste sites in minority communities. That study found that three of every five African Americans and Latinos nationwide lived in a community with an illegal or abandoned toxic dump and that communities with a hazardous waste facility had twice the percentage of residents who were minorities compared with communities with no hazardous waste sites.

BOX 7.1.   THE SUPERFUND PROGRAM.

The Superfund Program was created in 1980 to locate, investigate, and clean up the most hazardous chemical waste sites nationwide. The Environmental Protection Agency administers the Superfund Program in cooperation with individual states and tribal governments.

A 2002 study in Massachusetts found that nine of the fifteen "intensively over-burdened towns" had high proportions of minority residents, as did nine of the twenty "extensively overburdened towns"(Faber & Krieg, 2002). A 1992 review of fifteen studies examining the location of environment hazards found support for the United Church of Christ commission study (Commission for Racial Justice, 1987), and a later review by Dr. Phil Brown (1995), a Brown University researcher, concluded that "the overwhelming bulk of evidence supports the environmental justice belief that environmental hazards are inequitably distributed by class, and especially race."

Research demonstrating greater social risk factors in predominantly minority communities include studies that found minority communities are targeted for to-bacco consumption, more so than White communities (Luke et al., 2000; Balbach, Gasior, & Barbeau, 2003; Hackbarth, Silvestri, & Cosper, 1995; Hackbarth et al., 2001; Pucci, Joseph, & Siegel, 1998; Stoddard, Johnson, Boley-Cruz, & Sussman, 1997). LaVeist and Wallace (2000) demonstrated that liquor stores in Baltimore City had greater than eight times the odds of being located in a low-income African American community compared with other communities. Lillie-Blanton, Schuster, and Anthony (2002) found that race differences in rates of utilization of crack cocaine were a function of availability: among persons who lived in communities with availability of crack cocaine, there was no race difference in use; rather, race differences in crack cocaine use were a function of Blacks being more likely to live in communities with high levels of availability of the drug. This was an important discovery because until Lillie-Blanton's study it was widely believed that Blacks had a greater predisposition to use crack cocaine.

Resource Deprivation Theory

According to this theory, racial/ethnic disparities in health status exist because minorities are more likely than Whites to live in communities that are lacking in the necessary infrastructure to support a healthy lifestyle. One study demonstrated an association between the location of food stores and food service places and the racial composition of the community (Morland et al., 2002). That study found that compared with predominantly Black neighborhoods, supermarkets were 2.9 times more likely to be located in racially integrated neighborhoods and 4.3 times more likely to be located in predominantly White neighborhoods. Full-service restaurants were 3.4 times more prevalent in integrated neighborhoods and 2.4 times more prevalent in predominantly White neighborhoods (see Figure 7.2).

Morrison et al. (2002) conducted a survey of pharmacies in New York City to determine whether the availability of pain medications (opioids) was associated with the racial/ethnic composition of the neighborhoods that the pharmacies served. The results

**FIGURE 7.2.   DENSITY OF SUPERMARKETS AND
FULL-SERVICE RESTAURANTS BY NEIGHBORHOOD
RACIAL SEGREGATION CATEGORY.**

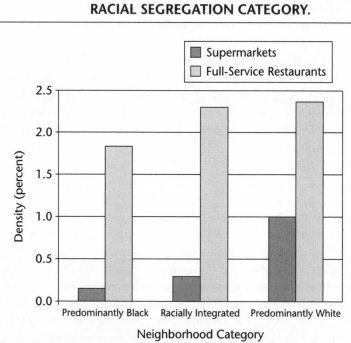

Source: Derived from data in Morland et al., 2002.

of their findings are summarized in Figure 7.3, which shows that where the proportion of each minority group is greater, the percentage of pharmacies with adequate supplies of pain medications is smaller.

Psychosocial/Behavioral Theories of Health Disparities

Psychosocial and behavioral theories are related to the aspects of the culture of specific racial/ethnic groups that influence the behavior of individuals.

The Weathering Hypothesis

Arlene Geronimus (2002) developed the weathering hypothesis to explain race differences in low birth weight and infant mortality. The hypothesis states that the health status of minorities begin to prematurely deteriorate in young adulthood. This premature

FIGURE 7.3. ADEQUACY OF OPIOID SUPPLIES BY RACIAL/ETHNICITY COMPOSITION OF THE NEIGHBORHOOD.

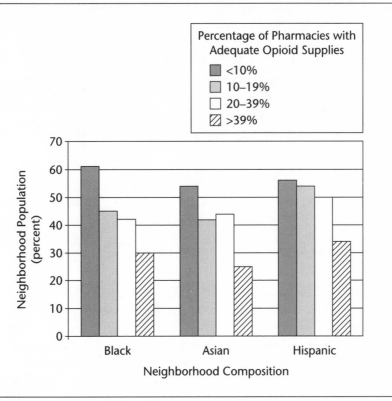

Source: Morrison et al., 2002, p. 467.

aging, which Geronimus refers to as weathering, occurs as a response to long-term exposure to social and financial stress and prolonged active coping with stressful circumstances. This premature aging could have negative effects on a woman's health status or health behaviors and, should she become a mother, on the health of her infant. By extension, the theory can be applied more broadly, beyond pregnancy outcomes. It can be applied to lower life expectancy and early onset of degenerative chronic conditions among racial/ethnic minorities, particularly African Americans.

Geronimus hypothesized that because of weathering, the Black-White disparity in low birth weight rates would widen as the age of the mother increased. This widening would occur because as African American women aged their health status would decline. As a consequence, their infants would have an increased risk of low birth weight. Geronimus's test of this hypothesis is displayed in Figure 7.4. The figure shows that low birth weight rates are *lowest* among African American mothers aged fifteen to

FIGURE 7.4. LOW BIRTH WEIGHT RATE BY RACE AND AGE AT BIRTH.

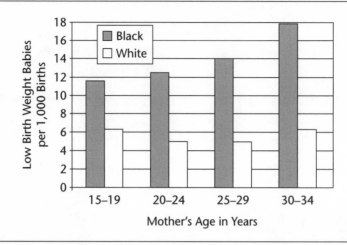

Source: Geronimus, 2002, p. 219.

seventeen. There is a gradual rise in low birth weight as maternal age increases. However, among Whites, mothers in their teens and thirties experience slightly higher low birth weight rates compared to White women in their twenties. Because of the different age patterns, the size of the race difference in low birth weight increases with maternal age.

Wildsmith (2002) conducted a study similar to Geronimus's study among Mexican-born and U.S.-born Mexican American women. That study found support for the weathering hypothesis as well. Wildsmith showed that for the foreign-born Mexicans, neonatal mortality rates were highest among younger mothers and lower for older mothers, and that the rate increased again in women at the oldest ages—similar to the patterns that Geronimus (2002) had found for White women. For the U.S.-born Mexican American women, the lowest neonatal mortality rates were found among women aged seventeen and eighteen years and twenty-seven to twenty-nine years. Levels for women aged nineteen to twenty-four years and thirty to thirty-four years are higher than those for seventeen- and eighteen-year-olds. Thus, the association between maternal age and pregnancy was not as strong as the association Geronimus found among African Americans; however, the patterns are suggestive of weathering.

John Henryism

The John Henryism hypothesis takes its name from the late-nineteenth-century legendary figure John Henry, the steel-driving man. As the legend goes, John Henry was widely known for his remarkable physical strength and skill at using a nine-pound hammer to drive the stakes that held the railroad tracks in place. One day, John Henry participated in a contest to determine if he could complete this task more quickly and efficiently than a mechanical steam drill. The test of man versus machine was close from beginning to end, but John Henry won. Moments after the contest ended, John Henry dropped dead from complete physical and mental exhaustion. Man had beaten machine, but at a great price.

According to Dr. Sherman James—the originator of the John Henryism hypothesis—John Henryism (an active response against difficult odds) emerged as a widespread behavioral phenomenon among Black Americans in the years following the Civil War; it was, in effect, a cultural adaptation to oppression. The hypothesis was developed in an attempt to explain why African Americans have a higher prevalence of hypertension compared to Whites. The John Henryism hypothesis states that individuals with lower social status (such as persons with low socioeconomic status or racial minorities) are routinely exposed to psychological and socioeconomic stressors (for example, chronic financial strain, job insecurity, and subtle or perhaps not so subtle social insults such as racial discrimination). These stressors require them to exert considerable energy daily to manage the psychological consequences generated by chronic exposure to stress.

The hypothesis assumes that not all individuals who are exposed to these stressors will respond in the same way. Some will respond with high-effort active coping (sustained cognitive and emotional engagement). Others will respond more passively or respond actively at first but then give up. The John Henryism hypothesis predicts that lower socioeconomic status individuals who persist with effortful active coping under

---

BOX 7.2.   JOHN HENRY.

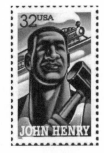

John Henry is an African American folk hero who symbolizes strength and determination. The stories about John Henry are not just "tall tales," for they are based on the life of a real person, a former slave working on the railroads after the Civil War, but time has blurred fact and fiction. In the stories, John Henry, a strong "steel-driving man," accepted the challenge of trying to outperform a steam-powered drill. Swinging a heavy hammer in each hand, he beat the machine but died soon after—some say from exhaustion, others say from a broken heart on realizing that machines would replace muscle and spirit.

Source: United State Postal Service, *African Americans on Stamps: A Celebration of African American Heritage* (Washington, DC: U.S. Postal Service, 2004).

difficult conditions will experience an increased heart rate and higher systolic blood pressure as they attempt to overcome the stressor. Thus, if individuals were categorized into two groups—those strongly predisposed to cope actively with psychosocial stressors (high John Henryism group) and those less predisposed to active coping (low John Henryism group)—the highest mean blood pressure level would be expected in those individuals who are simultaneously categorized by low socioeconomic status and high John Henryism.

John Henryism is measured using a questionnaire. Study participants respond to twelve questions designed to identify those that have a predisposition to an active coping style (John Henryism). Dr. James described the hypothesized relationship between John Henryism and hypertension as follows: "The inverse association between socioeconomic status and blood pressure will be much more pronounced (that is, more striking) for individuals who score high on John Henryism than for those who score low" (James, 2002). Figure 7.5 shows the results of a study testing the John Henryism hypothesis among a sample of African Americans in Pitt County, North Carolina. The study found that among individuals who were high in John Henryism there is a

FIGURE 7.5. ADJUSTED PREVALENCE OF HYPERTENSION IN BLACK ADULTS, AGED 25 TO 50 YEARS, BY SOCIOECONOMIC STATUS AND LEVEL OF JOHN HENRYISM, PITT COUNTY, NORTH CAROLINA, 1992.

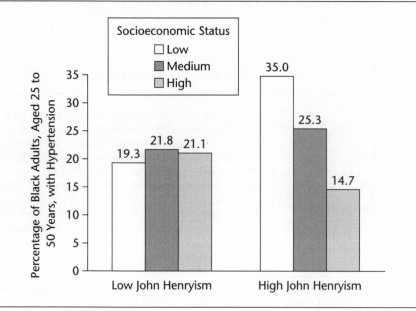

Source: James et al., 1992, p. 64.

BOX 7.3.   JOHN HENRYISM AND TYPE A PERSONALITY.

The John Henryism concept is sometimes confused with Type A personality, which is characterized by competitive, aggressive, and tense behavior. Such behavior as been associated with increased risk for heart disease (Rafanelli et al., 2003).

A 1988 study was conducted to determine if the Type A personality profile was the same as the John Henryism profile. A team of researchers from the University of South Carolina School of Nursing investigated the two concepts in a sample of persons in Charleston, South Carolina. They conclude that the Framingham Type A and John Henryism scales do in fact measure two quite different behavior patterns.

Weinrich, Weinrich, Keil, Gazes, and Potter, 1988.

---

strong dose-response relationship, whereby the highest percentage of individuals with hypertension was found among lower socioeconomic status individuals who scored high on John Henryism. Among persons with high levels of John Henryism, lower socioeconomic status was associated with an increased likelihood of having hypertension. By contrast, among those who scored low on John Henryism, socioeconomic status was not associated with hypertension (James, Keenan, Strogatz, Browning, & Garrett, 1992).

Although the John Henryism hypothesis was developed to explain variation in the prevalence of hypertension among African Americans, a test of the hypothesis in a White population in the Netherlands found "mixed" support for the hypothesis in that population. Duijkers, Drijver, Kromhout, and James (1988) conducted a test of the John Henryism hypothesis among a sample of residents of Zutphen, the Netherlands. The study found a significant association between John Henryism and systolic blood pressure among men, but did not find the association among women. The association was most pronounced for men of low educational background. Overall, however, John Henryism has mainly been studied in African American populations and has been applied as an explanation for racial disparities in hypertension.

Immigration and Acculturation

One of the most interesting phenomena regarding minority health is the finding that foreign-born persons have better health outcomes than their U.S.-born counterparts. Additionally, as the number of years that the foreign-born person lives in the United States increases, the person's health status begins to approximate the health status of U.S.-born counterparts. There are studies on this topic that have not previously been organized into a formal theory. The consistent finding can be summarized as follows: as the duration of time immigrants live in the United States increases, their health status begins to approximate the health status of those who were already living in the United States. Although the studies that examine this hypothesis are consistent for immigrants from various nations, most of the research that explores this issue has been conducted on U.S.-born and Mexican-born Mexicans (Frisbie, Cho, & Hummer, 2002). However, similar findings have been documented for other ethnic groups; for example, Frisbie et al. found a similar pattern in a comparison of U.S.-born and foreign-born Asians and Pacific Islanders. David and Collins (2002) found similar results in their comparison of African-born and U.S.-born Blacks. And Singh and Yu (2002) tested this pattern of findings among immigrants of nine different countries or regions.

Figure 7.6 summarizes the results of analysis by Singh and Yu, which illustrate infant mortality rates among U.S.-born and their foreign-born counterparts who gave birth in the United States. The figure shows a consistent pattern in which the foreign-born women have a lower infant mortality rate compared with their U.S.-born counterpart. The single exception to this pattern is for Central and South American women,

FIGURE 7.6. INFANT MORTALITY RATES FOR U.S.-BORN WOMEN AND THEIR FOREIGN-BORN COUNTERPARTS.

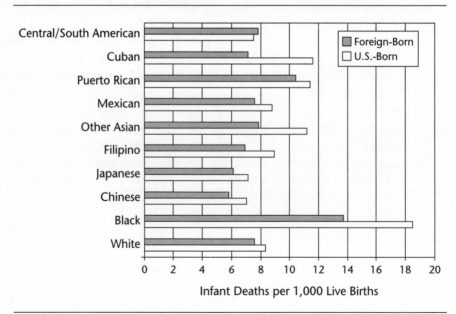

Source: Data from Singh and Yu, 2002, p. 269.

among whom the foreign-born women have a slightly higher infant mortality rate. Figure 7.7 summarizes the primary findings from the David and Collins 2002 study. This figure shows the well-known fact that African Americans have substantially lower average birth weights compared to White Americans. However, African-born Blacks who gave birth in the United States had infants with birth weights substantially higher than those of African Americans and only slightly below the average birth weight for White Americans.

Figure 7.8 summarizes analysis, originally conducted by Frisbie et al. (2002), which compares the odds that Asian immigrants will have a disability and the odds that they will spend at least one week in a hospital. The figure demonstrates that as the duration of time immigrants have lived in the United States increases, the odds of having a disability or a long-term hospitalization increases and begins to approach the odds for U.S.-born Asians.

Racial Discrimination: The Racism Biopsychosocial Model

Racism continues to be a controversial and contentious issue in the United States. Discussions of racism can often become quite emotional. The term *racism* itself has been defined in many different and sometimes contradictory ways. Some have attempted

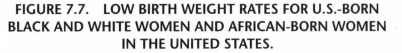

FIGURE 7.7. LOW BIRTH WEIGHT RATES FOR U.S.-BORN BLACK AND WHITE WOMEN AND AFRICAN-BORN WOMEN IN THE UNITED STATES.

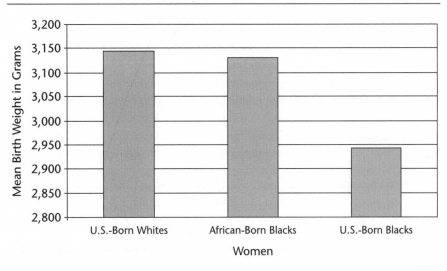

Source: Data from David and Collins, 2002.

FIGURE 7.8. ODDS OF HAVING A DISABILITY AND ODDS OF SPENDING A WEEK IN A HOSPITAL AMONG FOREIGN-BORN AND U.S.-BORN ASIANS, NATIONAL HEALTH INTERVIEW SURVEY, 1992–1995 COMBINED.

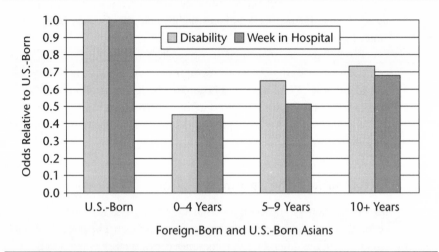

Source: Frisbie, Cho, and Hummer, 2002, p. 242.

to incorporate elements of power, oppression, or minority-versus-majority status into their definitions. However, in this chapter the term *racism* will be used as defined by Clark, Anderson, Clark, and Williams (2002): "beliefs, attitudes, institutional arrangements, and acts that tend to denigrate individuals or groups because of phenotypic characteristics or ethnic group affiliation."

Williams, Neighbors, & Jackson (2003) conducted a review of studies that assess the relationship between exposure to racism and health outcomes. That review found fifty-three studies that demonstrate an association between racism and health. Exposure to racism has been associated with negative mental health outcomes, physical health outcomes, and health behavior (such as smoking and alcohol consumption). However, although many studies have demonstrated an association between exposure to racism and health-related outcomes, only recently have scholars begun to specify the mechanisms that link racism and health. As of now those mechanisms are still theoretical. Most studies have hypothesized that racism is a stressor and as such leads to negative health outcomes. This perspective is described in the biopsychosocial model outlined by Clark et al. (2002).

The biopsychosocial model views racism as a stressor. Each individual has a unique set of characteristics (psychological, sociodemographic, and behavior) that comprise their individual constitution. When exposed to racism, individuals will vary in the degree to which they perceive that social stimulus. Obviously, those who do not perceive the stimulus will not suffer any negative health effects as a direct result of the racism stimulus. Also, some individuals may perceive the stimulus but not attribute it to racism. Those who perceive the stressor (whether as racism or some other stressor) will then filter the event through their individual coping resources. Those who have strong coping resources may be able to reduce or even eliminate any potential psychological or physiological response. Those whose coping resources are not able to blunt the impact will suffer psychological and physiological stress responses. Examples of these physiological stress responses are: (1) musculoskeletal stress response (Soderfeldt, Soderfeldt, Ohlson, & Warg, 1996), (2) cardiovascular stress response (Traustadottir, Bosch, & Matt, 2003), and (3) immune dysfunction (Padgett & Glaser, 2003). There is now substantial scientific evidence of a physiological response to stress (Padgett & Glaser, 2003).

Most studies of racism and health have measured racism by way of questionnaire. Such studies actually measure the perception of racism, not racism itself. As the model in Figure 7.9 suggests, different individuals can experience the same negative event, yet interpret the event differently. One person might perceive racism in a given situation; another person might interpret the situation differently. This reality sets up a problem that plagues research on racism and health: respondents who report on a questionnaire that they have experienced racism may be overreporting (or underreporting). However, whether or not an individual appraises an event as racism may, in itself, be an important aspect of the appraisal/coping mechanism that links racism to health—but how to measure it?

While most studies have measured racism (or more precisely, perceived exposure to racism) through questionnaires, other studies have measured racism through skin color. The notion is that darker skin color will be associated with greater exposure to discrimination. Some of these studies have allowed study respondents to self-rate their complexions (Klonoff & Landrine, 2002), while others have used objective means of measurement such as a reflectometer (Klag, Whelton, Coresh, Grim, & Kuller, 1991). In a 1991 study published in the *Journal of the American Medical Association*, Johns Hopkins Medical School researcher Dr. Michael Klag and his colleagues found that both systolic and diastolic blood pressure were higher among dark-complexioned Blacks compared with light-complexioned Blacks with low socioeconomic status.

Other studies have found an association between skin complexion and health outcomes. Knapp et al. (1995) studied skin complexion and cancer mortality among Black men in Charleston, South Carolina. The study found that among men with higher socioeconomic status, darker skin color was associated with a higher cancer mortality rate. Dressler (1991) conducted a study of skin color, socioeconomic status, and blood pressure in Brazil. That study found higher blood pressure among study participants with darker skin. Mosley et al. (2000) conducted a study of skin complexion and blood

FIGURE 7.9.   THE BIOPSYCHOSOCIAL RACISM MODEL.

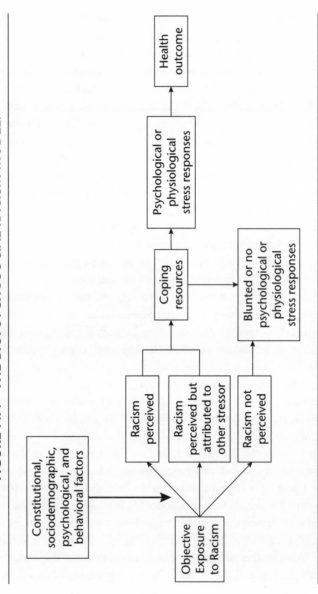

Source: Based on the model developed by Clark et al., 2002.

pressure in a national sample in Egypt; the study demonstrated higher blood pressure among darker-skinned Egyptians. And Gleiberman, Harburg, Frone, Russell, and Cooper (1993) examined the relationship between skin complexion and blood pressure among White non-Hispanic and White Hispanic residents in Erie County, New York. The skin color/health gradient was found in that population as well. It is not possible to rule out the possibility that the skin color/health status relationship may be a function of racial admixture. However, most researchers have argued that skin color is a marker for exposure to discrimination and therefore the relationship between skin color and health is a function of social and psychological factors associated with discrimination (Dressler, 1991).

The Hispanic Epidemiological Paradox

The Hispanic epidemiological paradox describes a pattern among mortality and morbidity rates in which Hispanics/Latinos tend to have more favorable health outcomes (in many causes of death) than non-Hispanics/Latinos (particularly Whites). This pattern is unexpected given the generally lower socioeconomic status of Hispanics/Latinos compared to Whites. Franzini, Ribble, and Keddie (2002) described four possible hypotheses to explain this pattern: (1) poor data quality, (2) the "salmon bias" hypothesis, (3) the healthy migrant hypothesis, and (4) differences in certain risk factors related to acculturation. The Hispanic epidemiological paradox is discussed in detail in Chapter Thirteen (Hispanic/Latino Health).

Biogenetic and Physiological Theories of Health Disparities

There are three possible ways in which biogenetic factors may play a role in explaining health disparities. First, there may be biological or genetic differences among racial and ethnic groups—differences that lead to varying levels of susceptibility to diseases. Second, there may be biogenetic or environmental interactions that account for different levels of disease. Exposure to environmental factors triggers biological processes that produce disease, and to the extent that minorities have greater exposure to environmental risks they will have higher rates of morbidity. The third possibility is outlined in the slavery hypertension hypothesis, which states that because of salt deprivation during the Atlantic slave trade (Middle Passage) and the excessive mortality rate of the Africans who were enslaved, the Africans who survived were those with a genetic predisposition to salt retention. Modern African Americans now live in a sodium-rich environment in which salt retention is no longer beneficial and, in fact, is harmful.

Biological or Genetic Differences Among Racial and Ethnic Groups

There has been much speculation about biological differences among race groups; however, in most cases the speculation is not supported with data. Over the past decade there have been tremendous advancements in genomic science. As a result, while it was widely believed that racial/ethnic groupings corresponded to underlying biological differences, few scientists still believe that human biogenetic variation can be adequately described by such categories (Garte, 2002). This is not to suggest that some scientists do not continue to support the idea that race has some biological relevance (Risch, Burchard, Ziv, & Tang, 2002), but that view is losing ground rapidly. For example, Dean et al. (1994) studied polymorphic admixture and its correlation to race/ethnicity. They examined 257 loci from each chromosome and found all variants present in Whites, Blacks, Chinese Americans, and Native Americans. They did find some differences in allele frequencies; however, no racial/ethnic-specific alleles were found. In fact, some researchers (such as Cavalli-Sforza, Menozzi, & Piazza, 1994) argue that if humans were grouped according to genetic characteristics, Africans and Europeans should be grouped into one genetic cluster apart from, for example, American Indians or Australian Aborigines. Similar arguments have also been made by other researchers (Garte, 2002; Weber, 1999; Mountain & Cavalli-Sforza, 1997).

Biogenetic-Environmental Interactions

Although most scientists believe the matter of the biological basis for racial/ethnic categories has been resolved, this does not mean that biogenetic factors do not play a role in health disparities. There are only a few studies of biogenetic and environmental interactions and health, so we still know relatively little about the role of biogenetic-environmental interactions in understanding racial/ethnic disparities in health. Virtually all such studies have examined the role of social stressors or personality characteristics, such as the studies conducted by James (2002) on John Henryism and by Klag et al. (1991) on skin color, previously discussed in this chapter. Simply put, there has not been adequate study of the hypothesis that social inequality leads to differential environmental exposures, and these different environmental factors interact with genes to produce health disparities. No scientific evidence exists to either support or refute this hypothesis.

The Slavery Hypertension Hypothesis

The slavery hypertension hypothesis was first mentioned by Blackburn and Prineas (1983); it was later developed by Grim and Wilson, first in a set of conference presentations in the late 1980s, later with publication in a scientific journal (Wilson & Grim,

1991). The hypothesis attempted to explain why African Americans had higher blood pressure and a higher prevalence of hypertension compared with Whites. However, native Africans (from the regions of Africa where African Americans were descended) have blood pressure and hypertension prevalence rates similar to those of White Americans (Kaufman & Barkey, 1993).

The slavery hypertension hypothesis argues that the higher prevalence of hypertension among African Americans is a result of selective survival. Salt (sodium) deprivation and brutal treatment during the Atlantic slave trade led to an extremely high mortality rate. Those who were predisposed to salt-saving renal-adrenal adaptation had a survival advantage. Because of the theory's seeming plausibility, it has enjoyed wide distribution and substantial popularity. However, there is little scientific evidence to support it. In fact, most rigorous examinations of the hypothesis have provided evidence that would tend to refute the hypothesis (Kaufman & Hall, 2003).

Summary

This chapter explored the various theories that seek to explain differences in the health status of racial/ethnic groups in the United States. The theories were organized into three categories based on the conceptual model of determinants of health. The three categories are (1) socioenvironmental or context, (2) psychosocial and behavioral, and (3) biophysiological. Socioenvironmental theories include context theories—racial/ethnic segregation, risk exposure theory, resource deprivation theory. Psychosocial theories include the weathering hypothesis, John Henryism, immigration and acculturation, and racial discrimination (racism). The biopsychosocial theories include the theory that there are true genetic differences between racial groups, the theory that differential gene environment interactions account for health disparities, and the slave hypertension hypothesis. (See Appendix B for additional readings.)

Key Words

Psychosocial

Context theory

Racial/ethnic segregation

Risk exposure theory

Resource deprivation theory

Weathering hypothesis

John Henryism

Immigration and acculturation

Racial discrimination

Racism biopsychosocial model

Hispanic epidemiological paradox

Biogenetic-environmental interactions

Slave hypertension hypothesis

CHAPTER EIGHT

SOCIOECONOMIC STATUS AND RACIAL/ETHNIC DIFFERENCES IN HEALTH

Outline

Introduction

People with low socioeconomic status (SES) due to factors such as limited education and low income, have higher rates of morbidity and mortality compared with those who have more economic resources. This is probably the best-documented finding in public health research (House & Williams, 2000). Studies conducted as early as the nineteenth and early twentieth centuries first found a relationship between social status and health (for example, Engels's book *The Condition of the Working Class in England*, originally published in 1845; Newsholme, 1910). And currently there is an impressive body of research, using various study designs, methods, measures of social status, and measures of health (see House & Williams, 2000, for a comprehensive review). In fact, the SES–health status relationship is so well documented that one author (Anderson, 1958) stated that any further research on the relationship is "a waste of time, money, and effort, because the gross relationship [has] been established conclusively enough." However, the many studies of low economic and social status (socioeconomic status) that have been published since Anderson made this comment suggest that his position is not a popular view. In fact, the social status–health status relationship is so complex and multifaceted that more than a half-century after Anderson's statement there is still a great deal that we do not understand about it.

What Is Socioeconomic Status?

Some people believe that racial and ethnic disparities in health are really just a reflection of socioeconomic status differences, since racial minorities generally have worse socioeconomic status than do most Whites. In this chapter we will explore this issue. But first I will provide a discussion of the definitions of socioeconomic status.

Socioeconomic status refers to a system of stratification whereby individuals are classified in a hierarchy along various dimensions of social class. The origins of the term can be found in Karl Marx's notion of social class. Marx viewed social classes as groupings of individuals who played similar roles in the economic system of a society. For example, classical Marxist theory classified individuals on the basis of their relationship to the *means of production*—that is, the economic system of the society. Marx argued that individuals living in capitalist societies were either owners of or workers in the economic system (he called the two groups the bourgeoisie and the proletariat, respectively). The class that a person belonged to determined the level of societal resources that person was able to access and whether the person benefited disproportionately or was exploited by the capitalist system. Marx argued that under capitalism the workers (the proletariat) were exploited because although their labor produces the

---

BOX 8.1.   SOCIOECONOMIC STATUS.

The term *socioeconomic status* (SES) was coined by American sociologist Lester Ward in 1883. Social and economic positions are combined to determine a person's SES status in society.

BOX 8.2.   SOCIAL CLASS.

Social classes are groupings of individuals based on their relationship to the economy.

---

company's profit, most of the profit goes to the owner (bourgeoisie), not the workers. Marx viewed class conflict as inevitable under such a system.

Max Weber advanced Marx's notion of social class by noting that although the individual's relationship to the means of production was important, there were other dimensions in society upon which individuals can be placed to form a hierarchy. Weber viewed classes as groupings of individuals who have similar life chances. He viewed a person's opportunities in life as resulting from multiple stratification dimensions (including, but not limited to, the person's relationship to the means of production); for example, religious affiliation, education, occupation, or birthrights and privilege from a "noble" family. Although Weber viewed stratification more broadly than Marx did, they were in basic agreement that societies place individuals within social stratification hierarchies.

A variety of measures are typically used as indicators of a person's socioeconomic status. These measures taken together form a composite picture of a person's position within a society's social stratification system. Research articles published in public health or medical journals often use income, education, or some other single measure as an indicator of socioeconomic status. Although this approach is rather common, it is less than ideal (this point will be further explained in the following section).

Measures of Socioeconomic Status

Identifying and measuring social stratification systems is one of the primary concerns of sociology. Nakao and Treas (1994) recount much of the history of this work in their article updating occupational prestige and socioeconomic status scoring. The six most frequently used measures of socioeconomic status are poverty, income, education, occupation, wealth, and various indexes that combine income, education, and occupational prestige. Beginning in the latter half of the twentieth century, increasing attention has been devoted to research on income inequality and health. Income inequality is a measure that compares the socioeconomic status of groups in relation to one another. In the next section, I will describe each of these approaches to measuring SES and briefly discuss their shortcomings and benefits, explore racial/ethnic patterns among these measures, and demonstrate how they are interrelated.

Income

Income measures attempt to stratify individuals on the basis of the amount of money the individual has at his or her disposal. Individuals use money to purchase goods and services that can aid in preventing ill health (such as good-quality nutritious food or good-quality housing) or resources that can be brought to bear to improve the individual's health status in a time of illness (such as access to medications). In studies of socioeconomic status and health that use income, income is sometimes measured as *individual income*—the income generated by the specific individual who is a participant in the study. However, more often income is measured as *family* or *household income,* because although individual income can be informative about some aspects of the individual being studied, family income is typically a better indicator of the actual amount of income the individual is able to access.

The primary benefit of using income as a measure of socioeconomic status is that it can be clearly defined and measured as the amount of dollars earned. Also, there are standardized ways to compute adjustments to income that will allow for comparisons over time, to compare groups of individuals or to compare societies. For example, one can adjust for inflation to compare income in different years, or one can adjust for differences in the exchange rate of countries to compare people in different countries. However, there are important shortcomings to using income as a measure. For one, often as many as 15 percent of study participants refuse to answer questions about income, so that in research on the effect of socioeconomic status on health there is often a significant amount of missing data. There can be important differences among individuals who report the same income as well. For example, a household income of $100,000 might mean very different things in the case of a household with one person working outside of the home compared with a multiearner household. The number of people the household comprises is also an important consideration. A household income of $50,000 for a two-person household is very different than for a seven-person household. Often, studies of income and health do not make the necessary adjustments to account for these considerations.

Another limitation of measuring by income is that it is especially subject to *downward drift* (also referred to as *reverse causation*). Downward drift refers to the phenomenon in which an individual whose health status declines may find their income also declining. Income can decline substantially over a relatively short period of time. The dynamic nature of income can also be a limitation. Since income fluctuates over time, the income data captured by the census or a researcher may not be a reflection of the person's long-term status.

Table 8.1 presents median household income for the U.S. population by racial and ethnic groups for the year 2002. The table shows that the median income for the country (all groups) was $42,409. Asian/Pacific Islanders have the highest median income of all racial/ethnic groups, $52,285. Hispanics had the lowest median income

---

BOX 8.3.   INCOME.

Income refers to money obtained from employment, transfer programs, or other sources.

- *Personal income:* Income generated by a specific individual
- *Family income:* The sum of all income generated by related individuals living in a household
- *Household income:* The sum of all income generated by all individuals living in a household, whether or not they are related

---

TABLE 8.1.   MEDIAN HOUSEHOLD INCOME IN CONSTANT 2002 DOLLARS, BY RACE AND HISPANIC ORIGIN.

Total U.S. Population	$42,409
White	$47,041
African American	$29,026
Hispanic	$33,103
Asian/Pacific Islander	$16,494

Source: U.S. Bureau of the Census, "Race and Hispanic Origin of Householder-Households by Median and Mean Income," http://www.census.gov/hhes/income/histinc/h0610.html.

of all groups, $33,103. Median income for African Americans and Whites was $29,026 and $47,041, respectively.

Poverty

Although the primary shortcoming of using income as a measure of socioeconomic status is the fact that it does not account for household size, this is precisely what poverty measure is designed to account for. The Census Bureau uses a set of income thresholds that vary by family size and composition to determine who is living in poverty. If a family's total income is less than the designated income threshold for that family size, then that family and every individual in it is considered poor.

For example, according to the U.S. Bureau of the Census, the poverty threshold for a family of five with one child for the year 2003 was $23,220. Suppose that each member had the following incomes in 2003:

Father	$12,750
Mother	$0

BOX 8.4. POVERTY.

The official measure of poverty was established by the Office of Management and Budget in Statistical Policy Directive 14. The poverty thresholds were originally developed in 1963–1964 by Mollie Orshansky of the Social Security Administration. She based her poverty thresholds on the economy food plan—the cheapest of four food plans developed by the Department of Agriculture. The actual combinations of foods in the food plans, devised by department dietitians using complex procedures, constituted nutritionally adequate diets; the department described the economy food plan as being "designed for temporary or emergency use when funds are low."

Grandmother	$6,200
Child	$0
Household total	$18,950

Because their total family income, $18,950, is below the poverty threshold for their family size, the family would be considered poor according to the official poverty measure. Table 8.2 shows the official poverty thresholds for all family sizes for the year 2003.

Poverty is typically conceptualized as a dichotomous variable: people are either in poverty or not in poverty. But this does not reflect the true level of variation among people. A family of four with an annual income of $100,000 can afford a different lifestyle than a family of four with an annual income of $50,000, but both families would simply be considered not to be poor. So poverty can also be conceptualized as a continuous variable, reflecting differences in the effects of income across different income levels. There can also be gradients of poverty. To demonstrate how this can be done, we continue the example with Table 8.3.

By computing poverty status as a ratio relative to the official federal poverty threshold, one can produce a gradient. For example, a family (or an individual) can be living at 50 percent of poverty if the household income is half of the official poverty level, or 75 percent of poverty if it is three quarters of the poverty level. Likewise, one would be at 150 percent of poverty with income 50 percent above the official poverty line, or at 200 percent above poverty with income double the poverty level. This is a particularly useful approach because of the controversial nature of poverty thresholds—official

TABLE 8.2. POVERTY THRESHOLDS FOR 2003, BY SIZE OF FAMILY AND NUMBER OF RELATED CHILDREN UNDER 18 YEARS OF AGE (IN DOLLARS).

Size of Family Unit	Related Children Under Age 18								
	None	One	Two	Three	Four	Five	Six	Seven	Eight or More
One person (unrelated individual)									
Under age 65	9,573								
Age 65 and over	8,825								
Two persons									
Householder under age 65	12,321	12,682							
Householder age 65 years and over	11,122	12,634	14,824						
Three persons	14,393	14,810	18,660	18,725					
Four persons	18,979	19,289	22,509	21,959	21,623				
Five persons	22,887	23,220	25,884	25,362	24,586	24,126			
Six persons	26,324	26,429	29,827	29,372	28,526	27,538	26,454		
Seven persons	30,289	30,479	33,560	33,021	32,256	31,286	30,275	30,019	
Eight persons	33,876	34,175	40,404	39,947	39,196	38,163	37,229	36,998	35,572
Nine persons or more	40,751	40,948							

Source: U.S. Bureau of the Census, "Poverty Thresholds, 2003," http://www.census.gov/hhes/poverty/threshld/thresh03.html.

TABLE 8.3.   PERCENTAGE OF POVERTY FOR A FAMILY OF FIVE WITH ONE CHILD, 2003.

Percentage of Poverty	Threshold
50	$11,610
75	$17,415
100	$23,220
125	$29,025
150	$34,839

poverty thresholds are widely regarded to be too low and as such tend to underestimate the true level of poverty. Furthermore, the official federal poverty thresholds do not vary by state or other geographic characteristics, even though there is substantial variation in cost of living across the country. A person with an annual income of $32,497.00 could afford a very different lifestyle in Mississippi than the lifestyle he or she could have living in San Francisco.

Table 8.4 lists trends in poverty rates by race/ethnicity for the United States for the years 1960 to 2000. Data for American Indians/Alaska Natives were only available for 1995; however, according to the poverty rates for that year, they have the highest poverty of all racial/ethnic groups. Although poverty rates have been declining for each racial/ethnic group, African Americans consistently have the highest poverty rate (22.0 percent) among groups with comparative data. The poverty rate for Hispanics

TABLE 8.4.   RATE OF POVERTY FOR THE U.S. POPULATION, 1960–2000.

Year	Total U.S. Population	White	African American	Hispanic	Asian/Pacific Islander	American Indian/ Alaska Native
2000	11.3	9.5	22.0	21.5	9.9	31.2 [a]
1990	13.5	10.7	31.9	28.1	12.2	N.A.
1980	13.0	10.2	32.5	25.7	N.A.	N.A.
1970	12.6	9.9	33.5	N.A.	N.A.	N.A.
1960	22.2	17.8	N.A.	N.A.	N.A.	N.A.

[a]Data are for 1995.

Sources: U.S. Bureau of the Census, "Poverty (Historical Table)," tab. 8.2, http://www.census.gov/hhes/poverty/histpov/hstpov2.html; "Selected Social and Economic Characteristics for the 25 Largest American Indian Tribes, 1990," http://www.census.gov/population/socdemo/race/indian/ailang2.txt.

is slightly lower than that of African Americans, at 21.5 percent. Whites have the lowest poverty rate, followed by Asians/Pacific Islanders: 9.5 percent and 9.9 percent, respectively.

Education

As a measure of socioeconomic status, educational attainment overcomes many of the shortcomings of income and poverty data. For example, missing data is not usually a significant problem with education. Educational attainment does have some nontrivial limitations; for one thing, educational attainment does not always do the best job of producing a hierarchy. A college graduate can be a bank teller or the bank president; a high school graduate can work as the janitor at Microsoft or he can also be Microsoft's founder. But in general education serves as a good measure for some aspects of socioeconomic status. Persons with higher levels of education generally enjoy a lifestyle that is more conducive to good health than the lifestyles of persons with less education. Most people complete their formal education by age twenty-five, so educational attainment is relatively stable in adulthood. Also, unlike income occupation or poverty, education does not fluctuate from year to year and does not decline as a person's health declines. Table 8.5 displays the percentage of high school graduates twenty-five years old or older, by race/ethnicity.

The table shows that the gap between African Americans and White Americans with at least a high school education narrowed significantly between 1959 and 2000. For Whites the percentage of high school graduates nearly doubled during that time period. For African Americans the rate of change from 1959 to 2000 has been much faster: the percentage of African American high school graduates has more than tripled. Hispanics have also seen great improvements in the percentage of high school graduates, but the Hispanic rate still lags behind those of the other groups.

TABLE 8.5. PERCENTAGE OF HIGH SCHOOL GRADUATES AGED 25 YEARS OR OLDER, BY RACE AND HISPANIC ORIGIN, 1959–2000.

Year	Total U.S. Population	White	African American	Hispanic	Asian/Pacific Islander
2000	84.1	84.9	78.9	57.0	84.7
1990	77.6	79.1	66.2	50.8	N.A.
1980	68.6	70.5	51.2	45.3	N.A.
1970	55.2	57.4	33.7	N.A.	N.A.
1959	46.3	46.1	24.8	N.A.	N.A.

Source: U.S. Bureau of the Census, http://www.census.gov/population/socdemo/education/tableA-2.txt.

As one might suspect, there is a relationship between education and income. People with more education generally have higher incomes. However, the relationship between education and income may not be as strong as one might think. As Figure 8.1 demonstrates, the relationship between education and income also varies by race or ethnicity. In other words, education influences income differently for people of different racial or ethnic groups and may therefore yield unreliable results in studies using education to measure SES.

Occupation

Job status is another factor for measuring socioeconomic status. We know that some occupations are held in higher regard than others—and along with this higher regard and prestige generally comes a higher income. The U.S. labor force has become increasingly concentrated in white-collar occupations: executive, professional, managerial, administrative, technical, clerical, and sales positions. As shown in Table 8.6, in 1996, 48 percent of male and 73 percent of female civilians aged twenty-five to sixty-four years held white-collar positions. Thirty-nine percent of civilian men in this age range held blue-collar jobs, compared with only 10 percent of women. By contrast, women were nearly twice as likely as men to be employed in service occupations (16 percent

FIGURE 8.1.   RELATIONSHIP BETWEEN EDUCATION AND INCOME AMONG MALES AGED 25 YEARS AND OVER.

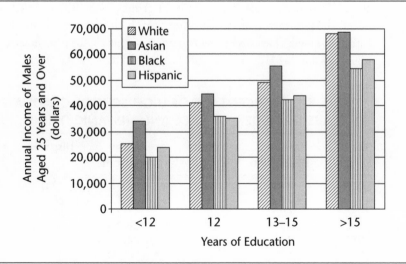

Source: U.S. Bureau of the Census, tab. O, "Total Money Income in 1996 of Persons 25 Years Old and Over, by Educational Attainment, Sex, Region, and Race, 1998."

compared with 9 percent). Only 4 percent of men and just 1 percent of women reported their major occupation as farm-related.

Asian or Pacific Islander men and non-Hispanic White men were much more likely to hold white-collar positions than Black or Hispanic men; three out of every five Asian or Pacific Islander men and over half of White men were employed in white-collar occupations, compared with one out of every three Black men and about one quarter of Hispanic men. For each race and ethnic group examined, the majority of employed civilian women between ages twenty-five and sixty-four held white-collar positions, from 52 percent of Hispanic women to nearly 78 percent of White women.

In 1996 the average compensation for persons holding blue-collar jobs was 81 percent of the average for white-collar workers. Nearly half of employed civilian Hispanic and Black men were working in blue-collar jobs in 1996, but only 28 percent of Asian or Pacific Islander men were in blue-collar employment. Only 8 percent of currently employed White women held blue-collar jobs, compared with between 15 and 18 percent of women in other racial and ethnic groups.

Occupational Prestige

Occupational prestige provides another measure of socioeconomic status through a ranking of the relative prestige of the individual's occupation. Although this approach has been used in sociological and economics research, it has not been widely used in health research. Occupational prestige scaling is a process in which occupations are

TABLE 8.6. CURRENT OCCUPATIONS FOR PERSONS 25–64 YEARS OF AGE.

Race	Men				Women			
	White-Collar	Blue-Collar	Service	Farm	White-Collar	Blue-Collar	Service	Farm
All races	48.4	39.2	8.7	3.8	72.9	10.2	15.8	1.1
White, non-Hispanic	52.6	37.4	6.7	3.4	77.6	8.3	13.0	1.1
Asian or Pacific Islander	60.9	27.7	8.9	2.5	68.5	15.7	15.4	0.4
Black, non-Hispanic	33.5	46.9	17.6	2.0	59.3	14.8	25.7	0.1
Hispanic	26.1	49.4	15.4	9.0	52.3	18.4	26.7	2.7

Source: U.S. Bureau of the Census, Current Population Survey, March 1996.

ranked on a scale from 1 to 100 in terms of their perceived prestige. The rankings are derived from surveys that ask respondents to attach a ranking to each occupation. Thousands of occupations are classified and the rankings are updated periodically (Nakao & Treas, 1994). Table 8.7 presents a sample of occupations from the Nakao and Treas occupational prestige rankings.

Typically, occupational prestige scales are used in conjunction with income and education to form a composite score. Several well-recognized socioeconomic status scales use this approach. Although there are some differences in the specific calculations for these indexes, they are all generally related. Examples of these scales are the Duncan SEI index (Duncan, 1961), the Featherman and Hauser scale (1976), Nam and Powers (1983), and Nakao and Treas (1994).

Wealth

Wealth has not received as much attention among health researchers as have other measures of socioeconomic status. Wealth refers to the accumulated assets (typically, income-generating assets) that an individual holds. Ownership of assets provides for additional resources beyond income from wages. Examples of such assets include investment real estate, automobiles, land, savings, royalties, and home ownership. Home equity is the major source of wealth for the average family. Often individuals accumulate these assets through inheritance as they are passed between generations of a family. Thus, when it comes to multigenerational accumulation of assets, persons who are the first generation of their family to advance out of poverty are greatly disadvantaged. Knowledge can also be considered an asset: consider the advantages that a fifth-generation college student has compared to a student who is the first in the family to ever go to college.

Some scholars have argued that when conducting research on racial or ethnic minorities, researchers should consider wealth as a more important factor than education and, to some extent, income. Witness the fact that although race differences

TABLE 8.7. SAMPLE OF OCCUPATIONAL PRESTIGE SCORES.

Occupation	Score
Physician	97
Dentist	96
School principal	85
Architect	84
Accountant	76
Real estate agent	64
Dancer	44
Receptionist	37
Toll collector	26

Source: Nakao and Treas, 1994.

in education levels have narrowed substantially since the 1960s, the wealth gap has been relatively unchanged.

Table 8.8 displays median net worth and median net worth excluding home equity of households, by race and Hispanic origin, as of 1995. Net worth is a measure of wealth that takes into account the net value of all assets after adjusting for liabilities. Although racial/ethnic differences in median income and education have narrowed substantially over the past four decades, there are still tremendous racial/ethnic differences in wealth. The median net worth for White Americans was $49,030; the figure for African Americans and Hispanics was $7,073 and $7,255, respectively. These great disparities in wealth are further borne out by differences in ownership of

---

BOX 8.5.   WEALTH.

Wealth is the accumulated value of all assets, including home equity, the value of savings and checking accounts, retirement accounts, stocks and mutual funds, rental property, businesses, and vehicles. According to the U.S. Bureau of the Census, home equity accounts for about 44 percent of a household's net worth.

BOX 8.6.   NET WORTH.

.Net worth is the total values of all assets minus the total values of all liabilities.

TABLE 8.8.   NET WORTH AND PERCENTAGE OWNING SELECTED ASSETS AMONG AFRICAN AMERICANS AND THE TOTAL U.S. POPULATION, 1995.

Asset	Total U.S. Population	White	African American	Hispanic
Median net worth	$40,200	$49,030	$7,073	$7,255
Interest-earning assets at financial institutions	69.1%	72.3%	46.4%	49.0%
Regular checking accounts	46.7%	48.9%	31.9%	38.1%
Stocks and mutual fund shares	20.8%	23.1%	5.2%	5.3%
Own business or profession	10.3%	11.3%	2.9%	6.2%
Motor vehicles	89.2%	91.5%	73.4%	80.8%
Own home	64.3%	67.4%	45.2%	41.4%
IRA or Keogh accounts	24.1%	26.5%	7.9%	8.5%

Source: Davern and Fisher, U.S. Bureau of the Census, Current Population Reports, Household Economic Studies, Series P70-71, "Household Net Worth and Asset Ownership: 1995," Table H.

interest-earning assets at financial institutions, stock or mutual fund ownership, ownership of businesses, and IRA or Keogh retirement accounts.

The Relationship Between Socioeconomic Status and Health

I have demonstrated the multiple ways in which SES is measured. Now I would like to describe the relationship between socioeconomic status and health status. As stated previously, one of the earliest research findings in public health illustrated that people in lower income groups have worse health outcomes than people who are more affluent. The relationship between socioeconomic status and health has been studied time and time again, and the relationship has been found to be the same in nearly every setting.

As socioeconomic status increases, health status improves in a linear fashion. The type of relationship is also called a dose-response relationship: the higher the "dose" of socioeconomic status, the better the health outcomes. Thus the relationship between socioeconomic status and health is sometimes referred to as the gradient because of the linear nature of the relationship.

The SES-Health Gradient

Figure 8.2 demonstrates the gradient (or dose-response) relationship between SES (as measured by income) and heart disease death rates among adults aged twenty-five to sixty-four years. The figure shows that among those whose income was less than $10,000 the heart disease death rate was greater than 300 deaths per 100,000 persons. However, as income increases we see a concomitant decrease in death rates, so that among those with incomes between $10,000 and $15,000 the heart disease death rate was lower than 250 deaths per 100,000 persons. For those with annual incomes between $15,000 and $25,000 the heart disease death rate was lower than 150 deaths per 100,000 persons. The lowest death rates were found among those with income over $25,000. A similar relationship can be found when looking at education and

---

BOX 8.7.   DOSE-RESPONSE.

Last (1988) defines *dose-response* as a relationship in which "a change in amount, intensity, or duration of exposure is associated with a change—either an increase or a decrease—in risk of a specific outcome."

health. Figure 8.3 demonstrates the relationship between educational status and health, as measured by selected causes of death, for all adult males aged twenty-five to sixty-four. Figure 8.3 demonstrates a similar gradient: increasing levels of education are associated with decreasing mortality rates for chronic disease, injuries, and communicable diseases.

The Social Causation and Social Selection Theories

There are two general theories that attempt to explain the relationship between socioeconomic status and health: the theories of social causation and social selection (also referred to as social drift). These two theories offer different perspectives on whether low socioeconomic status causes poor health—or poor health causes low socioeconomic status.

The social causation theory states that people with low socioeconomic status have worse health outcomes because low socioeconomic status places individuals at greater risk of exposure to factors that negatively impact health (see Table 8.9). For example, persons of lower socioeconomic status are more likely to live in communities with poor-quality housing, are more likely to be exposed to environmental health risks such as chemical toxins, and are more likely to have occupations that are hazardous. In

FIGURE 8.2.   THE RELATIONSHIP BETWEEN INCOME AND HEALTH: HEART DISEASE DEATH RATES AMONG ADULTS AGED 25–64 YEARS.

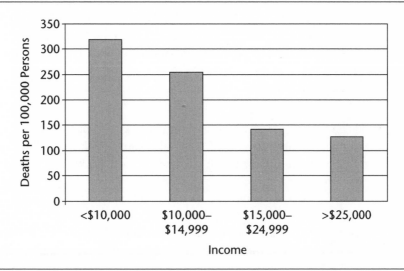

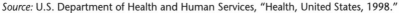

Source: U.S. Department of Health and Human Services, "Health, United States, 1998."

FIGURE 8.3.   THE RELATIONSHIP BETWEEN EDUCATION AND HEALTH: SELECTED CAUSES OF DEATH FOR ADULT MALES AGED 25–64 YEARS.

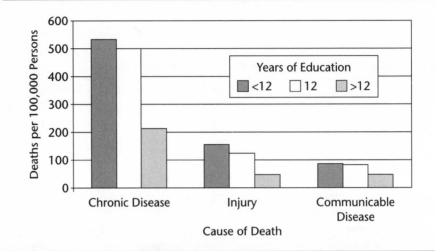

Source: U.S. Department of Health and Human Services, "Health, United States, 1998."

TABLE 8.9.   THE RELATIONSHIP BETWEEN SOCIAL CONTEXT AND HEALTH.

		Neighborhood SES	
		Low	**High**
Individual SES	**Low**	Worst health status	Poor health status
	High	Better health status	Best health status

addition to having greater exposure to health risks, persons of low socioeconomic status are also less likely to have the financial means and other resources to help to minimize the impact of these health risks; for example, health insurance or an ongoing relationship with a physician.

The social selection theory takes a different approach to explaining why people of lower socioeconomic status have worse health status. This theory states that people with worse health status are less able to develop the human capital (such as education or specialized training) that will make them competitive in the economic market. Moreover, people that have poor health status are also less able to work; thus their reduced productivity leads to lower wages and therefore lower socioeconomic status.

BOX 8.8.   THE SOCIAL CAUSATION AND SOCIAL SELECTION THEORIES.

Social causation: Exposure to low SES leads to worsening of health status.
Social selection: Poor health status leads to lower SES.

Many studies have examined these two theories. In general, the studies have found support for both perspectives. Lichtenstein, Harris, Pedersen, & McClearn (1993) conducted a survey of 724 pairs of twins (some reared apart and others reared together) that examined the effects of changes in socioeconomic status between childhood and adulthood on health status in adulthood. The study found support for both the social causation and the social selection theories. This suggests that the two theories are not necessarily contradictory.

All study findings suggest that the relationship between socioeconomic status and health status may be reciprocal, as depicted in Figure 8.4. Low socioeconomic status leads to worse health, and poor health also leads to lower socioeconomic status. Most of the studies that have been conducted have found support for both theories. However, in general social causation has a stronger impact than social selection—that is, the effects of low socioeconomic status on health in society are greater than the effects of health status on socioeconomic status.

Socioeconomic Context

Other studies have examined whether the socioeconomic context of the community in which a person lives has an effect on health, independent of the socioeconomic status of the individual. In other words, does a person with low socioeconomic status who lives in a neighborhood with other people who have low socioeconomic status have worse health than a person who has low socioeconomic status but lives in a more affluent neighborhood?

Of the handful of studies that have addressed this question, all have found support for the idea that the social context in which an individual lives has an impact on the individual's health status over and above the socioeconomic status of the specific individual. A research team from Erasmus University in the Netherlands conducted a study of 8,506 men and women between the ages of fifteen and seventy-four to determine the effect of neighborhood socioeconomic status on mortality. The study also accounted for the socioeconomic status of each individual. This study found that persons living in a low socioeconomic status neighborhood had a higher mortality rate

FIGURE 8.4.   THE RELATIONSHIP BETWEEN SOCIOECONOMIC STATUS AND HEALTH.

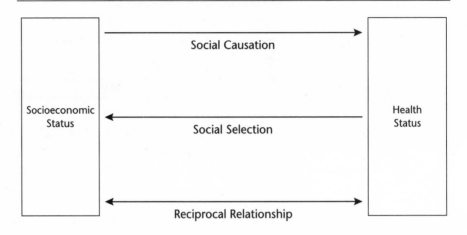

than those living in a higher socioeconomic status neighborhood (Bosma, van de Mheen, Borsboom, & Mackenbach, 2001). Research teams conducting studies in Stockholm, Sweden (Lundberg, 1993), and Rio de Janeiro, Brazil (Szwarcwald, Bastos, Barcellos, Pina, & Esteves, 2000), found similar results.

A U.S.-based study team examined the social context hypothesis in a sample of 2,482 adults living in Illinois (Ross & Mirowsky, 2001). This study found that residents of disadvantaged neighborhoods had worse health than residents of more advantaged neighborhoods. The daily stress associated with living in a neighborhood that is high in crime and "incivility" is believed to have damaging effects upon the health status of individuals. Another U.S.-based study (Wen, Browning, & Cagney, 2003) found similar results and concluded that "the presence of affluent residents is essential to sustain neighborhood social organization which in turn positively affects health." Another U.S.-based study found social context to be an important predictor of health behaviors among adolescents and teenagers. Living in a low socioeconomic status context was found to be associated with poorer dietary habits and a greater likelihood of smoking (Lee & Cubbin, 2002).

Taking into account these studies as well as studies of the effects of individual socioeconomic status on health, one can summarize the health effects of socioeconomic context and individual socioeconomic status as follows:

- An individual with low socioeconomic status living in a low socioeconomic status neighborhood would be expected to have the worst health status
- An individual with low socioeconomic status living in a high socioeconomic status neighborhood would be expected to have better but still poor health status
- An individual with high socioeconomic status living in a low socioeconomic status neighborhood would be expected to have better health status
- An individual with high socioeconomic status living in a high socioeconomic status neighborhood would be expected to have the best health status

Income Inequality and Health

Another aspect of the relationship between socioeconomic status and health is income inequality. Income inequality differs from socioeconomic status in several important respects. First, it is a measure not of an individual but of the social and economic status of *groups* of individuals in a geographic area, such as a city, state, or country. Income inequality refers to the income distribution in a geographic area. Thus, if 90 percent of the income in a country is owned by 10 percent of the population of the country, that country can be said to have a high degree of income inequality. In contrast, a country in which 90 percent of the income is controlled by 50 percent of the population can be said to have less income inequality.

There have been many studies of the effect of income inequality in a geographic area on the health status of that geographic area. Most of the best-known studies of this type were conducted across nations. These cross-national studies have shown that countries with a more equitable distribution of income have higher life expectancy and lower mortality rates. In contrast, countries with higher levels of income inequality tend to have lower life expectancy rates and higher mortality rates.

There have been several more regional studies conducted in U.S. cities, states, and metropolitan areas. Figure 8.5 shows the results from an analysis across U.S. states.

Some believe that income inequality has an effect on health that is independent of the actual socioeconomic status of individuals; that is to say, the income inequality of the social context in which the individual lives is said to have an impact on the health status of the individual, in addition to the individual's own income level. Since the early studies of income inequality and health, published mainly in the 1990s, other studies have been unable to find support for the relationship between income inequality and health status. At this time one must state that it is unclear whether or not there is a relationship between income inequality and health. (For a review of studies of income inequality and health, see Kawachi, Kennedy, and Wilkinson, 1999.)

Are Racial/Ethnic Disparities in Health Manifestations of SES Differences?

This chapter has demonstrated the relationship between socioeconomic status and health status. As we've seen, socioeconomic status is an important determinant of health status. Race/ethnicity is known to be a strong determinant of health status as well. Finally, it is well known that racial and ethnic minorities, in particular African Americans and Hispanics, have lower socioeconomic status compared with Asian Americans and Whites. This set of well-known relationships has led some to speculate that racial/ethnic differences in health status are really manifestations of racial/ethnic differences in socioeconomic status; that is, African Americans and Hispanics have worse health status than Asian Americans and Whites because on average they have lower socioeconomic status. However, although the available evidence does demonstrate that racial/ethnic disparities in health status are caused to some extent by socioeconomic status, it is not the case that socioeconomic status differences among racial/ethnic groups account for racial/ethnic differences in health outcomes. When the health of individuals from

FIGURE 8.5.   INCOME INEQUALITY IN 1999 VERSUS ALL-CAUSE AGE-ADJUSTED (2000 STANDARD) MORTALITY IN 1999.

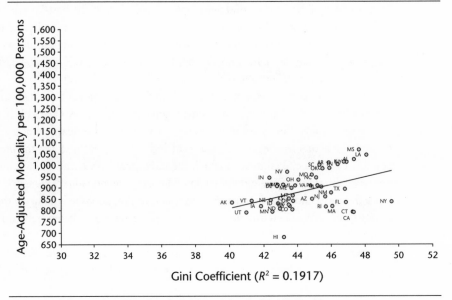

Source: Dr. John Lynch, University of Michigan School of Public Health.

various racial/ethnic groups with similar socioeconomic status is compared, we still find racial/ethnic differences in health for many health outcomes.

Figure 8.6 displays the percentage of people reporting that they have fair or poor health by income levels and race/ethnicity. The figure shows that in each racial/ethnic group there is a gradient relationship between income and health. As income increases the percentage of people reporting fair or poor health decreases. However, the figure also shows that at each level of income African Americans are more likely to report fair or poor health compared with Whites and Hispanics. Also, Hispanics are more likely than Whites to report their health as fair or poor.

This pattern can also be seen with blood lead levels. Figure 8.7 shows the percentage of men aged eighteen years or older with elevated blood lead levels among Whites, African Americans, and Mexican Americans. The figure shows that at each level of income African Americans have the highest percentage of men with elevated blood lead. The pattern comparing Whites and Mexican Americans is not as consistent as the pattern for African Americans; however, it is clear that higher rates of low socioeconomic status among African Americans do not account for racial/ethnic differences.

FIGURE 8.6.   FAIR OR POOR HEALTH AMONG ADULTS 18 YEARS OF AGE AND OVER.

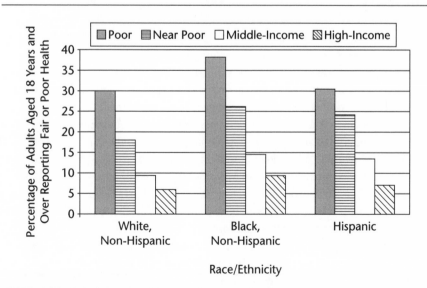

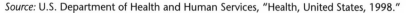

Source: U.S. Department of Health and Human Services, "Health, United States, 1998."

FIGURE 8.7.   ELEVATED BLOOD LEAD AMONG MEN 18 YEARS OF AGE AND OVER.

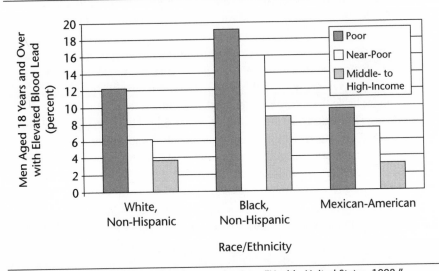

Source: U.S. Department of Health and Human Services, "Health, United States, 1998."

Summary

- Although the terms *socioeconomic status* and *social class* are often used interchangeably, each concept has a distinct definition.
- Socioeconomic status has proved to be a consistent predictor of health status. Persons with low socioeconomic status generally have worse health outcomes than persons that do not have low social economic status.
- Socioeconomic status is best measured by a combination of variables such as income, education, and occupational prestige. Studies that use only one variable as a measure of socioeconomic status run the risk of inadequately measuring socioeconomic status and may result in biased findings.
- There are several dimensions to the relationship between socioeconomic status and health. These dimensions include the social gradient, social mobility, social causation and social drift, social context, and income inequality.
- Although there are substantial differences in socioeconomic status by race/ethnicity, it is not the case that racial/ethnic differences in health status are merely the results of differences in socioeconomic status. (See Appendix B for additional readings.)

Key Words

Social class

Socioeconomic status

Income

Poverty

Poverty threshold

Occupational prestige

Wealth

Net worth

Social causation theory

Social selection theory (social drift)

Socioeconomic context

Income inequality

CHAPTER NINE

BEHAVIOR AND HEALTH

Outline

Introduction

In this chapter we will examine the role of behavior in preventing disease and contributing to illness. According to Last (1988), health behavior is "the combination of knowledge, practices, and attitudes that together motivate the actions we take regarding health." These actions can be either positive or negative, so we divide health behavior into two general categories: *risk behavior,* which can increase the risk of negative health outcomes, and *prevention behavior,* which can help prevent negative health outcomes. An additional concept related to health behavior is *illness behavior.* However, as we will see, illness behavior is to be distinguished from health behavior.

Risk Behavior

Risk behavior refers to actions individuals engage in that can *increase* the likelihood of developing a disease or sustaining an injury or disability at some time in the future. The most prevalent risk behaviors include failing to maintain a healthy weight, smoking cigarettes, abusing alcohol or other drugs, and driving recklessly.

Prevention Behavior

As the name implies, prevention behavior refers to actions individuals take to *reduce* the likelihood of developing a disease or sustaining an injury or disability. Health prevention is commonly classified into three categories: primary prevention, secondary prevention, and tertiary prevention. This classifies prevention activities based on the point along the disease continuum at which the activity occurs.

Primary prevention behavior reduces risk before the onset of disease. Exercising regularly to maintain a healthy body weight can be considered primary prevention behavior designed to prevent heart disease.

Secondary prevention behavior shortens the duration of disease. Getting regular blood pressure checks can be considered a secondary prevention behavior as this will help in early detection of hypertension, allowing for immediate treatment.

Tertiary prevention reduces potential complications of the disease and/or limits its progression to more serious conditions. If a person who has already been diagnosed with hypertension modifies the sodium in his or her diet, this can be considered tertiary prevention behavior. It is important to note that the three levels of prevention sometimes overlap. "For example, regular hypertension screening is considered secondary prevention behavior; however, identification of hypertension in an individual may motivate that person to increase physical activity, resulting in primary prevention benefits" (Brownson & Bal, 1996).

Illness Behavior

As was stated earlier, illness behavior must be distinguished from health behavior. Health behavior consists of actions that either prevent illness or make it more likely; illness behavior consists of actions that either promote or impede recovery from illness. Last (1988) defines illness behavior as "the conduct of persons in response to abnormal body signals. Such behavior influences the manner in which a person monitors

	BOX 9.1. PREVENTION BEHAVIOR.		
	Primary Prevention	**Secondary Prevention**	**Tertiary Prevention**
Smoking prevention program for teens	X		
School-based strategies to promote good nutrition and a healthy lifestyle	X		
Program of regular exercise to manage weight and prevent heart disease	X		
Starting a program of regular exercise to manage weight after you've had heart disease		X	
Liver transplant			X
Participating in Alcoholics Anonymous			X
Treating HIV with medication to prevent symptoms of AIDS		X	

Source: Paulina López.

his body, defines and interprets her symptoms, takes remedial actions, and uses the healthcare system." Thus, illness behaviors are actions taken in response to ill health.

Prevention Behavior and Risk Behavior

Let us examine racial/ethnic issues as they relate to prevention and health risk behavior.

Physical Inactivity

Vigorous physical activity is a health behavior well documented to aid in the prevention of disease. Even moderate-intensity physical activity, such as brisk walking, is associated with a variety of health benefits (Powell, Thompson, Caspersen, & Kendrick,

1987; U.S. Department of Health and Human Services, 1996; Pate et al., 1995). The benefits of physical activity include reduced morbidity and mortality associated with coronary heart disease; control of blood pressure, glucose levels, and cholesterol; and improved weight management. In contrast to the clear health benefits of physical activity, there are clear health risks associated with inactivity. Lack of physical activity is associated with musculoskeletal problems that can negatively affect functional ability, including loss of muscle mass (sarcopenia) and bone loss and osteoporosis (Wagner, LaCroix, Buchner, & Larson, 1992). The benefits of exercise are well known, yet less than 30 percent of the U.S. population engages in regular exercise (Jones et al., 1998; Yusuf et al., 1996).

Table 9.1 presents data on physical inactivity by race and gender from the CDC's Behavioral Risk Factor Surveillance System (BRFSS). The table shows that women are more likely to be inactive than are men. This pattern is consistent for all racial/ethnic groups. Black men have the highest percentage of inactivity among men, followed closely by Hispanic men. Black women have the highest percentage of inactivity among all groups.

Although the reasons for racial differences in physical activity are not clearly understood, researchers are increasingly moving away from the position that it is simply a lifestyle choice; they are beginning to think that differences in physical activity are caused by social and community factors that limit the range of lifestyle choices available to minorities. For example, minorities are more likely to live in communities that offer limited recreational opportunities and have higher rates of crime, thus creating disincentives for people to spend time outdoors (Kumanyika, 2002).

Nutrition

Since 1991, the U.S. Department of Health and Human Services has managed a national health educational program called 5 A Day. The 5 A Day program advocates that people eat five or more servings of fruits and vegetables daily. Diets rich in fruits

TABLE 9.1. PERCENTAGE OF ADULTS AGED 18 YEARS AND OVER REPORTING NO PARTICIPATION IN LEISURE-TIME PHYSICAL ACTIVITY, BY RACE/ETHNICITY AND SEX, 1992.

Race/Ethnicity	Male	Female
White	25.3	28.2
Black	33.1	42.7
Hispanic	30.2	39.0

Source: U.S. Department of Health and Human Services, 1996, p. 190.

and vegetables, which contain essential nutrients and vitamins, have been associated with a reduction in cardiovascular disease and some cancers (Gazino, Manson, Buring, & Hennekens, 1992; Block, Patterson, & Subar, 1992; Steinmetz, Potter, & Folsom, 1993). Fruits and vegetables are also associated with benefits to the gastrointestinal tract (Schaefer & Cheskin, 1998).

The Behavioral Risk Factor Surveillance System (BRFSS) is an annual national telephone survey conducted by the National Center for Chronic Disease Prevention and Health Promotion, a unit of the CDC. The BRFSS survey tracks health risks (specifically health behaviors) in the United States. The survey asks about diet, exercise, smoking, and other health behaviors. Table 9.2 displays the results from the 2002 BRFSS questions related to the 5 A Day program goals. The BRFSS found that there is relatively little variation among the various racial/ethnic groups in the percent of persons who consume the daily recommended amount of fruit and vegetables. For each group, a minority percentage eat five or more servings.

Overweight and Obesity

Over the past half century, rates of obesity have been increasing in the United States. Obesity has become widely regarded as a pandemic (a major worldwide outbreak) with no apparent end in sight (World Health Organization, 2000). As Figure 9.1 shows, the proportion of Americans who are overweight or obese has exploded, from about 50 percent in 1960 through 1962 to over two thirds in 1999 and 2000. Although not specifically a health behavior, obesity is the consequence of two of the most important health

TABLE 9.2. AVERAGE DAILY CONSUMPTION OF FRUIT AND VEGETABLES, BY RACE/ETHNICITY, 2002.

Race	*Median Percentage*			
	Zero to Less Than Once a Day	**One to Less Than Three Times a Day**	**Three to Less Than Five Times a Day**	**Five or More Times a Day**
White	4.0	34.8	37.9	23.4
Black	6.3	38.6	32.6	21.4
Hispanic	6.5	37.1	32.8	22.9
Other	4.2	32.1	34.3	29.1
Multiracial	2.8	33.3	32.7	25.3

Note: Respondents surveyed in all fifty states and the District of Columbia, Guam, Puerto Rico, and the U.S. Virgin Islands.

Source: Centers for Disease Control and Prevention, 2002b.

behaviors, diet and exercise—or more specifically, the consequence of consuming a high-calorie diet and being physically inactive. Obesity is the second largest behavior-related cause of death, and it is rapidly catching up with smoking, the number one behavior-related cause of death.

Obesity and overweight are typically measured by the body mass index (BMI), a ratio of a person's height to their weight. BMI equals a person's weight in kilograms divided by the person's height in meters squared ($BMI = kg/m^2$). Box 9.3 shows weight status for each level of BMI. A BMI between 18.5 and 25 is considered a healthy weight, a BMI of 25 to 30 is considered overweight, and a BMI above 30 is considered obese.

FIGURE 9.1.   OVERWEIGHT, OBESITY, AND HEALTHY WEIGHT AMONG PERSONS AGED 20–74 IN THE UNITED STATES, 1960–2000.

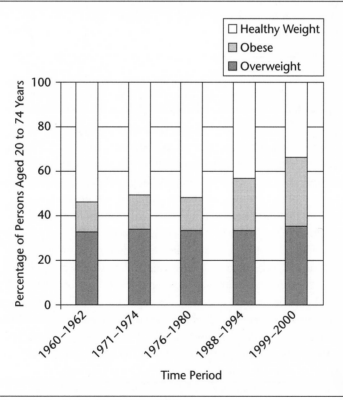

Source: National Center for Health Statistics, 2003.

BOX 9.2.   CALCULATING BODY MASS INDEX (BMI).

BMI can be converted to pounds by using the following formula:

$$BMI = \left[\frac{\text{weight in pounds}}{(\text{height in inches}) \times (\text{height in inches})} \right] \times 703$$

BOX 9.3.   LEVELS OF OBESITY.

BMI	Weight Status
Below 18.5	Underweight
18.5–24.9	Normal
25.0–29.9	Overweight
30.0–39.9	Obese
40.0 or more	Morbidly obese (clinically severe obesity)

Obesity is a major risk factor for a wide range of conditions, including many of the leading causes of death. Obesity is a risk factor for diabetes, cardiovascular disease, cancer, pulmonary diseases, osteoarthritis, hypertension, stroke, and many other diseases. Obesity and its related conditions are associated with a high burden of morbidity, mortality, disability, and rising health care costs. Obesity is also a significant complicating factor in many medical and surgical interventions for other diseases. Although obesity is associated with a great many negative health outcomes, the good news is that the converse is also true. A 10-kilogram reduction in body weight (about 22 pounds) can result in a substantial reduction of disease risk (Jung, 1997).

Figure 9.2 demonstrates that although rates of obesity and overweight are high among all groups, there are substantial differences by race/ethnicity. Of Black women ages 20 to 74, 77.7 percent are either overweight or obese, with 50.4 percent having a BMI greater than 30 (meaning they are obese). Of Mexican American males, 74.4 percent are overweight or obese. Mexican American women are slightly lower, with a combined overweight/obesity rate of 71.8 percent. The lowest rate of overweight and obesity was that of White women. Twenty-six percent of White women are overweight. Among males, Black men have the lowest rate of obesity at 28.9 percent with Mexican American men slightly higher (29.4 percent).

Data for Native Americans were not available from official U.S. government sources; however, other studies have examined obesity among Native Americans. For

BOX 9.4. HEALTH BENEFITS OF LOSING 10 KG (22 LB) OF WEIGHT.

Mortality	20%–25% decrease in total mortality
	30%–40% decrease in diabetes-related deaths
	40%–50% decrease in obesity-related cancer deaths
Blood pressure	Decrease of 20 mmHg systolic pressure
	Decrease of 20 mmHg diastolic pressure
Angina	91% reduction in symptoms
	33% increase in exercise tolerance
Lipids	10% decrease in total cholesterol
	15% decrease in LDL cholesterol
	30% decrease in triglycerides
	8% increase in HDL cholesterol
Diabetes	> 50% reduction in the risk of developing diabetes
	30%–50% decrease in fasting blood glucose
	15% decrease in HbA1c

Source: Jung, 1997.

BOX 9.5. ANOTHER MEASURE OF OBESITY: WAIST-TO-HIP RATIO.

Waist-to-hip ratio: Measure of the ratio of hip circumference to waist circumference. A ratio of 1.0 or higher is considered "at risk" for undesirable health consequences. For men, a ratio of 0.90 or less is considered ideal. For women, a ratio of 0.80 or less is considered ideal.

example, a survey of twenty- to seventy-year-old Pima Indians found that obesity/overweight ranged from 31 percent to 78 percent in men and from 60 percent to 87 percent among women (Broussard et al., 1991). And a survey of Navajo adults twenty to ninety-eight years old found that 30 percent of men and 50 percent of women were obese or overweight (Hall et al., 1992).

The reasons for racial/ethnic differences in obesity and overweight are not well understood. Although some have called for obesity to be considered a biomedical condition, most obesity researchers believe it to be a cultural issue. The cultural aspects of overweight and obesity relate to differences in standards of beauty and perceptions

FIGURE 9.2. OVERWEIGHT, OBESITY, AND HEALTHY WEIGHT AMONG PERSONS AGED 20–74, BY RACE/ETHNICITY, 1999–2000.

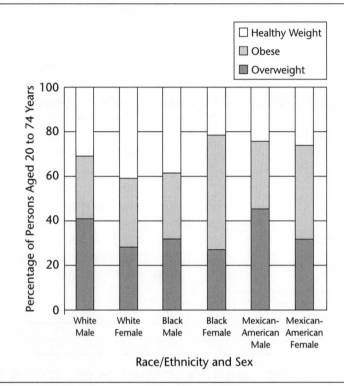

Note: Rates are age-adjusted.

Source: National Center for Health Statistics, 2003, tab. 68.

of fecundity for females, and perceptions of strength, wealth, and physical prowess for males (Kumanyika, 2002). An additional possible explanation is socioeconomic status (SES). There is a well-established relationship between SES and obesity (Drewnowski & Speter, 2004). SES and obesity have an inverse relationship, so that persons with higher SES (usually defined in terms of education and income; see Chapter Eight) have lower rates of obesity compared with persons with lower socioeconomic status. This is particularly the case among women in developed societies. The SES-obesity relationship for men is not as strong (Sobal & Stunkard, 1989). It may seem counterintuitive that less affluent persons would be more likely to be obese compared with more affluent persons, but most public health researchers conclude that the SES-obesity relationship reflects the lack of access to healthy foods, safe exercise locations, and sound nutritional knowledge among lower SES individuals (Jeffery & French, 1996).

Smoking

According to the U.S. surgeon general, cigarette smoking is currently the number one behavior-related cause of disease and death in the United States (U.S. Department of Health and Human Services, 1998). (Note, however, that the rate of overweight and obesity is increasing and may soon overtake cigarette smoking as the leading behavior-related cause of death.) This statement is true for all racial and ethnic groups in the United States. Blacks have the greatest health burden of cigarette smoking, and differences in rates of smoking-related disease among racial/ethnic minorities are directly related to racial/ethnic differences in smoking patterns (see Table 9.3).

Smoking-related diseases include cancer (especially lung cancer), coronary heart disease, stroke, and respiratory diseases such as bronchitis, emphysema, and other chronic airway obstruction diseases. Cancer is the most common smoking-related disease. Although lung cancer incidence and death rates vary widely among minorities, lung cancer is the leading cause of cancer death for all racial/ethnic minority groups. And though lung cancer is by far the most common smoking-related condition, other cancers are also quite prevalent among smokers; for example, cancer of the lip, esophagus, pancreas, stomach, and larynx.

When examining the pattern of cigarette smoking by race/ethnicity and age, we find a quite interesting phenomenon. The pattern is outlined in Figures 9.3 and 9.4. Figure 9.3 shows that Black and Hispanic male teens and young adults are far less likely to smoke cigarettes compared with White teens and young adults. However, as they enter middle age this pattern changes. White male cigarette smoking rates reach their peak during the teen and young adult years and decline with age. In contrast, smoking rates among Black males are relatively low in the teen and young adult years, but increase with age so that by the thirty-five to forty-four age period, the Black male smoking rate exceeds the White male rate.

TABLE 9.3.   CURRENT CIGARETTE SMOKING BY ADULTS ACCORDING TO SEX, 1999–2001.

Race/Ethnic Group	Male	Female	Male-to-Female Rate Ratio
Total	25.1	21.2	1.18
White	25.6	22.3	1.15
Black	27.3	19.7	1.39
American Indian/Alaska Native	30.4	34.7	0.88
Asian	20.3	6.7	3.03
Hispanic	22.3	12.1	1.84

Source: National Center for Health Statistics, 2003, tab. 61.

FIGURE 9.3. SMOKING PREVALENCE AND RACE/ETHNICITY AMONG U.S. MEN, 1999–2001.

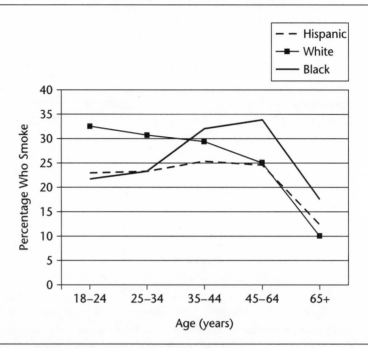

*Source:*National Center for Health Statistics, 2003, tab. 61.

For Hispanic males the rate of increase in cigarette smoking has been more gradual than for Black males. The Hispanic rate does not rise to equal the White male rate until the forty-five to sixty-four age group. Above age sixty-five smoking rates for all groups decline rapidly, probably for several reasons. For example, we know there are much higher death rates among smokers compared with nonsmokers. As such, some smokers die before reaching age sixty-five. It is also likely that as people develop chronic conditions in late middle age, they quit smoking as part of their treatment (as a secondary prevention).

Alcohol Use and Abuse

The use and abuse of alcohol continues to be a public health concern, although during the last quarter of the twentieth century there was a downward trend in the proportion of Americans who drink alcohol. Health consequences of alcohol use and abuse are substantial. They include increased risk for cardiovascular disease, cirrhosis of the liver, and death and injury due to alcohol-related motor vehicle accidents.

**FIGURE 9.4.   SMOKING PREVALENCE AND RACE/ETHNICITY
AMONG U.S. WOMEN, 1999–2001.**

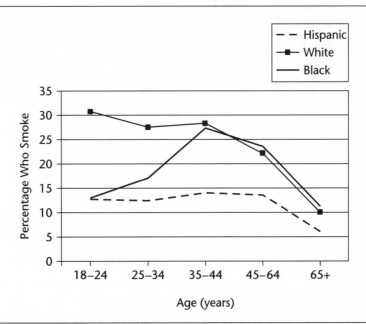

Source: National Center for Health Statistics, 2003, tab. 61.

Additional negative consequences of alcohol abuse include degradation of social networks, family conflict, threat to employment, and financial strain.

The pattern of alcohol use and abuse has been fairly consistent: men have higher rates of alcohol use and heavy drinking compared to women. Although the gap between men and women varies by race and age, the general pattern of higher rates of alcohol use and abuse among males is consistent (Dawson, Grant, Chou, & Pickering, 1995; Jones-Webb, Snowden, Herd, Short, & Hannan, 1997).

The pattern of alcohol use over the life course tends to be an inverted U-shaped curve. The lowest rates of use tend to be among persons under age eighteen. The rate gradually increases until it peaks in the twenty-five to forty-four age group and then declines rapidly after age fifty (Anthony & Echeagaray-Wagner, 2000; Dawson et al., 1995).

Empirical findings on rates of usage among racial/ethnic groups consistently show that Whites have higher rates of alcohol utilization across all age levels. However, problem drinking and alcohol-related consequences are more prevalent among African Americans, despite lower rates of use (National Institute on Drug Abuse, 1995; Bachman et al., 1991; Amey, Albrecht, & Miller, 1996; Wallace et al., 2002).

Figure 9.5 shows patterns of alcohol consumption among persons aged eighteen and above. The figure shows that Whites have the highest percentage of current drinkers—more than twenty percentage points greater than every other racial/ethnic group. However, although Whites have the highest rate of current drinkers, they are not the group with the highest consumption. For example, nearly 28 percent of American Indians/Alaska Natives reported that they had more than five drinks the last time they consumed alcohol. The next highest percentage is for Whites, with a rate of 21.3 percent, followed by Hispanics, with a rate of 17.9 percent. Blacks and Asians had rates of 12.5 percent and 12.9 percent, respectively.

Although Black rates of alcohol consumption are among the lowest, deaths related to alcohol abuse have been highest for Blacks. However, the trends over the latter half of the twentieth century illustrate a substantial decline in serious health consequences of long-term alcohol use, such as cirrhosis of the liver. As Figure 9.6 shows, although the mortality rate from liver cirrhosis for Black males was nearly double the rate for White males in 1970, by 2000 the gap had been eliminated (Yoon, Yi,

FIGURE 9.5.   ALCOHOL CONSUMPTION AMONG PERSONS AGED 18 YEARS AND OVER, BY RACE/ETHNICITY, 2001.

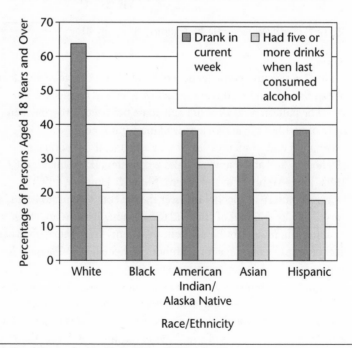

Source: National Center for Health Statistics, 2003, tab. 65.

Grant, Stinson, & Dufour, 2003). The rate for Hispanic males, however, remains more than double the rate for Black and White males. Because minority populations are so heterogeneous, generalizations about their patterns of abuse can be misleading. For example, these data do not distinguish between rates of alcohol consumption among different American Indian tribes or different Hispanic groups.

The prevalence of alcohol use and abuse among Native Americans is highly variable among different American Indian communities. In communities with high rates of alcoholism, an estimated 75 percent of all injuries—a leading cause of death among American Indians—are alcohol related. According to the Indian Health Service, the age-adjusted alcohol-related death rate in 1992 was 5.6 times higher than for the general population, with the peak ages for death between forty-five and sixty-four.

FIGURE 9.6. AGE-ADJUSTED DEATH RATES FROM ALCOHOL-RELATED LIVER CIRRHOSIS, 1970–2000.

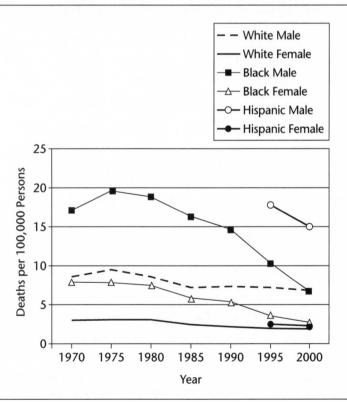

Source: National Center for Health Statistics, 2003.

Because Asian Americans and Pacific Islanders encompass many ethnic groups with distinctive cultural norms, heritage, and language, it is not surprising that drinking behaviors vary widely among Asian American subgroups. Japanese Americans, for example, have significantly higher rates for both alcohol use and heavy drinking than Chinese Americans, a phenomenon frequently attributed to genetic and physiological factors as well as sociocultural values pertaining to alcohol use. In contrast, the reported prevalence of binge drinking for Native Hawaiians is 20 percent compared with 15 percent for the state population as a whole. Binge drinking is defined as at least five drinks per occasion in a given month. According to the Hawaii Department of Health (2004), the percentage of adults in Hawaii reported to be chronic drinkers (at least sixty drinks in a given month) ranged from 5 to 6 percent compared with the national prevalence of 3 percent.

Illicit Drug Use

Many people believe that illicit drug use is more prevalent among African Americans and Hispanics. However, this popular belief is incorrect. According to the National Household Survey data, rates for the use of illicit drugs are highest among American Indians, followed by Whites and Hispanics. Blacks and Asian Americans (when combining all Asian subgroups) have the lowest drug utilization rates. (See Figure 9.7 and Table 9.4.) However, although substance abuse is a problem in all American racial/ethnic groups, it is true that the health and social consequences of illicit drug use (HIV/AIDS, lack of treatment access, emergency room visits, and death) seem to fall disproportionately on racial/ethnic minorities, especially African Americans.

According to the National Household Survey on Drug Abuse (NHSDA), in 1999 and 2000 an estimated 6.4 percent of Whites had recently used illegal drugs (use in the past month). The corresponding estimates for African Americans and Hispanic Americans are virtually indistinguishable from the White rate. The only Hispanic subgroup with a rate that was substantially higher than the White rate was Puerto Ricans, with a one-month illicit drug use rate of 9.2. Other than Puerto Ricans, the one-month illegal drug use prevalence rates for Hispanic subgroups are no different than the rate for Whites, and in some cases the Hispanic rate is lower.

Another noteworthy observation from Figure 9.7 is the high one-month prevalence estimate (11.2 percent) for American Indians/Alaska Natives compared with other subgroups. This is the only group with a one-month utilization rate greater than 10 percent. American Indian/Alaska Natives also have the highest lifetime use rate (54 percent). Their lifetime use rate is nearly ten percentage points higher than that of the second highest group (Whites) and more than four times the rate for the group with the lowest lifetime use rate (Asian Indians).

FIGURE 9.7. PERCENTAGES OF PERSONS AGED 12 YEARS AND OLDER REPORTING LIFETIME, PAST-YEAR, AND PAST-MONTH ILLICIT DRUG USE, 2000–2001.

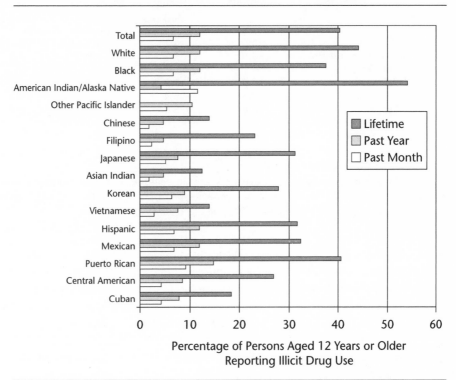

Percentage of Persons Aged 12 Years or Older Reporting Illicit Drug Use

Sources: Substance Abuse and Mental Health Services Administration, 2000, 2001.

Finally, there is noteworthy variation in illicit drug use among the Asian subgroups. In general, Asian Americans have the lowest rates of illicit drug use. Only one Asian American subgroup (Japanese Americans) has a lifetime rate greater than 30 percent, and no Asian American subgroup has a one-year use rate greater than 10 percent. However, this generalization does not hold true for Korean Americans, whose one-month illicit drug use rate is 5.0 percent.

Use of Preventive Medical Services

People often think of influenza as a mere nuisance, and for most people it is. However, the flu is also a major cause of morbidity and mortality. Influenza accounts for about 36,000 annual deaths in the United States. Pneumococcal disease (pneumonia)

TABLE 9.4.   CONSUMPTION OF ALCOHOL AND OTHER DRUGS AMONG PERSONS AGED 12 AND OLDER, BY RACE/ETHNICITY, 2001.

Race/Ethnicity	Alcohol[a]	Heavy Alcohol Use[b]	Marijuana[a]	Illicit Drugs[c]
Black	34.3	4.1	5.6	7.4
American Indian/ Alaska Native	33.9	7.1	8.0	9.9
Asian	30.7	1.5	1.7	2.8
White	50.3	6.4	5.6	7.2
Hispanic	38.6	4.4	4.2	6.4

[a]Use within the past thirty days.

[b]Heavy use is defined as drinking five or more drinks on the same occasion on each of five or more days in the past thirty days.

[c]Any illicit drug including: marijuana, cocaine (including crack), heroin, hallucinogens (including LSD and PCP), inhalants, or any prescription-type psychotherapeutic drugs used nonmedically.

Source: National Center for Health Statistics, 2003, tab. 62.

accounts for an additional 50,000 deaths annually (Egede et al., 2003). The economic impact of these diseases includes unnecessary hospitalizations and lost productivity at work. The influenza and pneumococcal vaccines are efficacious and cost-effective tools for preventing these diseases and decreasing the severity of symptoms. The Advisory Committee on Immunization Practices of the CDC recommends a yearly influenza inoculation for all adults aged sixty-five and older (Bridges et al., 2000). Americans in this age group are, with few exceptions, eligible for Medicare, which offers the vaccine at no cost to the patient.

Racial/ethnic disparities in utilization of immunizations have been well documented (Egede and Zheng, 2003; Marin, Johanson, & Salas-Lopez, 2002), as have disparities in use of childhood immunizations (Ehresmann et al., 1998; Flynn-Saldana, Kirsch, & Lister, 2003). Figure 9.8 displays racial/ethnic differences in utilization of the influenza and pneumococcal vaccination. The figure shows that Whites have the highest influenza vaccine utilization rate, followed by Asian Americans. African Americans have the lowest rate, at less than 50 percent. The White pneumococcal vaccine utilization rate of nearly 60 percent is more than a third higher than the ethnic group with the second highest rate (Asian Americans), and the White rate is nearly double the rate of the ethnic group with the lowest utilization rate (Hispanics).

Mammography (a screening procedure designed to detect breast cancer) and the Pap smear (a screening procedure for cervical cancer) are other health prevention behaviors with documented racial/ethnic disparities in use (Coughlin, Uhler, Bobo, & Caplan, 2004; Pearlman, Rakowski, Ehrich, & Clark, 1996; Ganesan et al., 2003;

FIGURE 9.8.   INFLUENZA AND PNEUMOCOCCAL VACCINATION
AMONG ADULTS AGED 65 YEARS AND OLDER, BY
RACE/ETHNICITY, 1999–2001.

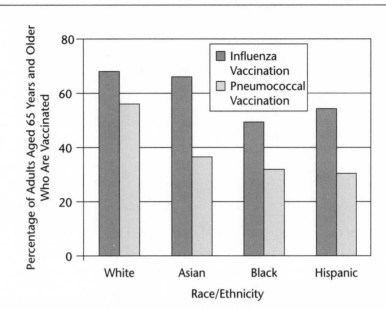

Source: National Center for Health Statistics, 2003, fig. 11.

Martin, Calle, Wingo, & Heath, 1996). Figures 9.9 and 9.10 show rates of utilization
of mammography and Pap smear by race/ethnicity. The figures show some racial/
ethnic variation in the use of the screening procedures among women under age sixty-
five; however, for women above age sixty-five there is essentially no difference in the
pattern of use of the procedures.

Illness Behavior

Illness behavior differs from prevention and risk behavior in that illness behavior deals
with the actions of individuals after they have developed symptoms of disease. Prevention and risk behavior refer to behaviors that cause or prevent disease. Illness behavior is perhaps the facet of health behavior that has received the least amount of
attention from researchers. Most research on illness behavior has focused on delay in
seeking care.

FIGURE 9.9.   PERCENTAGE OF WOMEN AGED 40 YEARS AND OVER WHO HAD A MAMMOGRAM WITHIN THE PAST TWO YEARS, 2000.

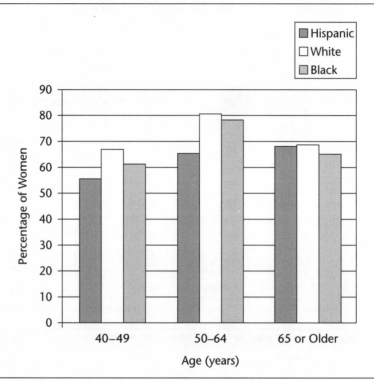

Source: National Center for Health Statistics, 2003, tab. 80.

Studies of racial/ethnic differences in treatment-seeking delay have found that racial/ethnic minorities are more likely to delay seeking care compared with Whites (Dracup & Moser, 1991). A study of racial/ethnic differences in delay in care-seeking among patients experiencing an acute myocardial infarction (heart attack) found that the total mean delay time differed significantly between Blacks and Whites: 16 hours versus 8.8 hours (Lee, Bahler, Chung, Alonzo, & Zeller, 2000). Another study examined care-seeking delay among a larger set of cardiac patients from a more diverse set of racial/ethnic groups and found that Hispanics delayed an average of 41.5 hours (median 9.2 hours), African Americans delayed an average of 30.8 hours (median 3.5 hours), Asian Americans delayed an average of 92 hours (median 12 hours), and Whites delayed an average of 31.6 hours (median 3.2 hours) (see Figure 9.11).

There is no consensus explanation for racial/ethnic differences in illness behavior; rather, researchers have proposed several possibilities. One is that certain minorities delay in seeking care because of culturally related differences in the way

FIGURE 9.10.   PERCENTAGE OF WOMEN AGED 18 YEARS AND OVER WHO HAD A PAP SMEAR WITHIN THE PAST THREE YEARS, 2000.

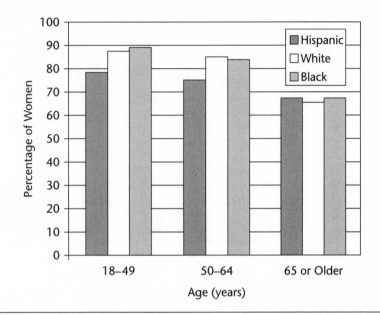

Source: National Center for Health Statistics, 2003, tab. 80.

they assess their symptoms; that is, they may be less likely to perceive their symptoms to be an indication that they need to seek medical care. In one study, patients who came to a hospital emergency room complaining of chest pain were interviewed to determine how symptom recognition and perception influenced their care-seeking (Klingler et al., 2002). The study found that 61 percent of African American patients attributed symptoms to a gastrointestinal source and 11 percent attributed their pain to a cardiac-related problem. The percentages for White patients making similar attributions were 26 percent and 33 percent, respectively. Another study examined patients' perceptions of symptoms and attribution of symptoms in an Alabama-based hospital (Raczynski et al., 1994). This study found that Black patients had a greater tendency to report fewer painful symptoms and to attribute their symptoms to noncardiac origins.

Fatalism, stigma, racism, and mistrust of hospitals have also been proposed as explanations for racial/ethnic differences in illness behavior. A small study of African Americans with type 2 diabetes found that fatalism was associated with the patient's ability to successfully carry out diabetes self-management (Egede & Bonadonna, 2003). In contrast, a study conducted by Mayo, Ureda, and Parker (2001) found that patients

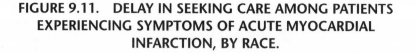

FIGURE 9.11. DELAY IN SEEKING CARE AMONG PATIENTS EXPERIENCING SYMPTOMS OF ACUTE MYOCARDIAL INFARCTION, BY RACE.

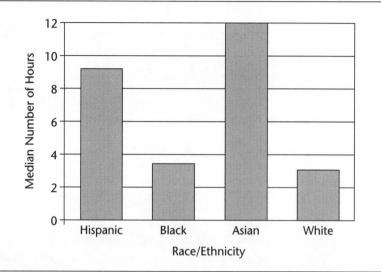

Source: Henderson, Magana, Korn, Genna, & Bretsky, 2002.

who were more fatalistic were more likely to be noncompliant with mammography screening.

The stigma associated with certain diseases has also been shown to impede the willingness of some patients to seek care. The role of stigma affecting the care process is significant. Patients often delay or fail to obtain care because of stigma, and in some cases delay can be life-threatening. The pervasiveness of the stigma associated with certain diseases is illustrated in Figure 9.12. The figure was produced based on a study by Herek, Capitanio, and Wildman (2002). The study examined the prevalence of HIV/AIDS stigma and misinformation and HIV in a national telephone survey. The study found that although the percentage of Americans who felt that AIDS patients should be quarantined has declined greatly, the proportion who felt that HIV patients "got what they deserve" had actually increased between 1991 and 1999. Among the most stigmatized conditions are schizophrenia (Ertugrul & Ulug, 2004; Hudson et al., 2004), depression (Halter, 2004), HIV/AIDS and other sexual-related diseases (de Bruyn, 2002; Clark, Lindner, Armistead, & Austin, 2003; Chng, Wong, Park, Edberg, & Lai, 2003), and substance abuse (Antai-Otong, 2002).

Patients' perception of racism and their mistrust of health care have also been shown to vary among persons of different racial/ethnic groups (LaVeist, Nickerson, & Bowie, 2000). A study of attitudes among cardiac patients asked patients to com-

FIGURE 9.12.   ATTITUDES TOWARD PATIENTS WITH HIV/AIDS, 1991–1999.

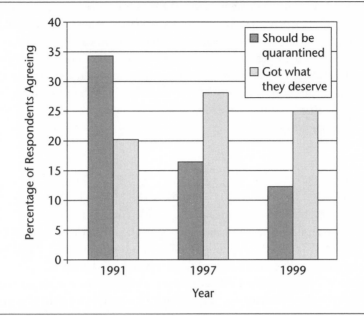

Source: Herek, Capitanio, and Wildman, 2002, p. 372.

plete a questionnaire that included a series of questions related to racism and mistrust. Patients were read four statements regarding racism in the health care system and asked to indicate their agreement using a four-point scale (strongly disagree, disagree, agree, strongly agree). Table 6.3 in Chapter Six displays race comparisons of the percentage of respondents who indicated that they strongly agree or agree. It shows a consistent racial disparity in reports of racism. Although about 67 percent of African American patients agreed or strongly agreed that "doctors treat African American and White people the same," nearly 87 percent of White patients felt that way. Thirty percent of African American patients endorsed the statement, "racial discrimination in the doctor's office is common," while only 7.3 percent of White patients endorsed that statement. Black patients were about 85 percent as likely as White patients to agree or strongly agree that African Americans and Whites received the same kind of care in hospitals. And although 88.1 percent of White patients agreed or strongly agreed that "African Americans can receive the care they want as equally as White people can," only 61.2 percent of Black patients felt that way.

Patients' attitudes of mistrust of the health care system are recorded in Table 6.2 in Chapter Six. Patients were asked to react to three statements regarding mistrust of the health care system on a four point scale (strongly disagree, disagree, agree, or strongly agree). The table reports responses of agree and strongly agree combined. When read the statement "patients have sometimes been deceived or misled at hospitals," 51.4 percent of Black patients agreed or strongly agreed compared to 42.4 percent of White patients. Nearly 40 percent of African American patients compared with about 25 percent of White patients felt that hospitals often wanted to know more about patients' personal affairs than they really needed to know. And African American patients were nearly twice as likely as White patients to agree or strongly agree that "hospitals have sometimes done harmful experiments on patients without their knowledge."

Summary

This chapter examined racial/ethnic difference in health behavior. Health behavior has several related subcomponents: prevention behavior, risk behavior, and illness behavior. Racial/ethnic differences in each subcomponent were discussed and possible reasons for these differences were outlined. The chapter discussed racial/ethnic differences in prevention behaviors, such as physical inactivity, nutrition, obesity, smoking, alcohol consumption, illicit drug use, and the utilization of preventive medicine. The chapter also outlined racial/ethnic differences in illness behaviors, such as delays in seeking care, and discussed some reasons for racial/ethnic differences in seeking healthcare. (See Appendix B for additional readings.)

Key Words

Risk behavior

Prevention behavior

Illness behavior

Primary prevention

Secondary prevention

Tertiary prevention

Obesity/overweight

Body mass index

PART FOUR

RACIAL/ETHNIC GROUP-SPECIFIC HEALTH ISSUES

CHAPTER TEN

AFRICAN AMERICAN HEALTH ISSUES

Outline

Introduction

This chapter will review major health-related issues faced by the African American population. According to the 2000 census, there are 36.4 million Americans of African descent. African Americans make up 12.9 percent of the U.S. population. In 2003 the U.S. Bureau of the Census announced that the Hispanic/Latino population had surpassed the Black American population, making African Americans the third largest racial/ethnic group in the country. More than one half (53.6 percent) of the African American population lives in the southern region. About 60 percent live in just ten states. The smallest proportions of African Americans (9.6 percent) live in the western states.

Death Rates and Causes of Death Among African Americans

Table 10.1 displays age-specific death rates for African Americans compared with other racial/ethnic groups. The table shows the African American death rate for each age group and the rate ratios for the other racial/ethnic groups compared with African Americans. A rate ratio of 1.0 indicates that African Americans and the comparison group have an equal death rate for the indicated age group. A rate ratio greater than 1.0 indicates that African Americans have a higher death rate than the comparison group (for example, a rate ratio of 1.5 would indicate that the African American death rate is one and one half times greater; 2.0 would indicate that the African American death rate is two times greater). If the rate ratio is less than 1.0, this indicates that African Americans have a lower death rate than the comparison group.

Table 10.1 shows that African Americans have a generally higher death rate compared to all other racial/ethnic groups. The magnitude of the disparity between African Americans and other racial/ethnic groups is substantial, reaching as high as 4.4 times (340 percent higher) than the API death rate for the forty- to forty-four-year-old age group. American Indians/Alaska Natives have comparably high death rates for some of the young age groups.

The largest disparities are found in comparisons with Asians/Pacific Islanders. The disparity between the groups increases into adulthood and reaches it peak in middle age. The disparities then decline gradually into the older ages. The smallest Black-API disparity is 1.5 for the over-eighty-five-year-old age group, indicating that African Americans have a death rate that is one and one half times (50 percent higher than) the Asian/Pacific Islander rate.

Comparing African Americans with Hispanics/Latinos, we find that Black death rates are in excess of two times the Hispanic/Latino rate for the adult ages twenty-five to sixty-nine. The largest disparity between African Americans and Hispanics/Latinos is 2.4, for the forty to forty-four age group. African American death rates for this group are also substantially higher than the rates for Whites. With the exception of three young age groups, the American Indian/Alaska Native death rate is consistently lower than the African American death rate.

It is instructive to note that African American death rates converge with death rates for Whites, and "cross over" around age eighty-five—a phenomenon first noted in Chapter Four. American Indians and Alaska Natives experience a similar crossover compared with Asian/Pacific Islanders and Hispanics/Latinos. These crossovers occur because of a phenomenon called selective survival, also discussed in Chapter Four. Selective survival leads to a crossover in death rates whereby African Americans and

TABLE 10.1. AGE-SPECIFIC DEATH RATES FOR AFRICAN AMERICANS COMPARED WITH OTHER RACIAL/ETHNIC GROUPS, 2001.

Age	African American Death Rate (per 100,000)	Rate Ratios			
		American Indian/ Alaska Native	Asian/Pacific Islander	Hispanic/ Latino	White
1–4	49.5	1.0	2.2	1.6	1.6
4–9	21.4	1.4	1.8	1.6	1.5
10–14	26.6	1.0	2.1	1.6	1.5
15–19	88.7	0.9	2.3	1.4	1.4
20–24	156.7	1.4	3.3	1.8	1.8
25–29	174.9	1.5	4.0	2.2	2.0
30–34	207.1	1.4	4.1	2.3	2.0
35–39	294.6	1.3	4.2	2.3	1.9
40–44	438.1	1.7	4.4	2.4	2.0
45–49	656.8	1.7	4.0	2.3	2.0
50–54	946.1	1.9	3.8	2.3	2.0
55–59	1,351.9	1.9	3.4	2.3	1.8
60–64	1,920.5	1.7	3.1	2.1	1.6
65–69	2,777.9	1.6	2.7	2.0	1.5
70–74	3,951.1	1.6	2.5	1.8	1.4
75–79	5,712.5	1.6	2.1	1.6	1.3
80–84	8,098.0	1.5	1.8	1.5	1.1
85+	14,660.8	1.6	1.5	1.2	1.0

Source: National Center for Health Statistics.

American Indian/Alaska Natives have *lower* death rates than other racial/ethnic groups at old ages (Markides & Machalek, 1984). High death rates among young African Americans reduce the proportion of frail elders, which results in lower death rates among older African Americans.

Table 10.2 displays the ten leading causes of death for African American males. The ten leading causes of death for African American females are listed in Table 10.3. In addition to showing the age-adjusted death rate and the percent of all African American deaths accounted for by each cause of death, the table also shows where that cause of death ranks among the other racial/ethnic groups. Heart disease and cancer are the two leading causes of death for African American men, as is the case for all men.

TABLE 10.2. LEADING CAUSES OF DEATH FOR AFRICAN AMERICAN MALES COMPARED WITH MALES OF OTHER ETHNIC GROUPS, 2001.

Rank for African American Males	Cause of Death	Percentage of Total Deaths	Age-Adjusted Death Rate	Rank for Males in Other Groups			
				American Indians	Asians/ Pacific Islanders	Hispanics/ Latinos	Whites
1	Heart disease	25.4	215.7	1	1	1	1
2	Cancer	22.5	190.8	2	2	2	2
3	Unintentional injury	5.8	49.5	3	4	3	5
4	Stroke	5.4	46.2	7	3	4	4
5	Homicide	4.6	39.3	10	—	5	—
6	HIV/AIDS	3.6	30.8	—	—	10	—
7	Diabetes mellitus	3.5	29.4	5	7	6	6
8	Respiratory disease	2.9	24.5	8	5	9	3
9	Nephritis	2.2	18.6	—	10	—	9
10	Influenza/pneumonia	1.9	16.3	9	6	—	7

Source: National Center for Health Statistics.

TABLE 10.3. LEADING CAUSES OF DEATH FOR AFRICAN AMERICAN FEMALES COMPARED WITH FEMALES OF OTHER ETHNIC GROUPS, 2001.

Rank for African American Females	Cause of Death	Percentage of Total Deaths	Age-Adjusted Death Rate	Rank for Females in Other Groups			
				American Indians	Asians/ Pacific Islanders	Hispanics/ Latinos	Whites
1	Heart disease	28.7	215.4	2	2	1	1
2	Cancer	20.8	156.5	1	1	2	2
3	Stroke	7.8	59.0	5	3	3	3
4	Diabetes mellitus	5.1	38.4	4	4	4	8
5	Nephritis	2.9	21.7	9	8	8	9
6	Unintentional injury	2.7	20.6	3	5	5	7
7	Respiratory disease	2.4	18.0	6	7	7	4
8	Septicemia	2.3	17.2	10	—	—	10
9	Influenza and pneumonia	2.1	15.6	8	6	6	6
10	HIV/AIDS	1.8	13.3	—	—	—	—

Source: National Center for Health Statistics.

BOX 10.1. CHRONIC AND ACUTE CONDITIONS.

Chronic conditions are conditions that are not cured once acquired (such as heart disease and diabetes).

An *acute condition* is a type of illness or injury that ordinarily lasts less than three months.

Together heart disease and cancer account for nearly 48 percent of all deaths in African American men.

Unintended injury (accidents) and stroke are third and fourth on the list in Table 10.2. Although the four leading causes of death for African American men are among the five leading causes of death for men of other racial/ethnic groups as well (with the exception of liver cirrhosis, which is number four for American Indian/Alaska Native men, but not in the leading ten for African Americans), the fifth leading cause of death for African American men (homicide) is among the top five causes only for Hispanic/Latino men. African American men also have a very high death rate from HIV/AIDS. Homicide and AIDS account for more than 8 percent of all deaths among African American males. Each of these issues will be discussed more fully later in this chapter.

The four leading causes of death for African American women are similar to those for women of other racial/ethnic groups: cancer, heart disease, diabetes, and stroke. There is one noteworthy departure from the leading causes of death for other women: the fifth leading cause of death for African American women is nephritis, which is not among the five leading causes of death for any other racial/ethnic group. Most noteworthy is the HIV/AIDS ranking: the tenth leading cause of death among African American women but not on the list for any other racial/ethnic group.

Table 10.4 presents the leading causes of death for African American adults (ages twenty to sixty-five). The leading causes of death for young adults are homicide, unintended injuries (accidents), and suicide. These causes of death are associated with psychosocial factors rather than biological factors. Among these psychosocial factors are violent/aggressive behavior, poverty, risk-taking, and depression. As African Americans progress through the life course, chronic conditions gradually rise to the top positions on the list. Chronic conditions include causes such as heart disease, cancer, diabetes, and stroke. It is also interesting to note the position of HIV/AIDS disease in the table: it is among the ten leading causes of death for African Americans in every age group.

TABLE 10.4. LEADING CAUSES OF DEATH ACROSS THE LIFE SPAN FOR AFRICAN AMERICAN ADULTS, 2001.

	Age Group				
Rank	20–24	25–34	35–44	45–54	55–65
1	Homicide	Homicide	Heart disease	Cancer	Cancer
2	Unintentional injury	Unintentional injury	HIV/AIDS	Heart disease	Heart disease
3	Suicide	HIV/AIDS	Cancer	HIV/AIDS	Stroke
4	Heart disease	Heart disease	Unintentional injury	Unintentional injury	Diabetes
5	Cancer	Cancer	Homicide	Stroke	Nephritis
6	HIV/AIDS	Suicide	Stroke	Diabetes	Unintentional injury
7	Congenital malformations	Diabetes	Diabetes	Chronic liver disease/ cirrhosis	Respiratory disease
8	Respiratory disease	Stroke	Chronic liver disease/ cirrhosis	Homicide	Septicemia
9	Anemia	Respiratory disease	Suicide	Nephritis	HIV/AIDS
10	Diabetes	Anemia	Nephritis	Septicemia	Chronic liver disease/ cirrhosis

Source: National Center for Health Statistics.

Health Care Access and Utilization

The dynamics of the interaction between African American patients and health care providers are not the same as for other racial/ethnic minorities. For APIs, American Indians/Alaska Natives, and Hispanics/Latinos, language is a significant barrier, as is the use of alternative medicines. For African Americans, these two factors are less of a problem. English is the primary language of the African American population, and although religion and spirituality have an important impact on care-seeking among African Americans (Dessio et al., 2004), African Americans have the lowest prevalence of use of complementary and alternative therapies (National Center for Complementary and Alternative Medicine, 2004).

Health care access and utilization issues for African Americans revolve mainly around access to and availability of health care resources (including access to health insurance), differential management of disease and illness, and racial discrimination within medical encounters.

Availability of Health Care Resources

Racial and ethnic differences in access and utilization of health services have been widely studied. Most of those studies have focused on demonstrating differences between Black and White Americans. For example, Shi (1999) showed that African Americans were 1.46 times more likely than Whites to identify their usual source of care as a facility rather than a person. Blendon et al. (1989) found that racial differences in access to care were found across all income groups and demonstrated severe underuse of services among African Americans. And Gregory, Rhoads, Wilson, O'Dowd, and Kostis (1999) found that underutilization of health services was caused, at least in part, by race differences in the medical care resources, such as opioid analgesics (pain medicine), available at the facilities where White and Black American patients receive care (Morrison et al., 2002).

Differential Medical Management of Conditions

Racial differences in the surgical and medical management of heart disease are perhaps the most studied health care situation (Ford & Cooper, 1995; Sheifer et al., 2000). The many studies of this topic have demonstrated that African American patients with similar needs as White patients are about half as likely to receive diagnostic and interventional treatments for heart disease. Although most studies of this type have been conducted on heart patients (Sheifer et al., 2000), similar findings have been demonstrated with other conditions as well. For example, differences in screening or treatment have been found in cancer (McMahon et al., 1999; Mandelblatt et al., 1999), asthma (Ali et al., 1997), participation in AIDS clinical trials (Stone et al., 1997), access to kidney transplantation (Eggers, 1995), access to long-term care (Wallace et al., 1998; Mui & Burnette, 1994), hormone replacement therapy (Marsh et al., 1999), knee replacement surgery (Wilson, May, & Kelly, 1994), and administration of pain medications (Todd, Deaton, D'Adamo, & Goe, 2002).

African Americans often face the prospect of obtaining care in facilities with fewer resources, and when they obtain access to similar facilities they often receive less optimal treatment.

Racial Differences in Patient/Provider Interaction

Several studies have demonstrated that the larger societal dynamics of race interactions play out in cross-cultural encounters in medicine, as they do in other aspects of society. A study by van Ryn and Burke (2002) showed that the race of the patient has an effect on physicians' perceptions of them (see Table 6.4 in Chapter Six). van Ryn and

Burke conducted a survey of physicians to obtain their attitudes toward patients. Their analysis showed that physicians tended to rate African-American patients more negatively than Whites on a number of health-related factors.

As Table 6.4 shows, the physicians held more negative attitudes toward Black patients on every question. Such perceptions may negatively influence the quality and type of care patients receive. And because doctors' attitudes may be perceptible to patients through nonverbal cues or verbal tone or inflection, they may create disincentives for patients to seek care or comply with a medical regimen. In this way, the negative attitudes of physicians may in fact become a self-fulfilling prophecy: (1) the doctor believes the African American patient will not follow through on advice; (2) the patient perceives the attitude and develops distrust for the physician; (3) as a result, the patient does not follow the doctor's advice. Other studies have also demonstrated less desirable treatment (in this case the word *treatment* is not being used to denote medical terminology). Flaherty and Meagher (1980) found that African American schizophrenia patients had shorter hospitalizations, were less likely to receive occupational therapy, were more likely to be placed in seclusion, and were more likely to be subjected to restraints.

Racial disparities have also been documented in doctor-patient communications. Cooper-Patrick et al. (2002) found that in cases in which the doctor and patient were of the same race (race concordant), the doctor tended to promote more patient participation in decision making. Although African Americans rated their medical encounters as less participatory than Whites overall, patients of all races saw their visits as more participatory when they were race concordant with their doctors. Saha, Komaromy, Koepsell, and Bindman (1999) found that African American race concordant patients were more likely to rate their physician as excellent and were more likely to report receiving preventive care.

However, there have not yet been rigorous studies that either prove or disprove that race concordance plays a role in the actual quality of care patients receive. The only such study is Chen, Rathore, Radford, Wang, and Krumholz (2002), which examined the effect of doctor-patient race concordance on racial disparities in utilization of diagnostic cardiac procedures. The study found that patients who were race concordant with their physician were not more likely to get referred for the procedure. However, that study had several significant limitations, which make it difficult to draw firm conclusions. Further study is needed before it is determined how important race concordance is for patient care.

Major Health Risks and Health Issues Among African Americans

Of the many health risk factors faced by African Americans, perhaps the greatest is poverty and low socioeconomic status (SES).

Poverty and Low Socioeconomic Status

According to the 2000 census, more than 22 percent of African Americans live below the official poverty level. Poverty and low SES are linked to living in communities with greater exposure to physical environmental risks (such as chemical and other toxins) and socioenvironmental risks (such as crime, illicit drugs, and poor quality housing) (Kawachi & Berkman, 2003). African Americans have a high rate of poverty and low SES. Consequently, they have greater exposure to poverty-related health risks.

HIV/AIDS

As of the end of 2002, an estimated 886,575 cases of AIDS had been diagnosed among adults and adolescents in the United States. Of these, 349,491 (39.19 percent) were among African American patients (see Figure 10.1). African Americans make up only 12.9 percent of the U.S. population, so their representation among AIDS cases is three times their proportion of the population (Centers for Disease Control and Prevention, 2002c).

FIGURE 10.1.   CUMULATIVE HIV CASES AS OF DECEMBER 2002, BY RACE/ETHNICITY.

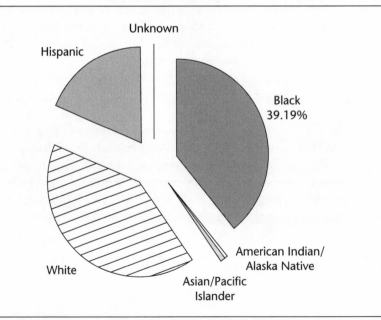

Source: Centers for Disease Control and Prevention, "Basic Statistics," http://www.cdc.gov/hiv/stats.htm#cumrace.

As staggering as that statistic is, it does not fully capture the degree to which HIV/AIDS has ravaged the African American population. Figure 10.2 displays HIV/AIDS age-adjusted death rates by race and sex for 2001. The figure shows that the death rate for African Americans far exceeds that of other racial/ethnic groups. The death rate is particularly high for African American males—more than three times the rate for Hispanic/Latino men, who have the second highest death rate. Black females have the highest death rate—more than double the rate for Hispanic/Latina women. For all racial/ethnic groups, the death rate for women is lower than the death rate for men. Between 1999 and 2002, African American men accounted for 49 percent of new HIV/AIDS cases among men in the United States. Black women accounted for 72 percent of new cases among women. The AIDS diagnosis rate for Black men is almost eleven times the rate among White men. And, the African American female rate is twenty-three times greater than the White female rate (CDC, 2002c).

The leading cause of HIV infection among African American women is heterosexual transmission, and the leading cause for African American men is homosexual sex and injection drug use (CDC, 2002c, 2000). The primary risk factors for HIV/AIDS infection are all highly prevalent among African Americans. Poverty is one such risk factor (Diaz et al., 1994): again, the African American poverty rate is over 22 percent. Diaz et al. posit that persons living below the poverty line have higher

FIGURE 10.2. AGE-ADJUSTED HIV/AIDS MORTALITY RATES, BY RACE/ETHNICITY, 2001.

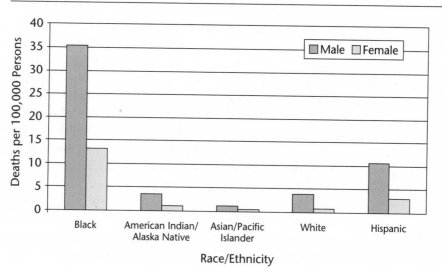

Source: National Center for Health Statistics.

risk of HIV infection due to reduced access to healthcare and less access to HIV prevention health education.

A second risk factor for HIV/AIDS is that the disease is highly stigmatized in the African American culture. African Americans have strong cultural taboos against male-to-male sex. This taboo is particularly strong within the Black church, a central feature of African American culture. One study found that church attendance was a strong predictor of antihomosexual attitudes (Schulte & Battle, 2003). As a result, Black men are less likely to disclose their homosexuality or bisexuality (CDC, 2003; Kennamer, Honnold, Bradford, & Hendricks, 2000). Consequently they are likely to be disinclined to heed HIV education messages targeted toward those communities.

A second consequence of the disinclination among African American men to disclose their sexual practices (whether bisexual or having multiple heterosexual partners without condom use) is that their female partners are not aware of their true health risk (Hader, Smith, Moore, & Holmberg, 2001). High rates of incarceration among low-income Black males are also a major contributor to HIV transmission (Braithwaite & Arriola, 2003). In prison, otherwise heterosexual men sometimes engage in homosexual sex, placing themselves at increased risk of infection.

Finally, injection drug use is the second leading mode of HIV transmission for African American men and women. Not only does HIV transmission occur by way of needle sharing, but it is well known that chronic drug users are also more likely to engage in unsafe sexual practices, such as having multiple partners and not using condoms (Leigh & Stall, 1993).

Homicide

Homicide is the sixth leading cause of death among African Americans. In 2001, the homicide death rate of 39.3 deaths per 100,000 African American men accounted for nearly 5 percent of all deaths of African American men. The Black female homicide rate was 7.1 homicides per 100,000 African American women. In 2000, homicides accounted for 8.5 percent of all years of potential life lost for African Americans. Comparisons with other racial/ethnic groups show that homicide takes a staggering toll on African Americans, especially males. As Figure 10.3 shows, the death rate for African American men was more than 39 deaths per 100,000 African American males. This rate was more than three times the rate for American Indians/Alaska Natives, who had the second highest homicide mortality rate. African American women have a homicide rate higher than that of women of every other racial/ethnic group. The Black female rate exceeds the rate for all males except for American Indian/Alaska Native men.

Figure 10.4 shows the distribution of homicide for Black males across the life span. The figure shows that the homicide rate reaches 85 deaths per 100,000 in the fifteen- to twenty-five-year-old age group. A high homicide rate persists into the

FIGURE 10.3.   AGE-ADJUSTED HOMICIDE RATES,
BY RACE/ETHNICITY, 2001.

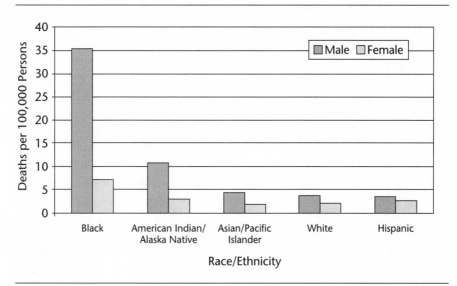

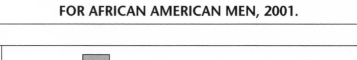

Source: National Center for Health Statistics, 2003, tab. 45.

FIGURE 10.4.   AGE-SPECIFIC HOMICIDE RATE
FOR AFRICAN AMERICAN MEN, 2001.

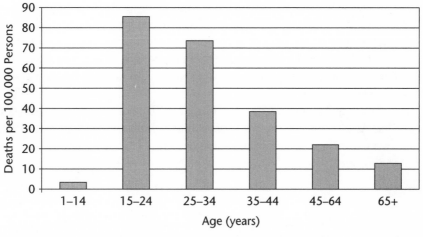

Source: National Center for Health Statistics, 2003, tab. 45.

BOX 10.2.   YEARS OF POTENTIAL LIFE LOST (YPLL).

Years of potential life lost is an estimate of the number of years of life lost due to premature deaths, assuming that all persons should live to be at least age seventy-five.

---

twenty-five- to thirty-year-old age group, for which the homicide rate is in excess of 70 deaths per 100,000. For ages thirty-five to forty-four the death rate declines to below 40 deaths; for ages forty-five to sixty-four it drops almost in half, to just over 20. Finally, for the sixty-five and older age group the Black male homicide rate remains in excess of 10 deaths per 100,000.

There are many reasons for these extremely high homicide rates among African Americans. A high poverty rate is one of them. Poverty exposes persons to social environments that foster social disorganization—conditions ripe for violence (Pridemore, 2002). African Americans disproportionately live in large urban areas, where homicide rates are highest. Such community environments foster gang violence as well as drug trafficking, which is associated with violence as well (Pridemore, 2002). Intimate partner violence is also a likely contributor (Campbell, Sharps, Gary, Campbell, & Lopez, 2002; Thompson, Kaslow, & Kingree, 2002).

Finally, Sikora and Mulvihill (2002) conducted an analysis of homicide from legal intervention between 1979 and 1997. Legal intervention refers to deaths due to law enforcement actions, regardless of their legality. Such deaths account for only 1.3 percent of all homicides; however, the importance of legal intervention lies not in the number of deaths, but the way those deaths are distributed by race. Sikora and Mulvihill found that 97 percent of all deaths due to legal intervention were among males and that 34 percent were among African Americans. Legal intervention varied greatly by age as well. For the twenty to twenty-four age group the Black male death rate from legal intervention was 1.4 deaths per 100,000, compared with 0.48 for White males in that age group (a nearly threefold disparity). To place the twenty- to twenty-four-year-old African American male legal intervention death rate into context, in 2001 the tenth leading cause of death for this group was diabetes, with a death rate of 1.5 per 100,000.

Obesity

Obesity is a major risk factor for many serious health conditions. It is one of the main risk factors for six of the ten leading causes of death in African Americans, including heart disease, cancer, stroke, diabetes, respiratory disease, and nephritis. It is also a primary risk factor for some of the most highly prevalent conditions in African Americans, such as hypertension. Obesity is also a significant complicating factor in many medical and surgical interventions for other diseases (Cossrow & Falkner, 2004). Obesity is the second leading behavior-related cause of death, and it is rapidly catching up with smoking, the number one behavior-related cause of death.

The prevalence of overweight and obesity (see Box 9.3 in Chapter Nine) is extremely high among all Americans and has been rising. This is especially true for African American women. As Figure 10.5 shows, 77.7 percent of Black women between ages twenty and seventy-four are either overweight or obese, with 50.4 percent having a body mass index (BMI; see Box 9.2 in Chapter Nine) greater than 30 (meaning obese). Black men have the lowest rate of obesity at 28.9 percent, but over 60 percent are at least overweight.

Most researchers believe that the high prevalence of obesity and overweight among African Americans is due to cultural factors, such as standards of beauty (Kumanyika, 2002; Padgett & Biro, 2003) and perceptions of "normal" weight (Gove, 1999). There is also a well-established relationship between SES and obesity (Drewnowski & Speter, 2004). Persons with higher SES have lower rates of obesity compared with persons with lower SES. (See Chapter Nine for further discussion of obesity and race/ethnicity.)

FIGURE 10.5. AGE-ADJUSTED PREVALENCE OF OVERWEIGHT AND OBESITY AMONG PERSONS AGED 20 YEARS AND OLDER, BY RACE/ETHNICITY AND SEX.

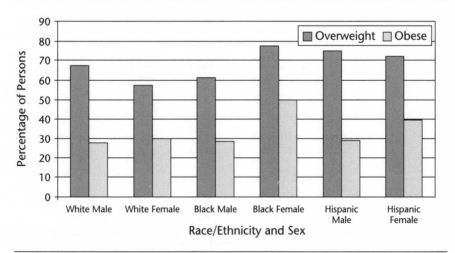

Source: National Center for Health Statistics, 2003, tab. 68.

Maternal and Child Health

Maternal and child health is another area of major concern for African Americans. Table 10.5 shows maternal mortality rates by race/ethnicity for the year 2000. Here we find that the maternal mortality rate for African American women greatly exceeds the rate for Hispanic/Latina and White women. The Black maternal mortality rate is more than three times the White rate and more than double the Hispanic/Latina rate.

Table 10.6 shows that African Americans have the highest infant mortality rate of all racial/ethnic groups in the United States. In 2001, the Black infant mortality rate (13.9 infant deaths per 1,000 live births) was more than double the rate for Hispanics/Latinos, Whites, and Asians/Pacific Islanders (all with rates below 6 deaths per 1,000 live births). When comparing racial/ethnic differences in infant mortality rates at different levels of maternal education, we find that the rate decreases with higher

TABLE 10.5. MATERNAL MORTALITY FOR COMPLICATIONS OF PREGNANCY, CHILDBIRTH, AND THE PUERPERIUM, BY RACE/ETHNICITY.

Race/Ethnicity	Deaths per 100,000
Black	20.1
White	6.2
Hispanic	9.0

Source: National Center for Health Statistics, 2003, tab. 43.

TABLE 10.6. INFANT MORTALITY RATES, BY EDUCATION AND RACE/ETHNICITY, 2001.

Race/Ethnicity	Total Mortem	< 12	12	> 12
Black	13.9	15.1	14.0	11.4
American Indian/Alaska Native	9.0	10.2	8.7	7.0
Asian/Pacific Islander	5.1	5.7	4.1	4.1
White	5.8	9.1	4.3	4.3
Hispanic	5.7	5.5	4.6	4.6

Source: National Center for Health Statistics, 2003, tab, 20.

levels of education. However, at each educational level the Black infant mortality rate far exceeds the other groups. In fact, the African American infant mortality rate among women with the highest educational level is higher than the rate for all other racial/ethnic groups at all educational levels, even the lowest.

Schoendorf, Hogue, Kleinman, and Rowley (1992) studied infant mortality among college-educated Black and White women to determine if race differences in SES account for race differences in infant mortality. That study found that infant mortality rates among college-educated African American women was still double the rate for college-educated White women. However, among those who had normal weight babies there was no race difference in infant mortality. Thus, the infant mortality race disparity appears to be caused by race differences in low birth weight. The reasons for race disparities in low birth weight are not well understood either. We know that prenatal care and maternal nutrition play a role, but these factors do not fully account for the disparities. Some have argued that the persistent race difference in infant birth weights is evidence of biological differences between race groups. However, studies in the military health system (where there are no disparities in living conditions, socioenvironmental exposures, or access to care) have found no race differences in pregnancy outcomes (Kugler, Connell, & Henley, 1990; Rawlings & Weir, 1992).

Smoking

According to the CDC (2002a), cigarette smoking remains the leading preventable cause of death in the United States, accounting for approximately one of every five deaths (440,000 people) each year. Chapter Nine outlined patterns of racial/ethnic differences in smoking, demonstrating that as adolescents, teens, and young adults, African Americans have substantially lower smoking rates compared with Whites, but as they reach middle age, smoking rates cross over until the Black rate exceeds the White rate. This pattern is demonstrated in Figure 10.6.

Wallace (1999) explains this phenomenon. As teenagers, African Americans have a low rate of tobacco use because of cultural norms that favor more authoritarian parenting styles (Sampson & Laub, 1994) and strong antismoking social norms. White teens smoke as experimentation. As African Americans age into adulthood, parental influences begin to wane. As they enter into the workforce, the stress of being a minority in the United States begins to take its toll. Smoking is then used as a coping mechanism. As African American smoking rates increase, the rate for Whites declines as they enter into adulthood and become more conscious of healthy living. As they enter middle age, smoking rates for both populations decline rapidly but the Black rate remains higher than the White rate.

**FIGURE 10.6.   CURRENT CIGARETTE SMOKING,
BY AGE AND RACE/ETHNICITY, 2001.**

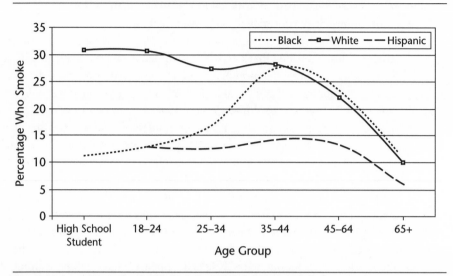

Source: National Center for Health Statistics, 2003, tabs. 61 and 63.

Summary

This chapter outlined the health status of African Americans and the major health issues affecting them. As African Americans are the second largest minority group in the United States, most of the research in minority health has been conducted on this population. African Americans have the highest mortality rates of any U.S. race/ethnic group. The pattern of high mortality rates persists throughout most of the life span. Among the very old, Black mortality rates are lower than White mortality rates. Black Americans have an extremely high death rate from homicide and HIV/AIDS. They face discrimination within health care settings. Obesity rates are also very high, especially for African American women. Compared with Whites, smoking rates are substantially lower for African American teenagers and young adults; however, in adulthood the rates reverse as the Black rate rapidly increases and exceeds the White rate. (See Appendix B for additional readings.)

Key Words

Mortality crossover

Doctor-patient race concordance

CHAPTER ELEVEN

AMERICAN INDIAN AND ALASKA NATIVE HEALTH ISSUES

Outline

Introduction

Progress on obtaining good-quality data on health care issues related to the American Indian and Alaska Native population has been severely hampered by a lack of data (LaVeist, 1995). This problem is well known. The U.S. federal government has taken steps to address this concern; however, the problem still remains. One of the most limiting issues is that often data systems within health care settings do not code a patient's race, or if they do, American Indian/Alaska Native (AIAN) is coded

"Other" and combined with Asian/Pacific Islander (API) (Garrett & Menke, 2001). In spite of this limitation, it is well known that there are a number of critical health care issues facing AIANs.

In the revised 1997 version of OMB Directive 15 (see Chapter One), American Indians and Alaska Natives were defined as "the original peoples of North and South America (including Central America)." According to the 2000 census, there are more than 4.1 million American Indians and Alaska Natives (1.5 percent of the total U.S. population). There are more than 550 federally recognized American Indian and Alaska Native tribes in the United States, ranging in size from fewer than 100 to more than 750,000. Tribes are sovereign nations that have a special relationship to the federal government and a unique legal status. Nearly 40 percent of persons who report being American Indian or Alaska Native also reported being a member of another racial or ethnic group. And about 74 percent of persons who indicated they were American Indians/Alaska Natives reported a specific tribal affiliation. Figure 11.1 displays the ten largest American Indian tribes; the largest Alaska Native tribes are displayed in Figure 11.2.

Figure 11.1 shows that the largest American Indian tribes were Cherokee (23.8 percent of the American Indian population), followed by Navajo (9.7 percent), Latin American Indian (5.9 percent), Choctaw (5.2 percent), Sioux (5.0 percent), and Chippewa (4.9 percent). Of the American Indians who reported a tribal affiliation, about 54 percent indicated one of these six tribes. As shown in Figure 11.2, among Alaska Natives the largest tribe was Eskimo (48.5 percent of those indicating an Alaska Native tribe).

Health Status

As we have seen in Chapter Four, the health profile of the AIAN population ranks very low among all the racial/ethnic groups in the United States. Disparities in the health of this population have a long history, going back to the arrival of the first European settlers. The European settlers brought with them diseases for which AIANs had little or no immunity. But although the poor health status of the AIAN population began there, it did not end there. The AIAN population has also endured inferior housing, education, and high rates of poverty.

Their long history of disenfranchisement, broken treaties, sterilization of American Indian women, placement of Indian children in boarding schools, and other experiences of oppression have established among American Indians "a deep-rooted intergenerational anger, intergenerational grief, and mistrust of the U.S. government that persists to this day" (U.S. Commission on Civil Rights, 2004). This history has had a negative impact on AIAN health and social status.

FIGURE 11.1.   THE TEN LARGEST AMERICAN INDIAN TRIBAL
GROUPINGS, 2000.

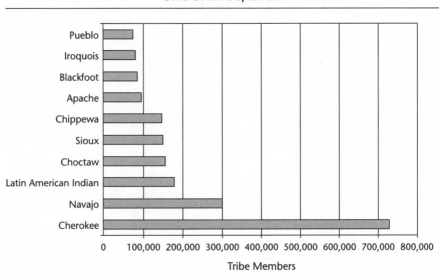

Source: U.S. Bureau of the Census, 2002, fig. 5.

FIGURE 11.2.   LARGEST ALASKA NATIVE TRIBAL GROUPINGS, 2000.

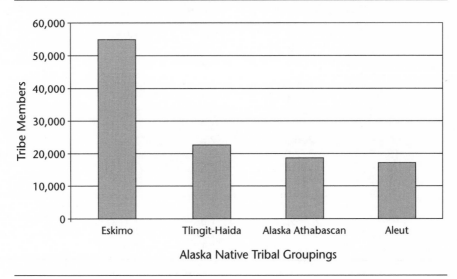

Source: U.S. Bureau of the Census, 2002, fig. 6.

Age-Specific Death Rates

Table 11.1 displays age-specific death rates for AIANs compared with other racial/ethnic groups. The table shows the AIAN death rate for each age group and the rate ratios for the other racial/ethnic groups compared with AIANs. A rate ratio of 1.0 indicates that AIANs and the comparison group have an equal death rate for the indicated age group. A rate ratio greater than 1.0 indicates AIANs have a higher death rate than the comparison group; for example, a rate ratio of 1.5 indicates that the AIAN rate is one and one half times greater; 2.0 indicates that the AIAN death rate is two times greater. If the rate ratio is less than 1.0, this indicates that AIANs have a lower death rate than the comparison group.

Table 11.1 shows that AIANs have a generally higher death rate compared to other racial/ethnic groups. Only African Americans have higher death rates for most age groups, but in some of the younger age groups, the AIAN death rates are equal

TABLE 11.1.   AGE-SPECIFIC DEATH RATES FOR AMERICAN INDIANS/ALASKA NATIVES COMPARED WITH OTHER RACIAL/ETHNIC GROUPS, 2001.

Age	American Indian/Alaska Native Death Rate (per 100,000)	Asian/ Pacific Islander	Hispanic/ Latino	White	African American
1–4	48.0	2.2	1.6	1.6	1.0
5–9	15.5	1.3	1.2	1.1	0.7
10–14	28.0	2.2	1.7	1.6	1.1
15–19	94.5	2.5	1.5	1.5	1.1
20–24	111.7	2.3	1.3	1.3	0.7
25–29	117.1	2.7	1.5	1.3	0.7
30–34	146.8	2.9	1.7	1.4	0.7
35–39	222.9	3.2	1.7	1.5	0.8
40–44	260.0	2.6	1.4	1.2	0.6
45–49	377.0	2.3	1.3	1.2	0.6
50–54	500.9	2.0	1.2	1.1	0.5
55–59	718.6	1.8	1.2	1.0	0.5
60–64	1,140.8	1.8	1.3	1.0	0.6
65–69	1,728.7	1.7	1.2	0.9	0.6
70–74	2,539.2	1.6	1.1	0.9	0.6
75–79	3,607.9	1.3	1.0	0.8	0.6
80–84	5,237.5	1.1	1.0	0.7	0.6
85 or older	8,897.1	0.9	0.8	0.6	0.6

Source: National Center for Health Statistics.

to or even higher than the African American rate. The magnitude of the disparity between AIANs and Asians/Pacific Islanders (APIs) is substantial, reaching as high as 3.2 times (220 percent higher than) the API death rate for the thirty-five to thirty-nine age group.

Comparing AIANs with Hispanics/Latinos, we find that the AIAN death rates are as much as 1.7 times (70 percent higher) for the ten to fourteen, thirty to thirty-four, and thirty-five to thirty-nine age groups. AIAN death rates are also substantially higher than the rates for Whites. However, with the exception of three young age groups, the AIAN death rate is consistently lower than the African American death rate.

It is instructive to note that AIAN death rates converge with death rates for APIs, Hispanics/Latinos, and Whites, and cross over at older ages. The AIAN/API and the AIAN/Hispanic crossover occur above age eighty, and the AIAN/White crossover occurs around age sixty-five. These crossovers occur because of a phenomenon called selective survival, discussed in Chapter Four. Selective survival leads to a crossover in death rates whereby AIANs and African Americans have lower death rates than other racial/ethnic groups at old ages (Markides & Machalek, 1984). High death rates among young AIANs reduce the proportion of frail elders, which results in lower death rates among older AIANs.

Leading Causes of Death

Table 11.2 displays the ten leading causes of death for AIAN males. The ten leading causes of death for AIAN females are listed in Table 11.3. In addition to showing the age-adjusted death rate and the percentage of all AIAN deaths accounted for by that cause of death, the tables also show where that cause of death ranks among the other racial/ethnic groups. Heart disease and cancer are the two leading causes of death for AIAN men, as is the case for all men. Together heart disease and cancer account for more than 38 percent of all deaths in AIAN men.

Unintended injury (accidents) and chronic liver disease (cirrhosis) are third and fourth on the list. Although the three leading causes of death for AIAN men are among the five leading causes of death for men of other racial/ethnic groups as well, liver cirrhosis is not among the ten leading causes for APIs, Whites, or African Americans. Cirrhosis of the liver is the seventh leading cause of death for Hispanic/Latino men. Liver cirrhosis is a cause of death associated with stigmatized behavior (Riston, 1999). Liver disease and cirrhosis are often associated with alcohol abuse. (The high AIAN death rate from cirrhosis of the liver will be discussed later in this chapter.)

The five leading causes of death for AIAN women are similar to those of women of other racial/ethnic groups—cancer, heart disease, accidents, diabetes, and stroke—with one noteworthy departure: the seventh leading cause of death is liver disease and

TABLE 11.2.   LEADING CAUSES OF DEATH FOR AMERICAN INDIAN/ALASKA NATIVE MALES COMPARED WITH MALES OF OTHER ETHNIC GROUPS, 2001.

Rank for AIAN Males	Cause of Death	Percentage of Total Deaths	Age-Adjusted Death Rate	Rank for Males in Other Groups			
				Asians/ Pacific Islanders	Hispanics/ Latinos	Whites	African Americans
1	Heart disease	21.0	89.1	1	1	1	1
2	Cancer	17.1	72.4	2	2	2	2
3	Accidents	14.0	59.6	4	3	5	3
4	Chronic liver disease/ cirrhosis	4.8	20.3	—	7	—	—
5	Diabetes mellitus	4.3	18.1	7	6	6	7
6	Suicide	4.0	17.0	8	8	8	—
7	Stroke	3.4	14.2	3	4	4	4
8	Respiratory disease	3.1	13.1	5	9	3	8
9	Influenza/pneumonia	2.5	10.5	6	—	7	10
10	Homicide	2.3	9.6	9	5	—	5

Source: National Center for Health Statistics.

TABLE 11.3. LEADING CAUSES OF DEATH FOR AMERICAN INDIAN/ALASKA NATIVE FEMALES COM-PARED WITH FEMALES OF OTHER ETHNIC GROUPS, 2001.

Rank for AIAN Females	Cause of Death	Percentage of Total Deaths	Age-Adjusted Death Rate	Rank for Feales in Other Groups			
				Asians/ Pacific Islanders	Hispanics/ Latinas	Whites	African Americans
1	Cancer	19.1	68.8	1	2	2	2
2	Heart disease	18.9	68.2	2	1	1	1
3	Accidents	8.2	29.6	5	5	7	6
4	Diabetes mellitus	6.7	24.1	4	4	8	4
5	Stroke	6.5	23.3	3	3	3	3
6	Respiratory disease	4.1	14.8	7	7	4	7
7	Chronic liver disease/ cirrhosis	4.1	14.6	—	10	—	—
8	Influenza/pneumonia	2.9	10.3	6	6	6	9
9	Nephritis	2.4	8.6	8	8	9	5
10	Septicemia	1.3	4.7	—	—	10	—

Source: National Center for Health Statistics.

cirrhosis, which accounts for more than four percent of all deaths of American Indian and Alaska Natives women. Hispanic/Latina women are the only other group of females with liver disease among the ten leading causes of death. However, in 2001 although Hispanic/Latina women accounted for 27 percent of all liver cirrhosis deaths among Hispanics/Latinos, AIAN women accounted for 42 percent of AIAN cirrhosis deaths.

Table 11.4 presents the leading causes of death for AIAN adults (ages twenty to sixty-five). The leading causes of death for young adults are accidents, homicide, and suicide. These causes of death are associated with psychosocial factors rather than biological factors. Among these psychosocial factors are violent and aggressive behavior, poverty, risk-taking, and depression. As American Indians and Alaska Natives progress through the life course, chronic conditions gradually rise to the top positions on the list. Chronic conditions include causes such as diseases of the heart, cancer, diabetes, and stroke (see Box 4.6 in Chapter Four).

TABLE 11.4. LEADING CAUSES OF DEATH ACROSS THE LIFE SPAN FOR AMERICAN INDIAN/ALASKA NATIVE ADULTS, 2001.

	Age Group				
Rank	20–24	25–34	35–44	45–54	55–65
1	Accidents	Accidents	Accidents	Cancer	Cancer
2	Suicide	Suicide	Chronic liver disease/cirrhosis	Heart disease	Heart disease
3	Homicide	Homicide	Heart disease	Accidents	Diabetes
4	Cancer	Cancer	Cancer	Chronic liver disease/cirrhosis	Chronic liver disease/cirrhosis
5	Heart disease	Heart disease	Suicide	Diabetes	Accidents
6	Congenital malformations	Chronic liver disease/cirrhosis	Homicide	Stroke	Respiratory disease
7	Diabetes	HIV/AIDS	HIV/AIDS	Suicide	Stroke
8	Chronic liver disease/cirrhosis	Influenza/pneumonia	Stroke	Nephritis	Nephritis
9	Septicemia	Stroke	Influenza/pneumonia	Septicemia	Influenza/pneumonia
10	Nephritis	Pregnancy	Diabetes	Homicide	Septicemia

Source: National Center for Health Statistics.

Health Care Access and Utilization

To understand the delivery of health care services to the AIAN population, it is necessary to understand the historic relationship between the U.S. government and America's native population. Before the arrival of European settlers, American Indians lived throughout North America. After settlers arrived, wars ensued, countless American Indians and Alaska Natives were killed (both by war and by settler-introduced diseases for which Indians had no immunity), and segregationist policies by the U.S. government led to the relocation of AIANs on reservations.

Over the years the U.S. government has signed many treaties with American Indian tribal governments but ignored many of the treaty provisions. The treaties commonly called for the U.S. government to provide education and health care. Initially, the U.S. Army was made responsible for carrying out this responsibility, but as one would imagine, the provision of health care was neither the expertise of nor a priority for the Army. The quality of care was inadequate.

Later the Bureau of Indian Affairs (BIA) was developed and took over the responsibility for providing health care to the American Indian population. Under the BIA the quality of health care improved. The BIA built health clinics and expanded the availability of health services. However, inadequate funding rendered the BIA incapable of meeting the level of health care needed. In 1955 the Indian Health Service (IHS) was formed and took over responsibility for the provision of care to American Indians. In 1959, Alaska became part of the United States, and eventually Alaskan tribes became eligible for IHS services.

Throughout the 1960s and into the 1980s the health status of the AIAN population drastically improved. The IHS brought expertise in public health to the reservations. They improved the quality of drinking water and sanitation. American Indians living on reservations underwent an epidemiologic transition (see Box 11.1), as the primary causes of death shifted from infectious diseases to chronic conditions. For example, since the creation of the IHS, AIAN tuberculosis incidence rates have decreased from 57.9 cases per 100,000 persons in 1955 to 2.2 cases per 100,000 in 1991. Other infectious diseases also declined drastically (Davis, 1999).

The Indian Health Service

Established in 1955, the Indian Health Service (IHS) is a federal agency (part of the U.S. Department of Health and Human Services) charged with fulfilling the U.S. government's treaty obligation to provide health services to American Indians and Alaska Natives. The IHS is a direct provider of health care though sixty-one health centers, thirty-six hospitals, forty-nine health stations, five residential treatment centers, and

---

BOX 11.1.   THE EPIDEMIOLOGICAL TRANSITION.

The *epidemiological transition* concept holds that as societies become more economically developed, the leading causes of death shift from infectious diseases
(which are indicative of unhealthy environmental and social conditions) to degenerative or chronic conditions (which are indicative of lifestyle choices or
old age).

---

thirty-four urban Indian health projects. The IHS also provides health services through
tribally contracted and operated health programs and more than nine thousand private providers annually. Persons are eligible to use Indian Health Service facilities if
they are of American Indian or Alaska Native descent (or both) and are recognized by
the community in which they live as an American Indian or Alaska Native (the complete eligibility criteria are presented in Box 11.2). About 16 percent of American
Indians/Alaska Natives rely on the Indian Health Service as their sole source of health
care (Zuckerman, Haley, Roubideaux, & Lillie-Blanton, 2004).

Although the Indian Health Service can be credited for improving access to
care for American Indians and Alaska Natives, this does not mean the population has
no health care access problems. Access to Indian Health Service facilities is limited
due to geography and funding (Korenbrot, Ehlers, & Crouch, 2003). The facilities tend
to be located in highly remote areas and cover vast geographic areas. Also, because of
funding limitations, services are rationed so that some services are not available at all
facilities. The IHS facilities are aging: according to the U.S. Commission on Civil
Rights (2004), "the average age of current IHS facilities is thirty-two years, compared
with nine years for private sector facilities." The IHS also has difficulty recruiting and
retaining high-quality health care providers.

Health Insurance Status

Zuckerman et al. (2004) conducted an analysis of the National Survey of America's
Families to assess the role of the Indian Health Service in improving health services
access, use, and insurance coverage among AIANs. The study concluded that "The
IHS partially offsets lack of insurance for some uninsured AIANs, but important needs
were potentially unmet." Although 16 percent of AIANs reported the IHS as their
usual source of health care, another 19 percent did not report the IHS as a source of
health care coverage. Among low-income AIANs, the reliance on the IHS was even
greater. Twenty-three percent relied on the IHS as their sole source of care and an additional 25 percent were uninsured (lacking even access to IHS facilities).

BOX 11.2. WHO IS ELIGIBLE TO USE THE INDIAN HEALTH SERVICE?

A person may be regarded as within the scope of the Indian Health program if he is not otherwise excluded therefrom by provision of law and

A. Is of Indian and/or Alaska Native descent as evidenced by one or more of the following factors:
1. Is regarded by the community in which he lives as an Indian or Alaska Native;
2. Is a member, enrolled or otherwise, of an Indian or Alaska Native Tribe or Group under federal supervision;
3. Resides on tax-exempt land or owns restricted property;
4. Actively participates in tribal affairs;
5. Any other reasonable factor indicative of Indian descent, or

B. Is an Indian of Canadian or Mexican origin recognized by any Indian tribe or group as a member of an Indian community served by the Indian Health program; or

C. Is a non-Indian woman pregnant with an eligible Indian's child for the duration of her pregnancy through post partum (usually 6 weeks); or

D. Is a non-Indian member of an eligible Indian's household and the medical officer in charge determines that services are necessary to control a public health hazard or an acute infectious disease which constitutes a public health hazard.

Source: U.S. Department of Health and Human Services, Indian Health Service, http://www.ihs.gov/generalweb/helpcenter/customerservices/elig.asp.

Major Health Risks

Efforts to reduce disproportionate exposure to hazardous environmental pollutants among racial/ethnic minorities and low-income people are called *environmental justice.* The U.S. Environmental Protection Agency defines environmental justice as "fair treatment for people of all races, cultures, and incomes, regarding the development of environmental laws, regulations, and policies."

Environmental exposures are a major health risk faced disproportionately by American Indians and Alaska Natives. American Indians are at increased risk for ill health effects associated with living near nuclear weapon test sites (Frohmberg, Goble, Sanchez, & Quigley, 2000). Radioactive iodine exposures threaten American Indians through certain culturally related behaviors such as eating small game, drinking the milk of cattle that graze in exposed area, and eating vegetables grown in exposed soil (Frohmberg et al., 2000; Quigley, Handy, Goble, Sanchez, & George, 2000). Studies have also demonstrated elevated exposure to PCBs (Fitzgerald et al., 2004), lead (Howell & Russette, 2004), and toxins from solid waste sites (Wolf, Spitz, Olson, Zavodska, & Algharaibeh, 2003).

Poverty and Low Socioeconomic Status

Poverty and low socioeconomic status (SES) are linked to living in communities, both urban and rural, with greater exposure to physical environmental risks (such as chemical and other toxins) and social environmental risks (such as crime, illicit drugs, and poor-quality housing) (Kawachi & Berkman, 2003). Although American Indians and Alaska Natives as a combined group have a high rate of poverty and low SES, a closer examination of AIAN subgroups (tribes) reveals substantial variation among them.

Figure 11.3 shows poverty rates among the ten largest American Indian tribes for 1995. Figure 11.4 shows per capita income. Poverty varies among the tribes, ranging

FIGURE 11.3.   PERCENTAGE OF AMERICAN INDIANS IN POVERTY, 1995.

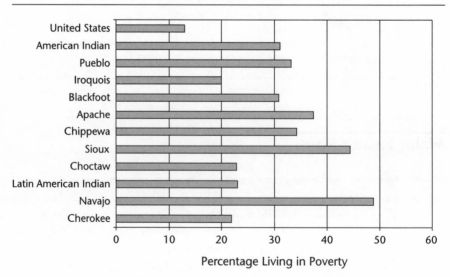

Source: U.S. Bureau of the Census, http://www.census.gov/population/socdemo/race/indian/ailang2.txt.

from about 20 percent among the Iroquois to nearly 50 percent among the Navajo. The Sioux also had a poverty rate greater than 40 percent. The other large tribes had poverty rates between 23 percent (Cherokee) and 37.5 percent (Apache). Poverty rates for all tribes combined were 31.2 percent—2.38 times greater than the poverty rate of the U.S. population as a whole (13.1 percent).

Although per capita income for the general U.S. population was over $14,000, per capita income for American Indians as a whole was just over $8,000. Consistent with their poverty rates, Navajo and Sioux have the lowest per capita income of the ten largest tribes. The highest per capita incomes were found among the Cherokee and Iroquois.

Language and Culture as Barriers to Care

As is the case with the Hispanic/Latino and Asian/Pacific Islander populations, language presents a barrier to obtaining quality care for AIANs. Non-English-proficient and limited-English-speaking patients receive less information about the process of

FIGURE 11.4.   PER CAPITA INCOME AMONG AMERICAN INDIANS, 1995.

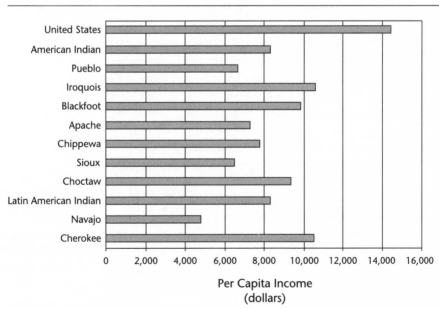

Per Capita Income
(dollars)

Source: U.S. Bureau of the Census, http://www.census.gov/population/socdemo/race/indian/ailang2.txt.

care for their condition and have more difficultly understanding instructions related to medication. They are less likely to keep follow-up appointments and more likely to make emergency room visits (Robert Wood Johnson Foundation, 2004). Figure 11.5 shows the percentage of American Indians who speak languages other than English and the percentage that "don't speak English well." The figure shows wide variation in the percentage of American Indians who speak a language other than English, ranging from a low of 7 percent among the Cherokee and Chippewa to a high of 75 percent among the Navajo. More than 60 percent of Pueblo speak another language.

How well one speaks English is perhaps more important than whether one speaks a language other than English. Slightly fewer than 40 percent of all American Indians indicate that they do not speak English well. More than 50 percent of Latin American Indians and more than 40 percent of Choctaw and Navajo report that they do not speak English well. English proficiency is highest (that is, the percentage of poor English speakers is lowest) among the Blackfoot, Chippewa, and Iroquois.

In addition to the practical advantages of being able to interact with the U.S. health care system in English, English proficiency is a marker for acculturation and the related concept, traditionalism. Most studies of traditionalism and health among AIANs have focused on the use of traditional healing practices (Novins, Beals, Moore, Spicer, & Manson, 2004; van Sickle, Morgan, & Wright, 2003). However, some have examined the relationship between traditionalism and health outcomes or behaviors. For example, Coe et al. (2004) conducted a study of 559 randomly selected women living on the Hopi reservation to determine whether women who were more traditional in their attitudes and behaviors had a different disease risk profile compared with less traditional women. That study found that women who were more traditional had *fewer* disease risks, including a greater likelihood of exercising regularly, lower rates of smoking, and a lower likelihood of obesity. Similar results were found in a study of Lakota men and women (Han et al., 1994). One study (Napholz, 2000) showed a positive effect of traditionalism among women living in an urban environment.

Cultural insensitivity among health care providers is an additional problem. Western providers tend not to accept traditional healing practices and traditional medicine. This can create barriers to receiving care. When AIAN patients see Western physicians whom they perceive to be culturally insensitive, this can lead to lower-quality health care. This can occur in several ways. AIAN patients may be less inclined to disclose their use of traditional healing practices, leaving the physician to diagnose and treat without information that might be important to prevent dangerous drug interactions or to properly diagnose disease. Also, such communications barriers can lead to distrust, which increases the likelihood that the patient will not follow the doctor's prescribed regimen.

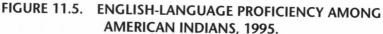

FIGURE 11.5.   ENGLISH-LANGUAGE PROFICIENCY AMONG
AMERICAN INDIANS, 1995.

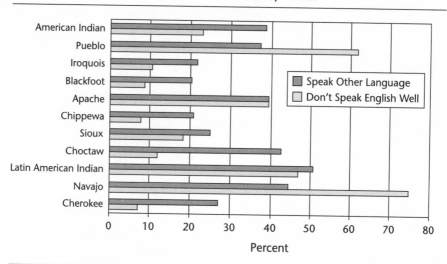

Source: U.S. Bureau of the Census, http://www.census.gov/population/socdemo/race/indian/
ailang2.txt.

Racial/Ethnic Group–Specific Health Issues

The two most important sources of health problems for AIANs are accidents and alcohol consumption.

Accidents (Unintentional Injuries)

The AIAN population experiences a disproportionate amount of morbidity and mortality from accidents (unintentional injuries). Unintentional injuries are the leading cause of death for AIANs under the age of forty-four and the third leading cause of death overall. The age-adjusted injury death rate for AIANs is approximately 250 percent higher than the rate for the total U.S. population. And AIANs sustain injuries at rates one and a half to five times the rates for other Americans. This translates into more than 1,300 deaths and more than 10,000 hospitalizations each year. Annually, the IHS spends more than $150 million to treat unintentional injuries. Injuries result in 46 percent of all years of potential life lost (YPLL) for the AIAN population. This is five times greater than the YPLL due to the next highest cause, heart disease (8 percent) (CDC, 2002c).

Figure 11.6 shows age-specific unintentional injury death rates for ages twenty to sixty-four by race/ethnicity. The figure shows the magnitude of the disparity in deaths

FIGURE 11.6   AGE-SPECIFIC DEATH RATES DUE TO ACCIDENT (UNINTENTIONAL INJURY), BY RACE/ETHNICITY, 2001.

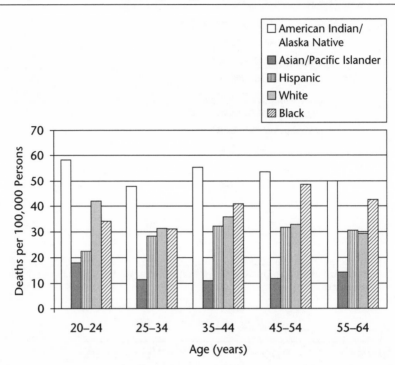

Source: National Center for Health Statistics.

caused by unintentional injury for AIANs compared with other racial/ethnic groups. The AIAN death rate is higher than the rate for all other racial/ethnic groups for each age group. Reasons for the high AIAN unintended injury mortality rate include alcohol abuse and poorly engineered (or unpaved) roads on tribal lands.

Alcohol

Alcohol use and abuse has taken a heavy toll on the health and social functioning of American Indian and Alaska Native communities. The high rate of alcohol use has many consequences, including a high death rate from alcohol-related causes such as liver cirrhosis and alcohol-related accidents. These alcohol-related issues are displayed in Table 11.5. The table shows racial/ethnic differences in the percentage of persons who exceed the National Institute on Alcohol Abuse and Alcoholism (NIAAA)

TABLE 11.5.   ALCOHOL USE, CIRRHOSIS DEATHS, AND ALCOHOL-RELATED MOTOR VEHICLE DEATHS, BY RACE/ETHNICITY, VARIOUS YEARS.

Race/Ethnic Group	Percent Exceeding Alcohol Consumption Guidelines[a]		Death Rate per 100,000 from Cirrhosis[b]	Death Rate per 100,000 from Alcohol-Related Vehicle Crashes[c]
	Male	Female		
American Indian/ Alaska Native	97	85	25.9	19.2
Asian/Pacific Islander	53	64	3.5	2.4
Black	74	65	10.2	6.4
White	74	72	8.8	6.0
Hispanic/Latino	80	72	15.4	N.A.

[a]National Longitudinal Alcohol Epidemiological Survey, 1992.

[b]National Vital Statistics System, 1998.

[c]Fatality Analysis Reporting System, 1998.

BOX 11.3.   ALCOHOL

What Defines a Drink?
The National Institute on Alcohol Abuse and Alcoholism (NIAAA) defines a drink as one 12-ounce bottle of regular beer, a 5-ounce glass of wine, or 1.5 ounces of 80-proof distilled spirits.

Guidelines for Alcohol Consumption
Males may be at risk for alcohol-related problems if they drink more than fourteen drinks per week or more than four drinks per occasion. Females may be at risk if they drink more than seven drinks per week or more than three drinks per occasion.

Source: National Institute on Alcohol Abuse and Alcoholism, 1995.

guidelines for alcohol consumption, death rates from cirrhosis of the liver, and death rates from alcohol-related motor vehicle crashes.

The table shows that AIAN men and women are more likely to exceed the NIAAA's alcohol consumption guidelines. An exceptionally high percentage of AIAN males (97 percent) indicate that their drinking patterns exceed the guidelines. The second highest percentage of men who exceed the guidelines were Hispanics/Latinos. The males of no other racial/ethnic group have a rate higher than 74 percent. Eighty-five percent of female AIANs report exceeding the NIAAA guidelines. Women of all other racial/ethnic groups had rates that were lower.

One consequence of a high rate of alcohol use is cirrhosis of the liver. The AIAN age-adjusted death rate from cirrhosis far exceeds the rate for all other racial/ethnic groups. The group with the second highest death rate is Hispanics/Latinos, but although their rate is high it is still more than 10 percentage points lower than the AIAN death rate. The AIAN cirrhosis mortality rate is more than double the African American rate, and it is three times the White rate. Finally, at 19.2 deaths per 100,000 persons, the AIAN alcohol-related automobile accident death rate is more than three times the rate of any other racial/ethnic group. AIANs also have a high death rate from intentional injuries (suicide) (Novins, Beals, Roberts, & Manson, 1999; Shaughnessy, Doshi, & Jones, 2004; Freedenthal & Stiffman, 2004; Borowsky, Resnick, Ireland, & Blum, 1999). Suicide is known to be associated with depression, alcohol abuse, and poverty.

Cruz (1999) described two competing theories to explain the high rates of alcoholism among AIANs: (1) the theory of anomie and (2) the aboriginal social pathology theory. The theory of anomie maintains that AIANs continue to mourn the loss of historic tradition, and their drinking habits are a reaction to stress associated with acculturation into mainstream American society. The loss of freedom and low social status causes some to "assert their Indianness" by fulfilling the "firewater" myth.

The aboriginal social pathology theory maintains that social pathology predates the introduction of alcohol into Indian cultures. It posits that the cultures were not robust enough to incorporate alcohol without its having severe destructive affects. But as Cruz (1999) cautions, these theories have not been rigorously tested. A third theory argues for a genetic linkage to alcohol dependence (Long et al., 1998).

Summary

This chapter provided an overview of issues in the health of the American Indian/Alaska Native population. There are more than 550 federally recognized AIAN tribes in the United States, ranging in size from fewer than 100 to more than 750,000. About half of the AIAN population lives on tribal lands; most of the others live in urban areas. The Indian Health Service (IHS) is the agency of the federal government that is responsible for the provision of health care to AIANs. Since the creation of the IHS the health status of the AIAN population has improved, but AIANs still have a higher all-cause mortality rate across the life span than all other racial/ethnic groups except African Americans. The AIAN population has a high mortality rate from causes of death associated with alcohol abuse, including unintentional accidents, automobile fatalities, and cirrhosis. (See Appendix B for additional readings.)

Key Words

Mortality crossover

Indian Health Service

Environmental justice

CHAPTER TWELVE

ASIAN AND PACIFIC ISLANDER HEALTH ISSUES

Outline

Introduction

The Asian and Pacific Islander (API) population is often referred to as the "model minority" because members of this group have relatively few health risks and numerous protective factors. The API population has the best overall health profile—longer life expectancy and lower mortality rate—of all ethnic groups in the United States, including Whites. However, the "model minority" moniker belies a complex reality for this highly heterogeneous population from diverse cultures and ethnic backgrounds. Commonly we discuss all Asian Americans and Pacific Islanders as a monocultural group. However, the API population is an extremely diverse population of different ethnic groups including native and foreign-born persons. These "subethnic" groups differ substantially in customs, language, and their integration into American life and culture (Braun, Yee, Browne, & Mokuau).

According to the 2000 census, 12,773,242 people (4.23 percent of the total population) identified themselves as Asians or Pacific Islanders (including individuals with ancestry from China, Korea, Japan, Taiwan, and other nations of Southeast Asia), Native Hawaiians, and Other Pacific Islanders. However, when these numbers are disaggregated, the data reveal a great deal of variability in their social and health status (Lin-Fu, 1988; Tanjasiri, Wallace, & Shibata, 1995).

The census identified twenty-four subethnic groups of Asians. Of the nearly twelve million census respondents who classified themselves as Asian American (see Figure 12.1), more than 88 percent were either Chinese, Filipino, Asian Indian, Korean, Vietnamese, or Japanese. Chinese (23.1 percent) and Filipino (18.5 percent) made up more than 40 percent of all Asian Americans in the census.

The Native Hawaiian/Pacific Islander population encompasses more than twenty-five groups with unique histories, languages, and cultures. Among the 874,414 people counted by Census 2000, some 46 percent are Native Hawaiian, 15 percent are Samoan, and 11 percent are Chamorro/Guamanian (see Figure 12.2). Other Pacific Islanders in the United States trace their ancestry to one or more of the Melanesian, Micronesian, and Polynesian cultures that settled in one of thousands of islands.

FIGURE 12.1   DIVERSITY OF THE ASIAN/PACIFIC ISLANDER POPULATION OF THE UNITED STATES, 2000.

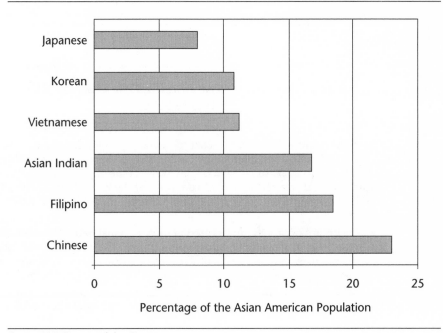

Percentage of the Asian American Population

Source: U.S. Bureau of the Census.

**FIGURE 12.2.   DIVERSITY OF THE NATIVE HAWAIIAN AND PACIFIC
ISLANDER POPULATION OF THE UNITED STATES, 2000.**

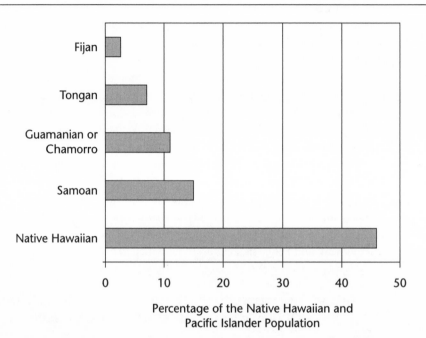

Percentage of the Native Hawaiian and
Pacific Islander Population

Source: U.S. Bureau of the Census.

**BOX 12.1.   DATA AVAILABILITY FOR ASIANS/PACIFIC
ISLANDERS.**

The federal data systems began collecting and reporting data for the API category in 1980, after the adoption of OMB Directive 15, which defined Asian/Pa-
cific Islander as "a person having origins in any of the original peoples of the Far
East, Southeast Asia, the Indian subcontinent, or the Pacific Islands. This area includes, for example, China, India, Japan, Korea, the Philippine Islands, and
Samoa."

The number of APIs represented in most national data collections is typically too small to allow for computation of statistics. As a result the API population is often overlooked in health research. Most rigorous studies of this
population have been smaller studies or studies in limited geographic areas.

A second problem is having sufficient data on the subgroups that the API
category comprises, especially Pacific Islanders. Data availability is a significant
limitation.

Asians make up more than 56 percent of the world's population (China, with 21 percent, and India, with 16.6 percent, account for more than one-third of the world population). Within the United States, however, Asian Americans are a minority. We have established that the API population is highly diverse, comprising more than fifty identifiable subethnic groups (including national and ethnic groups). The substantial variation within this population sometimes makes it difficult to study their health because of a lack of data that is not aggregated among these groups. Accordingly, the public health, medical, and nursing research literature on Asians/Pacific Islanders is more limited compared with research on other racial/ethnic groups. This chapter reviews studies and data that are in some cases aggregated and in other cases specific to a subethnic group. In each case we use the lowest level of aggregation available.

Health Status

In 2002 the National Institutes of Health (NIH) released its *Women of Color Health Data Book*, which, among other things, compiled multiple data sources to estimate life expectancy among Asian/Pacific Islander subethnic groups. The NIH data book reported that life expectancy for each API subethnic group for which data were available compared favorably to that of Whites and all other American racial/ethnic groups (Leigh & Jimenez, 2002). Male life expectancies for API subethnic groups were 79.5 years for Japanese Americans, 79.8 years for Chinese, 71.5 years for Hawaiians, 71.0 years for Samoans, and 72.4 years for Guamanians. This compared to a male life expectancy of 74.8 for Whites and 68.2 for African Americans in the year 2000.

Female life expectancy for API subethnic groups also compares favorably with other racial/ethnic groups. Female life expectancy rates are as follows: Japanese, 84.5 years; Chinese Hawaiian, 86.1 years; Hawaiian, 77.2 years; Samoan, 74.9 years; and Guamanian, 76.1 years. This compares with female life expectancy rates for White (80 years) and Black (74.9 years) Americans.

Age-Specific Death Rates

Table 12.1 shows the API death rate for each age group and the rate ratios for the other racial/ethnic groups compared with APIs. A rate ratio of 1.0 indicates that APIs and the comparison group have an equal death rate for the indicated age group. If the rate ratio is greater than 1.0, then APIs have a higher death rate than the comparison group (for example, a rate ratio of 1.5 would indicate that the API death rate is one and one half times greater; 2.0 would indicate that the API death rate is two times greater). If the rate ratio is less than 1.0, this indicates that APIs have a lower death rate than the comparison group.

TABLE 12.1.   AGE-SPECIFIC DEATH RATES FOR ASIANS/PACIFIC
ISLANDERS COMPARED WITH OTHER RACIAL/ETHNIC
GROUPS, 2001.

| Age | Asian/Pacific Islander Death Rate | *Rate Ratios* | | | |
		American Indian/ Alaska Native	Hispanic/ Latino	White	African American
1–4	22.3	0.5	0.7	0.7	0.5
5–9	11.6	0.7	0.7	0.8	0.5
10–14	12.8	0.5	0.7	0.7	0.5
15–19	38.0	0.4	0.6	0.6	0.4
20–24	47.6	0.4	0.5	0.6	0.3
25–29	43.9	0.4	0.4	0.5	0.3
30–34	50.8	0.3	0.4	0.5	0.2
35–39	69.9	0.3	0.4	0.5	0.2
40–44	99.7	0.4	0.4	0.5	0.2
45–49	164.2	0.4	0.5	0.5	0.3
50–54	247.6	0.5	0.5	0.5	0.3
55–59	395.5	0.6	0.5	0.5	0.3
60–64	624.1	0.5	0.5	0.5	0.3
65–69	1,012.3	0.6	0.5	0.6	0.4
70–74	1,606.0	0.6	0.6	0.6	0.4
75–79	2,683.3	0.7	0.6	0.6	0.5
80–84	4,579.6	0.9	0.6	0.6	0.6
85 or older	9,714.8	1.1	0.6	0.6	0.7

Source: National Center for Health Statistics.

Table 12.1 shows that at all ages APIs generally have a lower death rate than all other American racial/ethnic groups. In nearly every comparison, we find a rate ratio of less than 1.0. The single exception to this pattern is the comparison with American Indian/Alaska Natives (AIAN) aged eighty-five and older. The reasons for this pattern are not well understood but may result from a phenomenon similar to the mortality crossover first discussed in Chapter Four. This pattern may be the result of selective survival among the AIAN population, in which high death rates among young AIANs eventually reduce the proportion of frail elders, which results in lower death rates among older AIANs. It is important to point out that this explanation, while plausible, is speculative and has not been examined using rigorous research methods.

Leading Causes of Death

Table 12.2 displays the ten leading causes of death for API males. The ten leading causes of death for API females are listed in Table 12.3. The tables also show the rank for each cause of death for the other racial/ethnic groups. Table 12.2 shows that heart disease and cancer are the two leading causes of death for API men. Together heart disease and cancer account for more than 50 percent of all deaths for API men. Stroke and accidents are the third and fourth leading causes of death. Each of these causes is among the top five for other minority men as well (with the exception of stroke, which is the seventh leading cause of death for American Indian/Alaska Native men).

Among API women the leading causes of death are similar to those for women of other racial/ethnic groups—cancer, heart disease, stroke, diabetes, and accidents (unintentional injury). However, the ninth and tenth leading causes of death for API women are unique: hypertension and Alzheimer's disease are not among the ten leading causes of death for any other racial/ethnic group (see Table 12.3).

Table 12.4 presents the leading causes of death for API adults across the life span (ages twenty to sixty-five). The leading causes of death for young adults are accidents, suicide, and homicide. These are causes of death associated with psychosocial factors rather than biological factors. Among these psychosocial factors are violent and aggressive behavior, poverty, risk-taking, and depression. As APIs age, chronic conditions gradually rise to the top positions on the list. Chronic conditions include causes such as diseases of the heart, cancer, diabetes, and stroke.

TABLE 12.2. LEADING CAUSES OF DEATH FOR ASIAN/PACIFIC ISLANDER MALES COMPARED WITH MALES OF OTHER ETHNIC GROUPS, 2001.

				Rank for Males in Other Groups			
Rank for API Males	Cause of Death	Percentage of Total Deaths	Age-Adjusted Death Rate	American Indian/ Alaska Native	Hispanic/ Latino	White	African American
1	Heart disease	26.0	87.3	1	1	1	1
2	Cancer	26.0	87.0	2	2	2	2
3	Stroke	8.2	27.5	7	4	4	4
4	Accidents	5.7	19.0	3	3	5	3
5	Respiratory disease	3.8	12.7	8	9	3	8
6	Influenza/ pneumonia	3.2	10.6	9	—	7	10
7	Diabetes mellitus	3.0	10.1	5	6	6	7
8	Suicide	2.3	7.7	6	8	8	—
9	Homicide	1.9	6.3	10	5	—	5
10	Nephritis	1.6	5.4	—	—	9	9

Source: National Center for Health Statistics.

TABLE 12.3. LEADING CAUSES OF DEATH FOR ASIAN/PACIFIC ISLANDER FEMALES COMPARED WITH FEMALES OF OTHER ETHNIC GROUPS, 2001.

Rank for API Females	Cause of Death	Percentage of Total Deaths	Age-Adjusted Death Rate	*Rank for Females in Other Groups*			
				American Indian/ Alaska Native	Hispanic/ Latina	White	African American
1	Cancer	27.0	74.0	1	2	2	2
2	Heart disease	24.8	67.9	2	1	1	1
3	Stroke	10.9	29.8	5	3	3	3
4	Diabetes mellitus	3.7	10.3	4	4	8	4
5	Accidents	3.6	10.0	3	5	7	6
6	Influenza/ pneumonia	3.2	8.7	8	6	6	9
7	Respiratory disease	2.5	6.8	6	7	4	7
8	Nephritis	1.8	4.9	9	8	9	5
9	Hypertension and hypertensive renal disease	1.4	3.7	—	—	—	—
10	Alzheimer's disease	1.1	3.0	—	—	5	—

Source: National Center for Health Statistics.

Cardiovascular Disease and Stroke. Native Hawaiians have a relatively high rate of hypertension, which contributes to high death rates for heart disease and stroke (Curb et al., 1996). One study (Taira, Seto, & Marciel, 2001) found evidence that Native Hawaiians had a lower likelihood of undergoing aggressive surgical interventions compared to their White counterparts. That study also showed that Native Hawaiians were more likely to undergo coronary artery bypass graft surgery. The authors suggested that this finding could be the result of delays in seeking care, which can lead to Native Hawaiians being diagnosed at later stages of disease, when the prognosis is not as good. This tends to suggest that Native Hawaiians had less access to care or they are less apt to use health services when such services are available to them. Samoans and Chamorros also suffer from high rates of hypertension, heart disease, and stroke (Wergowske, Blanchette, & Diaz, 1999).

One somewhat unexpected finding is that Japanese American men in the United States have a high stroke death rate (Kiyohara et al., 2003). Most other APIs have

TABLE 12.4. LEADING CAUSES OF DEATH ACROSS THE LIFE SPAN FOR ASIAN/PACIFIC ISLANDER ADULTS, 2001.

Rank	20–24	25–34	Age Group 35–44	45–54	55–65
1	Accidents	Accidents	Cancer	Cancer	Cancer
2	Suicide	Cancer	Heart disease	Heart disease	Heart disease
3	Homicide	Homicide	Accidents	Stroke	Stroke
4	Cancer	Suicide	Suicide	Accidents	Diabetes
5	Heart disease	Heart disease	Homicide	Diabetes	Accidents
6	Congenital malformations	Stroke	Stroke	Suicide	Respiratory disease
7	Septicemia	HIV/AIDS	Liver disease/ cirrhosis	Homicide	Nephritis
8	Influenza/ pneumonia	Septicemia	HIV/AIDS	Liver disease/ cirrhosis	Liver disease/ cirrhosis
9	Stroke	Congenital malformations	Diabetes	Viral hepatitis	Suicide
10	Respiratory disease	Influenza/ pneumonia	Viral hepatitis	Respiratory disease	Viral hepatitis

Source: National Center for Health Statistics.

stroke rates similar to those of White Americans. Among Filipino Americans, high blood pressure is a significant public health problem (Ryan et al., 2000). The problem is particularly severe among Filipino American women, who are substantially more likely to have poorly controlled hypertension compared with other racial/ethnic groups (Liu, 1985). This finding is somewhat puzzling, as APIs in general have a lower prevalence of some of the best-understood cardiovascular and stroke risks (such as obesity, smoking, and high cholesterol) (Office of Minority Health Resource Center, 1988).

Cancer. The diversity of the API population leads to variation in cancer incidence rates. These dissimilarities reflect environmental and culturally influenced factors (such as diet) that differ across the various countries of origin and ethnic groups that this population comprises. For example, Japanese and Chinese patients diagnosed with bladder cancer have higher survival rates than Whites; however, Filipino and Hawaiian patients have lower survival compared with Whites (Hashibe, Gao, Li, Dalbagni, & Zhang, 2003). Native Hawaiians have the highest stomach cancer mortality rates among all racial/ethnic groups and the third highest for breast cancer (Miller et al., 1996).

In a comparative study between Native Hawaiian and American Samoan males, Mishra, Luce-Aoelua, & Wilkens (1996) found higher rates of lung, prostate, thyroid, and liver cancers and lower rates of colorectal cancers among American Samoan men. They also found that Samoan women have higher rates of leukemia, thyroid, and pancreatic cancers, and lower rates of colorectal cancers. Finally, incidence rates of thyroid cancer are higher among female Southeast Asians immigrants compared with other women living in the United States (Haselkorn, Stewart, & Horn-Ross, 2003).

Diabetes. Diabetes is highly prevalent among some of the subgroups that the API population comprises. The diabetes prevalence rate is particularly high among the Guamanian and Chamorro populations. These populations are four to seven times more likely to develop diabetes than Whites. They also are more likely to develop secondary complications from the disease and to die prematurely (Papa Ola Lokahi, 1998; Wergowske et al., 1999). A study conducted by Pinhey, Rubinstein, and Colfax (1997) found that the Guamanian and Chamorro population had higher rates of diabetes than other APIs and Whites.

Mental Health. As was discussed in Chapter Five, good-quality data on mental health are limited. This is particularly true for Asian/Pacific Islanders. Much of what is known about mental health in the API population comes from hospital or medical records, which record patterns of use of mental health services (Takeuchi et al., 1998). This is a severe limitation because such data can only assess those persons who seek and obtain health care. Because APIs are more likely than others (except Hispanics/Latinos) to lack adequate health insurance, research based on hospital records would likely significantly underestimate the level of need of mental health services for APIs.

Moreover, in some Pacific Islander subgroups mental health is considered to be integrated holistically with biological, social, cognitive, and spiritual functioning (Lee & Mokuau, 2002). Some API cultures do not even have a word that directly translates into *mental illness*. For example, Native Hawaiians typically use the general word for trouble, *pilikia,* for an emotional or psychological problem (Rezentes, 1996).

Furthermore, a large proportion of APIs are immigrants, and immigrants are known to have a higher prevalence of mental health problems associated with difficulty adjusting to a new society. Immigrants are also less likely to seek mental health services. As such, it is likely that available estimates of mental illness are underestimated (Yamashiro & Matsuoka, 1997). Thus the true prevalence of mental illness in the API population is very difficult to determine. Takeuchi et al. (1998) suggested two hypotheses regarding the true prevalence of psychiatric disorders in this population. The first hypothesis is that APIs would have a high prevalence of mental disorders due to the stress of adjusting to a new country. A second, somewhat contradictory hypothesis is that APIs would have a low prevalence of mental disorders (especially mood disorders) because of culturally related modes of expression of psychiatric distress. APIs are known to be more likely to express their problems behaviorally or somatically (by way of physical bodily symptoms).

BOX 12.2.   CULTURE-BOUND SYNDROMES.

Culture-bound syndromes are psychological conditions that are confined to certain cultures or cultural groups.

BOX 12.3.   SELECTED CULTURE-BOUND SYNDROMES IN ASIAN/PACIFIC ISLANDER POPULATIONS.

Amok	Southeast Asian males showing sudden assaultive behavior
Hwa-byung	A Korean response to prolonged suppressed anger, causing epigastric distress and fears of death
Latah	An exaggerated startled response to minimal stimuli in Japanese and Southeast Asian women
Taijin kyofusho	Intense fear among Japanese that one's bodily functions give offense to others
Dhat	Southeast Asian anxiety over the loss of semen

Culture-bound syndrome is a term used to describe the uniqueness of some mental syndromes in specific cultures (see Chapter Five). There are no accurate data on the prevalence of psychopathology in APIs. However, culture-bound syndromes—although rare—are an important aspect of the mental health profile of the API population. Culturally unique syndromes of mental illness associated with APIs include *amok* and *dhat* (Southeast Asia), *hwa-byung* (Korea), *taijin kyofusho* (Japan), and *latah* (Japan and Southeast Asia) (Sumathipala, Siribaddana, & Bhugra, 2004; Park et al., 2001; Lin, 1983).

In general, suicide rates for APIs in the United States are lower than the rates for other groups. However, among older API individuals the suicide rate is higher. In a large study of patients of the Department of Veterans Affairs Medical Centers, Bartels et al. (2002) screened patients for suicidal and death ideations. The study found that API patients had the highest rate of both death ideation and suicide ideation of all racial/ethnic groups (see Figure 12.3).

Furthermore, several studies have found that Native Hawaiians have high rates of depression, have lower self-esteem than other racial/ethnic groups, and are more than other groups likely to commit suicide (Crabbe, 1998; Marsella, Oliveira, Plummer, & Crabbe, 1995; Kaholokula, Grandinetti, Crabbe, Chang, & Kenui, 1999).

FIGURE 12.3.   SUICIDAL AND DEATH IDEATIONS AMONG PATIENTS IN VA MEDICAL CENTERS.

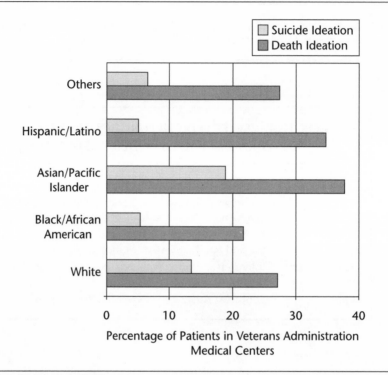

Source: Bartels et al., 2002.

Health Care Access and Utilization

The Asian/Pacific Islander population of the United States has been growing at a rapid rate over the past two decades. Much of this growth has come by way of immigration, and in many cases Asian immigrants enter the United States with limited proficiency in English. This has predictable implications for accessing health care. Limited English proficiency is a severe impediment to obtaining quality care. However, although language and cultural barriers have been severe problems for Hispanic/Latino immigrants, one might think that the problem would be less severe for APIs because of the larger proportion of API physicians. One study found that APIs who have a usual source of health care are more likely to have a physician who is of the same racial/ethnic group compared with other racial/ethnic groups (with the exception of Whites) (LaVeist & Nuru-Jeter, 2002).

However, this perception would be misleading. In fact, there are significant health and health care concerns for several API subgroups. Specifically, Southeast Asian refugees tend to underuse health care services (Uba, 1992). A study conducted by Uba found that underutilization of health services is caused by cultural factors such as attitudes toward suffering (such as beliefs that suffering is inevitable or that one's life span is predetermined). Such attitudes can make one disinclined to seek health care.

Traditional Medical Practices

One important complication in the quality of care received by APIs is the coexistence of traditional and Western medicine. According to the National Center for Complementary and Alternative Medicine (2004), a center of the National Institutes of Health, more than 43 percent of Asians use "alternative medicines" (excluding megavitamin therapy). The use of traditional medicine can affect the efficacy of Western medicine in several ways. Some traditional medical practices may be harmful. For example, one report from the Centers for Disease Control and Prevention (2004) found that Ayurveda, a traditional form of medicine practiced in India and other South Asian countries, could result in lead poisoning in adults. According to the CDC, "Ayurvedic medications can contain herbs, minerals, metals, or animal products and are made in standardized and nonstandardized formulations."

Traditional medicine can also affect Western medicine's efficacy by influencing patients' treatment-seeking behavior. Ngo-Metzger and colleagues (2003) found that most Chinese and Vietnamese participants in their focus groups reported delaying seeking care and trying traditional medicine before seeking care from a Western medicine provider. An additional limitation identified by Ngo-Metzger and colleagues was that Asian immigrants reported that they encountered negative attitudes from physicians when they disclosed that they have used traditional Asian medicine. This makes patients less likely to disclose their use of traditional medical remedies to their Western physicians, and it can serve to hinder the development of a trusting doctor-patient relationship that is important for the provision of good-quality care.

Language and Culture as Barriers to Care

Language limitations are also an important barrier to obtaining good-quality care. Often API immigrants rely on relatives to serve as language interpreters during medical encounters. However, this practice can have problematic consequences, such as difficulty maintaining the privacy of the patient's health information. It is also difficult to determine the accuracy of the translation and whether the patient is receiving good-quality information about their health. Even in the presence of good-quality language interpretation services, the language barrier may make the patient less likely to ask all of the questions they might have or to fully disclose information that might be important for the physician to know.

Johnson, Saha, Arbelaez, Beach, and Cooper (2004) conducted an analysis of the Commonwealth Fund Minority Health Survey (a national sample of Whites, African Americans, Hispanics, and APIs) to examine patients' perceptions of quality of care. In that survey APIs consistently reported less communication with their health care providers compared with all other racial/ethnic groups. For example, as Figure 12.4 reveals, APIs were less likely to report that their doctor listened to what they said, and were more likely to report that they did not have as much input into decision-making as they would have liked. API respondents to the survey were also less likely than White, African American, or Hispanic respondents to report that their doctor understands them, and were more likely to agree with the statement, "I often feel as if my doctor looks down on me and the way I live my life."

FIGURE 12.4. PATIENT-DOCTOR COMMUNICATION IN THE COMMONWEALTH FUND MINORITY HEALTH SURVEY, 2001.

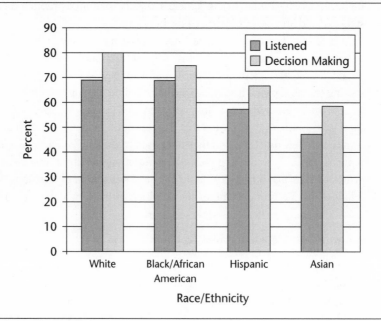

Source: Based on Johnson et al., 2004.

Major Health Issues Among Asians/Pacific Islanders

In health behavior, as in other aspects of health, the lack of good-quality data limits the conclusions that one can make about Asians/Pacific Islanders. However, a review of the literature reveals a handful of studies (many of them small) that present a picture of the API population as highly diverse, with many cultural aspects that have direct implications for health and illness behaviors.

One study challenged the commonly held beliefs that there are few if any heavy drinkers among Asian Americans, and that Asian subgroups would exhibit similar patterns of drinking (Chi, Lubben, & Kitano, 1989). The study team conducted a survey of Chinese, Japanese, and Korean Americans in Los Angeles. Their data found heavy drinkers in each group. They also found variation among the groups: Japanese Americans had the highest proportion of heavy drinkers, and Chinese Americans had the lowest.

Wong, Klingle, and Price (2004) demonstrated higher rates of alcohol, cigarette, and illicit drug use among Pacific Islanders compared with Chinese, Filipino, and Japanese American study participants. As Figure 12.5 demonstrates, rate of use of alcohol, tobacco, and other drugs (ATOD) were substantially higher among Pacific Islanders compared with the other groups. In some cases the Pacific Islander ATOD utilization rate was greater than three times the rate of the comparison groups.

Chinese and Japanese Americans living in the United States have a greater risk (compared with Whites) of developing two cancers that are closely associated with smoking and heavy alcohol consumption: cancer of the esophagus and cancer of the pancreas (Makimoto, Oda, & Higuchi, 2000). The incidence rate for esophageal cancer is 2.5 times higher for Japanese American men, 1.8 times higher for Chinese American men, and 1.6 times higher for Chinese American women than for their White counterparts. Cancer of the pancreas is 20 percent higher among Chinese American women than among White women, and this cancer is increasing in both Chinese American men and women.

Culturally Related Beliefs and Values

Some Southeast Asian refugees maintain beliefs that ancestral spirits or supernatural powers (such as the spirits of nature, trees, and the forest) can influence health both negatively and positively (Eisenbruch & Handelman, 1990). Most Pacific Islander cultures also place a great deal of importance on the spirit realm. Such cultures exhibit respect for nature and emphasize collective over individual needs—a characteristic called *allocentrism* (Mokuau & Tauili'ili, 1998; Palafox & Warren, 1980). Also, these cultures place great importance on respect for the wisdom of elders (Harden, 1999;

FIGURE 12.5.   CURRENT USE OF ALCOHOL, TOBACCO, AND OTHER
DRUGS AMONG CHINESE, FILIPINO, JAPANESE, PACIFIC ISLANDER,
AND WHITE NINTH GRADERS.

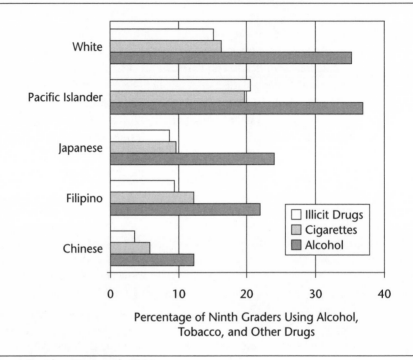

Percentage of Ninth Graders Using Alcohol,
Tobacco, and Other Drugs

Source: Based on Wong et al., 2004.

Mokuau & Browne, 1994). Each of these values can influence patterns of health services use, including use of preventive health services, curative care, and long-term care
for seniors.

Because mental impairment is viewed as an integrated part of the balance among
humanity, the environment, and the spiritual realm (Mokuau, Lukela, Obra, & Voeller,
1997; Mokuau, Reid, & Napalapalai, 2002), in API populations mental disability
can go untreated. For example, many Hawaiians view dementia symptoms as a normal part of the aging process (Braun & Browne, 1998). As such, they may feel no need
to seek health care for this devastating disease.

Furthermore, families are expected to provide care for sick or disabled family
members, because such caregiving is believed to have important spiritual significance (Braun, Mokuau, & Tsark, 1997). People are expected to have cared for those
who have died, and the spirits of the dead are expected to watch over the living
(McLaughlin & Braun, 1998). Because of the cultural imperative to care for sick family

---

BOX 12.4.   ALLOCENTRISM.

Allocentrism is a characteristic of cultures that emphasizes the needs, objectives, and points of view of the group over the individual. Allocentrism is a feature of most Asian/Pacific Islander cultures (Schaubroeck, Lam, & Xie, 2000) as well as most Hispanic cultures (Bassford, 1995).

---

members, it is not uncommon for families to attempt to take on care responsibilities that—in Western societies—are typically handled in health care facilities. The Hawaiian word for this concept is *kokua* (cooperation)—reciprocity among people, especially family. Family members are expected to anticipate each other's needs and help each other without being asked.

Although in general most would probably consider *kokua* to be a desirable familial value, it can also have the unintended negative consequence of undermining efforts by health care providers to have patients benefit from self-care, rehabilitation, and end-of-life planning (Braun et al., 1997; Braun & Nichols, 1996). However, if the health care provider understands the culture and works through the patient's *haku* (decision maker), they can incorporate the family into the care process and decision making. *Kokua* can be used as a positive force for improving health care outcomes, by increasing the odds that the patient will be compliant (Braun et al., 1997; Braun & Browne, 1998).

One study examined knowledge about cancer risks among Samoans living in American Samoa, Hawaii, and Los Angeles (Mishra, Luce-Aoelua, & Hubbell, 2000). Some believed that cancer can be caused by *aitu* (spirits), that cancer is a punishment from God, and that cancer can be cured by *fofo* (traditional Samoan healers). Samoans residing in American Samoa and Hawaii were more likely to hold these beliefs compared to those living in Los Angeles. Some Samoan women expressed feelings of embarrassment after allowing a physician to touch their body. This can discourage some women from consenting to certain health exams (Ishida, Toomata-Mayer, & Braginsky, 2001; Braun, Yee, Browne, & Mokuau, 2004).

"Coining," "coin rubbing," or *cao gio* is an ancient Vietnamese folk remedy that is practiced by many Vietnamese Americans to treat minor ailments. The back, neck, head, shoulder, and chest are common sites of application. The procedure is usually harmless; however, there have been some documented negative health effects, such as severe burns (Amshel & Caruso, 2000), but these complications are atypical. Even though there are usually no serious complications, the resulting burns and lesions resemble trauma and can lead to misunderstandings. For example, teachers, medical personnel, and social workers may misinterpret the lesions as resulting from abuse (Buchwald, Panwala, & Hooton, 1992).

BOX 12.5.   COINING AND CUPPING.

Coining: the practice of rubbing the spine and sternum with oil and a coin to release the "wind" or "cold" element.

Cupping: the practice of heating air in a cup with a flame and placing the cup onto the skin to pull out the cold air.

Source: Pachter, 1994.

Acculturation and Health

It is well known that the degree to which Asian and Pacific Islanders are acculturated to American culture (Americanized) can be associated with health status and health behavior. (The effects of acculturation on health are discussed in more detail in Chapter Seven.) However, the relationship between acculturation and health and health behavior can operate in multiple directions.

There are two somewhat contradictory propositions regarding acculturation and health among the API population. The first proposition is that immigrants who are *more* acculturated into American culture can have better health outcomes and behaviors, because as they become more Americanized they become more effective users of health care services (for example, they are better able to communicate with providers, better able to advocate for themselves, and have greater appreciation for preventive health measures). The second proposition is that immigrants who are *less* acculturated into American culture can have better health outcomes and behaviors because as yet they have not adopted a high-fat diet and sedentary American lifestyle, which would increase their risk for chronic diseases such as heart disease, cancer, and diabetes.

There is evidence to support both of these propositions. For example, Yi (1995) conducted a survey of Vietnamese women to examine the effect of acculturation on access and use of preventive health services. The study found that the more acculturated Vietnamese women were more likely to report having a "routine place for health care and a regular provider." They were also more likely than less acculturated women to have had a Pap smear and clinical breast examination. On the other hand, Pinhey, Heathcote, and Rarick (1994) found higher rates of obesity among more acculturated Chamorro women. However, although there is empirical support for both propositions, the overall evidence that acculturation leads to worse health consequences among Asians seems to have more empirical support (Frisbie et al., 2002).

Summary

This chapter provided an overview of issues in the health of the Asian/Pacific Islander population. This is a highly diverse group with many subgroups. The health issues vary widely across these groups. Some of the subgroups that the API category comprises are emigrants from countries that have some of the best health statistics in the world (such as Japan), but others come from countries or territories that have many health challenges (such as Samoans, Kanaka Maoli, and Hmong). When all of these groups are combined together, the variation among the subgroups is masked. And since the mortality and morbidity rates for the combined group are very good, there is a risk that the underlying health issues that affect some API subpopulations will be overlooked. For this reason one must be very careful when making general statements about Asians/Pacific Islanders.

For a case study, see Appendix A. See Appendix B for additional readings.

Key Words

Culture-bound syndrome

Complementary and alternative medicine

Allocentrism

Acculturation

CHAPTER THIRTEEN

HISPANIC/LATINO HEALTH ISSUES

Outline

Introduction

In the last decades of the twentieth century the Hispanic/Latino population of the United States expanded rapidly. According to the U.S. Bureau of the Census, in 1980 there were approximately 14.6 million Hispanics/Latinos living in the United States. By 2000 that number had exploded nearly 142 percent to 35.3 million. The Hispanic/Latino population has now displaced African Americans as the largest minority group in the United States. And the Census Bureau projects that by the middle of the twenty-first century, largely because of the growth of the Hispanic/Latino population, the U.S.-based racial/ethnic minority population will exceed the White population. These statistics make an impression; however, they suggest that Hispanics/Latinos are a monolithic ethnic group. This is certainly not the case; the term *Hispanics* or *Latinos* describes a large group of people of different nationalities, ethnicities, and races (Falcon, Aguirre-Molina, & Molina, 2001).

Table 13.1 and Figure 13.1 show the diversity of the Hispanic population in the 2000 census. Mexican Americans are the largest subgroup—nearly 60 percent of all Hispanics/Latinos. Puerto Ricans are the second largest group. Together Mexican Americans and Puerto Ricans account for over two thirds of the Hispanic/Latino population.

The Hispanic/Latino population is young relative to other racial/ethnic groups. In 2000 some 25.7 percent of the total U.S. population was under age eighteen, but 35 percent of the Hispanic population was under age eighteen. Hispanics also have the highest fertility rate. This combination of demographic facts—a large proportion of young persons and a high fertility rate—leads to a high "natural increase" in the Hispanic/Latino population. Additionally, Hispanics/Latinos have a high rate of immigration (rivaled only by Asians).

Although Mexico still contributes the largest number of immigrants to the United States, increasingly Hispanic/Latino immigration is coming from Central and South America. Between 1980 and 2000 the Central and South American population in the United States doubled, from 7 percent to more than 14 percent. During the same time span the proportion of Mexicans, Puerto Ricans, and Cubans remained essentially unchanged (Falcon, Aguirre-Molina, & Molina, 2001). Salvadorians are the largest Central American subgroup, making up nearly 39 percent of all immigrants from that region. The South American nation with the largest percentage of Hispanic expatriates is Colombia: nearly 35 percent of South Americans living in the United States are from Colombia.

BOX 13.1.   HISPANIC OR LATINO: WHAT'S IN A NAME?

There is no universally accepted term for describing and defining the population we call Hispanic or Latino. In 1995 the U.S. Bureau of the Census conducted a survey to determine which term was preferred by most Americans of Latin American descent. The survey found that the majority (57.88 percent) preferred Hispanic, whereas only 11.74 percent preferred Latino. For this book I decided to use both terms because there are compelling arguments in favor of Latino as well. For a complete discussion of Hispanic/Latino terminology, see Chapter Nine of the companion reader to this textbook (Hayes-Bautista & Chapa, 2002).

TABLE 13.1.   HISPANIC POPULATION BY NATIONALITY, 2000.

Nationality	Number	Percent
All Hispanics	35,305,818	100.0
Mexican	20,640,711	58.5
Puerto Rican	3,406,178	9.6
Cuban	1,241,685	3.5
Dominican Republic	764,945	2.2
Spanish	100,135	0.3
All other Hispanics	10,017,244	28.4
Central American (excluding Mexican)	1,686,937	4.8
Costa Rican	68,588	0.2
Guatemalan	372,487	1.1
Honduran	217,569	0.6
Nicaraguan	177,684	0.5
Panamanian	91,723	0.3
Salvadoran	655,165	1.9
Other Central American	103,721	0.3
South American	1,353,562	3.8
Argentinean	100,864	0.3
Bolivian	42,068	0.1
Chilean	68,849	0.2
Colombian	470,684	1.3
Ecuadorian	260,559	0.7
Paraguayan	8,769	0.0
Peruvian	233,926	0.7
Uruguayan	18,804	0.1
Venezuelan	91,507	0.3
Other South American	57,532	0.2

Source: U.S. Bureau of the Census, Census 2000.

Death Rates and Causes of Death Among Hispanics/Latinos

Table 13.2 displays age-specific death rates for Hispanics/Latinos compared with other racial/ethnic groups. The table shows the Hispanic death rate for each age group and the rate ratios for the other racial/ethnic groups compared with Hispanics/Latinos. A rate ratio of 1.0 indicates that Hispanics/Latinos and the comparison group have an equal death rate for the indicated age group. A rate ratio greater than 1.0 indicates Hispanics/Latinos have a higher death rate than the comparison group; for example, a rate ratio of 1.5 indicates that the Hispanic/Latino death rate is one and one half times greater; 2.0 indicates that the Hispanic/Latino death rate is two times greater. If the rate ratio is less than 1.0, this indicates that Hispanics/Latinos have a lower death rate than the comparison group.

FIGURE 13.1 COUNTRY OF ORIGIN OF THE U.S. HISPANIC POPULATION, 2000.

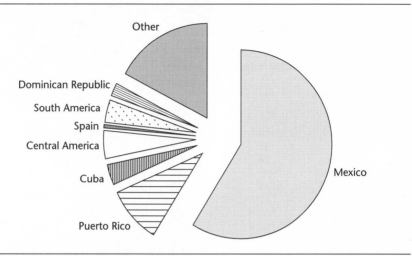

Source: U.S. Bureau of the Census, Census 2000.

Table 13.2 shows that Hispanics/Latinos generally have a lower death rate compared with American Indians/Alaska Natives (AIANs). The Hispanic/Latino death rates are lower for nearly every age group into middle age, but by age forty-five the rates converge and then the Hispanic/Latino death rate exceeds the death rate for AIANs. This pattern results from the phenomenon of selective survival, discussed in Chapter Four, which leads to a crossover in death rates whereby American Indians/ Alaska Natives and African Americans have lower death rates than other racial/ethnic groups in old age (Markides & Machalek, 1984).

When comparing Hispanics/Latinos to Asian/Pacific Islanders (APIs), the pattern is quite different. Across all age groups, the Hispanic/Latino age-specific death rates are higher than the death rates for APIs. The rate ratios range from 1.4 to 2.5, with the largest disparities occurring during adulthood and middle age. This pattern is in stark contrast with comparisons of Hispanics/Latinos and Whites. The rate ratios for these comparisons show a nearly uniform pattern, with similar death rates at all ages. Finally, comparisons of Hispanics/Latinos with African Americans show substantially lower death rates for Hispanics/Latinos across the age spectrum. Only in the oldest age groups (beginning around age eighty and continuing into the eighty-five and above age group) do the rates converge.

TABLE 13.2. AGE-SPECIFIC DEATH RATES FOR HISPANICS/LATINOS COMPARED WITH OTHER RACIAL/ETHNIC GROUPS, 2001.

Age	Hispanic/Latino Death Rate	Rate Ratios			
		American Indian/ Alaska Native	Asian/ Pacific Islander	White	African American
1–4	33.8	0.7	1.5	1.1	0.7
5–9	15.8	1.0	1.4	1.1	0.7
10–14	19.6	0.7	1.5	1.1	0.7
15–19	67.3	0.7	1.8	1.1	0.8
20–24	96.2	0.9	2.0	1.1	0.6
25–29	99.2	0.8	2.3	1.1	0.6
30–34	117.5	0.8	2.3	1.1	0.6
35–39	170.6	0.8	2.4	1.1	0.6
40–44	245.8	0.9	2.5	1.1	0.6
45–49	360.4	1.0	2.2	1.1	0.5
50–54	519.3	1.0	2.1	1.1	0.5
55–59	783.7	1.1	2.0	1.1	0.6
60–64	1,228.7	1.1	2.0	1.1	0.6
65–69	1,896.2	1.1	1.9	1.0	0.7
70–74	2,908.7	1.1	1.8	1.0	0.7
75–79	4,528.0	1.3	1.7	1.0	0.8
80–84	7,201.4	1.4	1.6	1.0	0.9
85 or older	15,199.0	1.7	1.6	1.0	1.0

Source: National Center for Health Statistics.

Table 13.3 displays the ten leading causes of death for Hispanic/Latino males. The ten leading causes of death for Hispanic/Latina females are listed in Table 13.4. In addition to showing the age-adjusted death rate and the percentage of all Hispanic/Latino deaths accounted for by that cause of death, the tables also shows where that cause of death ranks among the other racial/ethnic groups. Heart disease and cancer are the two leading causes of death for Hispanic/Latino men, as is the case for all men. Together heart disease and cancer account for more than 41 percent of all deaths of Hispanic/Latino men. Unintended injury and stroke are third and fourth on the list. Each of these causes is among the top five for men of other racial/ethnic groups as well (with the exception of stroke, the seventh leading cause of death among Native American men).

TABLE 13.3. LEADING CAUSES OF DEATH FOR HISPANIC/LATINO MALES COMPARED WITH MALES OF OTHER ETHNIC GROUPS, 2001.

Rank for Hispanic/ Latino Males	Cause of Death	Percentage of Total Deaths	Age-Adjusted Death Rate	Rank for Males in Other Groups			
				White	African American	American Indian/ Alaska Native	Asian/ Pacific Islander
1	Heart disease	22.4	74.6	1	1	1	1
2	Cancer	18.7	62.2	2	2	2	2
3	Accident (unintentional injury)	11.3	37.6	3	3	3	4
4	Stroke	4.7	15.7	5	4	7	3
5	Homicide	4.4	14.5	—	5	10	9
6	Diabetes mellitus	4.1	13.6	6	7	5	7
7	Liver disease/ cirrhosis	3.8	12.7	10	—	4	—
8	Suicide	2.5	8.3	8	—	6	—
9	Respiratory disease	2.3	7.8	4	8	8	5
10	HIV/AIDS	2.3	7.6	—	6	—	—

Source: National Center for Health Statistics.

For Hispanics/Latinos, the homicide rate stands out from other racial/ethnic groups. Homicide is the fifth leading cause of deaths among Hispanic/Latino males, but is not in the top five for any other group except for African Americans. Perhaps the most noteworthy causes of death to make the top ten for Hispanics/Latinos are liver disease (or cirrhosis of the liver) and HIV/AIDS. Both causes of death are associated with stigmatized behavior (de Bruyn, 2002; Riston, 1999): liver disease and cirrhosis is often associated with alcohol abuse, and HIV is associated with the use of injection drugs (such as heroin) and unsafe sexual behavior.

Four of the five leading causes of death among Hispanic/Latina women are similar to those of their male counterparts: heart disease, cancer, stroke, and unintentional injury. This pattern also resembles those for other women. There are, however, two noteworthy departures in the leading cause of death for Hispanic women compared with women of other racial/ethnic groups: the tenth leading cause of death is liver disease and cirrhosis, which accounts for nearly 2 percent of all deaths of Hispanic/Latina women. American Indian/Alaska Native females are the only other group of females for which liver disease is among the ten leading causes of death. A study conducted by the National Institute on Alcohol Abuse and Alcoholism found that among the Hispanic subgroups, Mexican Americans had the highest death rate from liver cirrhosis (Stinson, Grant, & Dufour, 2001).

The ninth leading cause of death for Hispanic/Latina women is maternal mortality or pregnancy-related death; the number of pregnancy-related deaths per 100,000 live births is called the pregnancy-related mortality ratio (PRMR; see Table 13.5). The Centers for Disease Control and Prevention (2001) define pregnancy-related death as "a death that occurred during pregnancy or within 1 year after the end of pregnancy and resulted from 1) complications of pregnancy itself, 2) a chain of events initiated by pregnancy, or 3) aggravation of an unrelated condition by the physiologic effects of pregnancy."

BOX 13.2.   FERTILITY RATE VERSUS BIRTH RATE.

The difference between fertility rate and birth rate is that when calculating fertility rate, the denominator is restricted to the number of women of childbearing age (usually considered to be ages fifteen to forty-four); when calculating the birth rate, the denominator is the total population.

TABLE 13.4. LEADING CAUSES OF DEATH FOR HISPANIC/LATINA FEMALES COMPARED WITH FEMALES OF OTHER ETHNIC GROUPS, 2001.

Rank for Hispanic/ Latino Females	Cause of Death	Percentage of Total Deaths	Age-Adjusted Death Rate	Rank for Females in Other Groups			
				White	African American	American Indian/ Alaska Native	Asian/ Pacific Islander
1	Heart disease	25.7	71.8	1	1	2	2
2	Cancer	21.1	58.7	2	2	1	1
3	Stroke	6.9	19.1	3	3	5	3
4	Diabetes mellitus	6.1	17.1	8	4	4	4
5	Accident (unintentional injury)	4.7	13.2	7	6	3	5
6	Influenza/ pneumonia	2.8	7.9	6	9	8	6
7	Respiratory disease	2.7	7.5	4	7	6	7
8	Nephritis	1.9	5.4	9	5	9	8
9	Maternal mortality (childbirth)	1.9	5.3	–	–	–	–
10	Liver disease/ cirrhosis	1.8	5.0	–	–	7	–

Source: National Center for Health Statistics.

TABLE 13.5.   PREGNANCY-RELATED MORTALITY RATIOS AMONG HISPANIC, ASIAN/PACIFIC ISLANDER, AMERICAN INDIAN/ALASKA NATIVE, NON-HISPANIC BLACK (BLACK), AND NON-HISPANIC WHITE (WHITE) WOMEN, UNITED STATES, 1993–1997.

Pregnancy-Related Mortality Ratio (PRMR)	Hispanic	Asian/ Pacific Islander	American Indian/ Alaska Native	Non-Hispanic Black	Non-Hispanic White	Total
U.S.-born women[a]	8.0	6.1[b]	13.2	30.0	7.6	11.6
Foreign-born women	11.8	12.7	—[c]	29.5	6.2	12.4

Note: N = 2,334.

[a]Born in the fifty states and the District of Columbia.

[b]Fewer than seven pregnancy-related deaths; considered unreliable (relative standard error >38%).

[c]Point estimates based on seven to nineteen deaths are highly variable (relative standard error = 23% to 38%).

Source: Centers for Disease Control and Prevention, 2001.

Hispanic/Latina women have a high fertility rate and high teen birth rate combined with a low abortion rate. Motherhood is venerated in Latin American cultures, due in large part to the strong Catholic influence (Portugal & Claro, 1993). Women who are mothers enjoy a higher social standing than those who are not, and women who have abortions are stigmatized. These social influences may be partly responsible for encouraging pregnancies and discouraging the termination of high-risk pregnancies. It is possible, therefore, that the ranking of pregnancy-related death among the ten leading causes of death among Hispanic/Latina women is the result of a higher proportion of high-risk pregnancies going to term rather than ending in abortion.

Figure 13.2 presents data on birth outcomes of Mexican-born, U.S.-born Mexican American, and White non-Hispanic/Latina women in California. The figure shows that the Mexican-born women have lower infant mortality, neonatal mortality, postneonatal mortality, and low birth weight rates than both comparison groups.

FIGURE 13.2.   BIRTH OUTCOMES OF MEXICAN-BORN, U.S.-BORN MEXICAN AMERICAN, AND WHITE NON-LATINA WOMEN IN CALIFORNIA.

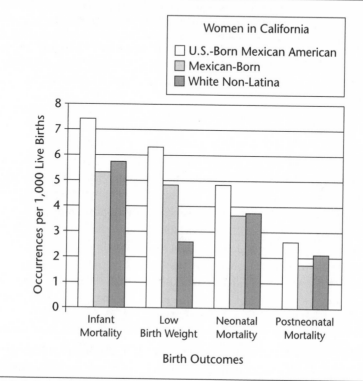

Source: Data from Iannotta, 2002.

Health Care Access and Utilization

The United States has the highest per-person spending on health care among the members of the Organization for Economic Cooperation and Development (OECD), which comprises thirty highly industrialized nations with market economies. Yet the United States ranks below many other OECD nations on health status indicators such as infant mortality and life expectancy (Woolhandler & Himmelstein, 1991). Access to health care is not the only reason for this, but it is certainly one of the reasons, and access to healthcare is closely related to health insurance. In the United States health insurance is largely tied to employment. Although many Americans have access to very high-quality health care, many others have only limited or no access to care.

BOX 13.3. WHAT IS THE "USUAL SOURCE OF CARE"?

Usual source of care was measured in the National Health Interview Survey (NHIS) by asking the respondent, "Is there a place that you usually go to when you are sick or need advice about your health?" Persons who report an emergency department as their usual source of care are defined as having no usual source. The NHIS is conducted by the National Center for Health Statistics.

Nearly 31 percent of Hispanics/Latinos do not have a usual source of health care. This is compared with Asians (18.5 percent), Blacks (16.7 percent), American Indians/Alaska Natives (15.9 percent), and Whites (13.9 percent). This is largely due to a high number of uninsured among Hispanics/Latinos (34.8 percent). Only American Indians/Alaska Natives (33.4 percent) have a proportion of persons without health insurance that approaches the Hispanic/Latino rate. There is, however, significant variation among Hispanic/Latino subgroups. Data from the National Health Interview Survey showed that although 17 percent of U.S.-born Cuban Americans and 12.0 percent of Puerto Ricans did not have health insurance, the rate for some other Hispanic subgroups was much higher. The rate for U.S.-born Central/South Americans was 23 percent and for U.S.-born Mexican Americans, 25 percent.

There are several reasons that Hispanics have less access to health care compared with other racial/ethnic groups. Again, the U.S. health care system operates under the assumption that most individuals will obtain health care insurance through their employer (Carrillo, Trevino, Betancourt, & Coustasse, 2001). A large proportion of Hispanics are immigrants (legal as well as undocumented). Immigrant status places significant limitations on employment options. Additionally, Hispanics tend to have fewer years of formal education compared with other American racial/ethnic groups. Among Hispanics there is also a higher proportion of individuals who have limited English proficiency, which also creates employment limitations. As such, many Hispanics have jobs that do not offer health insurance benefits. According to a study published by the Commonwealth Fund (Quinn, 2000), nearly nine million of the eleven million Hispanics who do not have health insurance live in a household in which at least one person is employed.

Variation in health insurance status is likely due to differences in legal status among the groups. For example, Puerto Ricans are U.S. citizens and as such have access to Medicare and Medicaid and can be legally employed. And U.S. immigration policy favors legalization for Cuban immigrants, which makes it less difficult for them to obtain health care benefits from either government sources or an employer. However, immigrants from Central/South America or Mexico are more likely to be in the country illegally without access to citizenship rights or protections such as government-funded health care. They are also less able to obtain employment in companies that offer health insurance benefits.

Major Health Issues Among Hispanics/Latinos

Although lack of health insurance is a major barrier to obtaining care, it is not the only barrier that impedes Hispanics from accessing good-quality health care. There are several important nonfinancial barriers as well. Language is one such barrier. In one study (Doty, 2003), 44 percent of Latinos reported that they "always, usually, or sometimes have a hard time speaking with or understanding the doctor because of language barriers." Forty-nine percent of Latinos reported that they "always or usually use an interpreter" when they seek medical care. And 30 percent reported that even with an interpreter they still do not fully understand what the doctor is telling them about their health.

Spanish-speaking patients typically obtain health care from a doctor who does not speak Spanish, and they most often receive care from a non-Hispanic provider. In addition to not speaking the patient's language, these health care providers may not understand the patient's cultural beliefs that influence their health and illness behavior (Rutherford & Roux, 2002). Many studies have shown that language barriers—even relatively minor ones—can be a major impediment to the delivery of good-quality care (Kirkman-Liff & Mondragon, 1991; Perez-Stable et al., 1997; Flores, Rabke-Verani, Pine, & Sabharwal, 2002). Compared with English speakers, patients who are primarily Spanish speakers are less likely to understand their diagnosis, medications, special instructions, and plans for follow-up care (Crane, 1997). Carrasquillo, Orav, Brennan, and Burstin (1999) found that Spanish-speaking patients were more likely to be dissatisfied with their care (see also Lee et al., 2002; Baker, Hayes, & Fortier, 1998) and to report that they were unwilling to return if they had a problem with their care. Studies show that professional language interpreter services can be cost effective (Jacobs, Shepard, Suaya, & Stone, 2004) and improve quality of care (Jacobs et al., 2001). However, such services are not widely available.

Good doctor-patient communication is essential to good-quality care. A study by LaVeist and Nuru-Jeter (2002) demonstrated that patients from all racial/ethnic groups were more satisfied with their care if their doctor was from the same group. However, such opportunities are rare for Hispanics, as only two percent of all physicians in the United States are Hispanic (Carrillo et al., 2001).

Poverty and Low Socioeconomic Status

Perhaps the greatest health risk factor faced by Hispanics is poverty combined with low socioeconomic status (SES). Poverty and low SES are linked to living in communities with greater exposure to physical environmental risks (such as chemical and other toxins) and social environmental risks (such as crime, illicit drugs, and poor quality housing) (Iannotta, 2002). Hispanics/Latinos have a high rate of poverty and low SES, so they have greater exposure to poverty-related health risks. When considering risk behavior among the poor, one often overlooked issue is that people living at the economic margins of society are forced to weigh health behavior against other competing priorities. Abating hunger may be more important than nutrition; paying for shelter may be more important than purchasing pharmaceuticals. This reality is exacerbated among those who are in the country illegally, who have the added fear of deportation even as they face language and cultural barriers and other limitations on their activities (such as driving, signing contracts, or, in some states, accessing health and social services).

Occupational Health

Hispanics/Latinos are more likely to be employed in occupations with high rates of unintentional injuries and exposures to health hazards. These occupations include farming and agricultural (largely seasonal and migrant farm workers), construction trades, and work in the garment industry. Among the most prevalent heath hazards among agricultural workers are chemical exposures, repetitive motion (such as bending or stooping), falls, and contact with objects or equipment (such as tools).

By definition, sweatshops are hazardous working environments (Moure-Eraso & Friedman-Jimenez, 2001). The General Accountability Office defines sweatshops as "businesses that regularly violate both safety or health and wage or child labor laws . . . chronic labor law violators." Although we typically associate sweatshops with the garment industry, a sweatshop can actually exist in any industry, including construction, agriculture, or piecework (such as in the manufacturing or assembly of apparel or electronics). The occupational health hazards associated with working in sweatshops include airborne hazards (such as dust, cleaning solvents, or other inhalants), ergonomic hazards (such as repetitive motion injuries, falls, or vibrating machinery), and hazards associated with extreme temperatures.

A related occupational concern are the so-called *maquiladora* industries (manufacturing or assembly plants located across the Mexican border). These factories primarily produce products for the U.S. market while taking advantage of the environmental, occupational health, and wage laws of Mexico. A study of females working in *maquiladoras* found musculoskeletal disorders and chemical exposures (Moure-Eraso, Wilcox, Punnett, Copeland, & Levenstein, 1994; Moure-Eraso et al., 1997).

HIV/AIDS

Hispanics/Latinos comprise about 13 percent of the U.S. population, yet they comprise more than 18 percent of all HIV/AIDS cases in the country (CDC, 2002c). And Hispanic/Latina women comprise more than 20 percent of females diagnosed with HIV/AIDS since records have been kept (Amaro, Vega, & Valencia, 2001). The HIV/AIDS case rate for Hispanics/Latinas is 16.6 cases per 1,000 women, nearly seven times the rate for non-Hispanic White women (2.4 per 1,000 women). Hispanic/Latino men comprise about 18 percent of all males ever diagnosed with the disease, and their incidence rate is more than three times the rate for Whites (58.2 and 17.8, respectively) (Amaro et al., 2001; CDC, 1998). HIV/AIDS is also highly prevalent among Hispanic/Latino children. According to Amaro et al. (2001), "Cumulative AIDS cases among Latino children and youth ages zero to nineteen represent 32.2 percent of all cases in this age group." HIV/AIDS incidence and prevalence rates are not reported for individual Hispanic/Latino subgroups; however, rates in Puerto Rico are substantially higher than the national average for the United States (the Puerto Rican rate is 29.5 compared with the U.S. national rate of 14.8) (CDC, 2002c).

The primary modes of HIV/AIDS transmission among Hispanics/Latinos are male-male sex, male-female sex, and injection drug use. Hispanics/Latinos have the lowest rate of condom use among all American racial/ethnic groups (Catania, Kegeles, & Coates, 1990). In one study, almost half of the sample of Hispanic/Latina women reported that they would not use condoms with their primary partner even if aware that the partner was HIV positive (Harrison et al., 1991). A study of female partners of male injection and non-injection drug users confirmed this finding (He, McCoy, Stevens, & Stark, 1998). Compared with women of other racial/ethnic groups, Hispanic/Latina women have fewer sexual partners (Romero, Wyatt, & Singer, 1998), yet they are at increased risk of acquiring HIV/AIDS because of multiple sex partners among Hispanic/Latino males (Choi et al., 1994; Romero-Daza, Weeks, & Singer, 1998). Also, male-male sex is highly stigmatized in Latin American cultures. This probably decreases the likelihood that Hispanic/Latino men would disclose their bisexuality to their female sex partners, so those partners may not be aware that they are at increased risk (Flaskerud, Uman, Lara, Romero, & Taka, 1996).

Injection drug use among Hispanics/Latinos is another major HIV/AIDS risk behavior. Amaro et al. (2001) report that Hispanics/Latinos (particularly those of Mexican and Puerto Rican descent) have the highest levels of drug-related risks for HIV/AIDS because of a higher prevalence of several high-risk behaviors: attending "shooting galleries," sharing needles, and having sex partners who are injection drug users (Sufian, Friedman, Curtis, Neaigus, & Stepherson, 1991). Higher rates of use of other drugs may also indirectly contribute to the high prevalence of HIV/AIDS among Hispanics/Latinos. Use of alcohol, crack cocaine, and other drugs may suppress inhibitions, leading individuals to make poor judgments related to risky sexual behavior (Romero-Daza et al., 1998).

Acculturation and Health

Franzini and colleagues (2002) define acculturation as "the process by which an individual raised in one culture enters the social structure and institutions of another, and internalizes the prevailing attitudes and beliefs of the new culture." Several studies have demonstrated a link between acculturation and health. Most of these studies have found that as individuals become more acculturated, they experience *worse* health effects (Coonrod, Bay, & Balcazar, 2004). Hispanics/Latinos who are more highly acculturated into mainstream U.S. culture have been found to have higher proportions of low birth-weight infants (Peete, 1999; Scribner & Dwyer, 1989) and are less likely to have their children immunized (Anderson, Wood, & Sherbourne, 1997), and females are more likely to be smokers (Balcazar, Castro, & Krull, 1995). It is possible that Hispanic/Latino immigrants have better health outcomes compared with U.S.-born Hispanics/Latinos because they are less acculturated into the U.S. culture and have not yet adopted its health risk behaviors, nor have they had extended exposure to the social stress and physical environmental health risks associated with growing up and living as a Hispanic/Latino in the United States. A handful of studies have found acculturation to be associated with better health outcomes (Ramirez et al., 2004; Yi, 1995).

Moreover, the acculturation hypothesis suggests that foreign-born Hispanics/Latinos have better health outcomes than non-Hispanic Whites because there are aspects of the Hispanic/Latino culture that are protective of health. Franzini et al. (2002) propose two possible contributing aspects: *confianza* (confidence), *familismo* (the centrality of the family), and *respeto* (respect for elders or individuals with experience). One can envision how these features of Hispanic/Latino cultures may be protective of health outcomes; for example, a pregnant woman who places great value on family would seek advice and support from other mothers, limit potentially harmful health behaviors during pregnancy (such as smoking and alcohol consumption), and obtain prenatal care.

Because acculturation is generally associated with negative health outcomes, as Hispanics/Latinos become more acculturated their health status would be expected to decline. Although this general pattern is true, the reality is more complicated. Several studies have found that Hispanics/Latinos who are less acculturated are at increased risk for several negative health outcomes. For example, Flaskerud et al. (1996) found that Hispanic/Latina females who were more acculturated tended to have more sex partners, but they were also more likely to use condoms (Marin, Tschann, Gomez, & Kegeles, 1993). Also, less acculturated Hispanics/Latinos are more likely to use alternative medications that may be harmful to health (CDC, 2004). A review of medical cases in one pediatric clinic found that more than one third of Spanish-speaking patients had used metamizole (a anti-inflammatory agent banned in the United States, but in wide use in Mexico and other Latin American countries), and in 25 percent of those cases of metamizole use they had purchased the drug in the United States (Bonkowsky, Frazer, Buchi, & Byington, 2002).

The Hispanic Epidemiological Paradox

Hispanics/Latinos tend to have more favorable health outcomes (mainly mortality rates, but not necessarily morbidity rates) than non-Hispanics/Latinos. This finding is considered paradoxical because Hispanics/Latinos tend to have higher rates of poverty, less educational attainment, and less access to health care services. Each of these factors is known to be associated with poorer health outcomes. Moreover, Hispanics/Latinos immigrate to the United States from countries that have generally worse health outcomes than in the United States.

The term *Hispanic epidemiological paradox* was coined by Markides and Coreil in their 1986 study. (The phenomenon is also referred to as the *epidemiological paradox*, the *Latino paradox*, and the *Latino epidemiological paradox*.) The first studies of the Hispanic epidemiological paradox examined pregnancy outcomes; however, subsequent studies have demonstrated the phenomenon in other health outcomes, including adult mortality (Bradshaw & Frisbie, 1992), heart disease (Goff, Ramsey, Labarthe, & Nichaman, 1994), stroke (Sacco et al., 1998), and cancer (Davis et al., 1995). A 2001 review of studies of the Hispanic epidemiological paradox by Franzini et al. is summarized in Table 13.6.

BOX 13.4. THE HISPANIC EPIDEMIOLOGICAL PARADOX

The Hispanic epidemiological paradox was described by Franzini et al. (2002) in this way: "Hispanics, as a group, have mortality (but not morbidity) outcomes equal [to] or surprisingly better than non-Hispanics in the United States, even though they rank low in most socioeconomic indicators."

TABLE 13.6. EVIDENCE FOR THE HISPANIC EPIDEMIOLOGICAL PARADOX.

Life Stage	Finding
Infancy	Hispanic infant mortality rate is lower than expected.
Youth	Excluding HIV and homicide deaths, Hispanic males have a lower mortality rate than White males aged 15 to 44.
Adulthood	For males aged 55 and older, Hispanics have lower mortality rates than Whites. These lower rates reflect lower mortality rates for most of the major chronic conditions.

Source: Adapted from Franzini et al., 2002.

BOX 13.5. THE HISPANIC EPIDEMIOLOGIC PARADOX: FOUR HYPOTHESES.

Data Reliability Hypothesis	Differences in the coding of ethnicity on birth and death records lead to misclassification, resulting in an artificially low death rate.
"Salmon Bias" Hypothesis	Migrants return home when they become seriously ill or reach old age. Their deaths are not recorded in the United States, thus producing a lower death rate for Hispanics.
Healthy Migrant Hypothesis	Selection bias leads to a healthier Hispanic population because migration requires relatively good health.
Risk Factors Hypothesis	Certain characteristics of Hispanic cultures place Hispanics at reduced health risk.

Figure 13.3 shows death rates from selected causes, with computed rate ratios for Hispanic/Latino compared with Whites for selected causes of death. The rate ratio is 1.0 if the Hispanic and White rates are the same, less than 1.0 if the Hispanic/Latino rate is lower than the White rate, and greater than 1.0 if the Hispanic rate is higher. The pattern of death rates demonstrates the Hispanic epidemiological paradox. The figure shows that with the exception of homicide, HIV, and alcohol-related liver disease, the Hispanic/Latino mortality rate is lower than the White rate. Each cause of death for which Hispanics/Latinos have higher rates is directly related to health behaviors.

Franzini et al. (2002) presented four possible hypotheses to explain the Hispanic epidemiological paradox.

The Data Reliability Hypothesis. This hypothesis posits that the Hispanic epidemiological paradox stems from poor-quality data; that is, the findings result from misclassification or errors in the reporting of data. In computing mortality rates, numerator data come from death certificates and denominator data from census data. Until 1978 death records did not include a code for Hispanic ethnicity; thus Hispanic death rates had to be estimated from last names. This procedure inevitably resulted in some misclassification of deaths and may have underestimated the number of deaths that occurred among Hispanics. Two studies have been able to address this problem by enrolling individuals and

FIGURE 13.3.   HISPANIC/WHITE MORTALITY RATE RATIOS FOR SELECTED CAUSES OF DEATH, 2001.

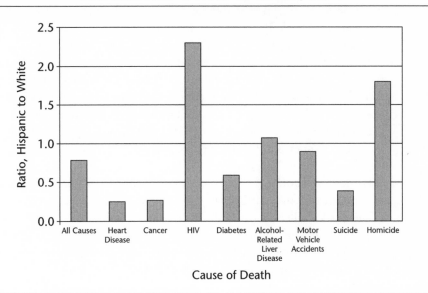

Source: National Center for Health Statistics.

following them up to their deaths (Liao et al., 1998; Sorlie, Backlund, Johnson, & Rogot, 1993). Both studies found support for the Hispanic epidemiological paradox.

The "Salmon Bias" Hypothesis. This hypothesis takes its name from the phenomenon of salmon swimming upstream to spawn before their death. The hypothesis maintains that migrants return home when they become seriously ill or reach old age. Those individuals would most likely die in their country of origin, not in the United States, so these deaths would go unrecorded in U.S. statistics. This would have the effect of producing artificially lower Hispanic mortality rates. Abraido-Lanza, Dohrenwen, Ng-Mak, and Turner (1999) tested this hypothesis among Cubans (most of whom cannot return home) and Puerto Ricans (whose deaths in Puerto Rico would be recorded in U.S. vital statistics). That study found the Hispanic epidemiological paradox present in these populations as well—which tends to refute the "salmon bias" hypothesis.

The Healthy Migrant Hypothesis. This hypothesis is based on the notion that only healthy and vigorous people migrate to other countries. Several studies have found that migrants tend to have better health status than persons in their country of origin (Marmot, Adelstein, & Bulusu, 1984), and migrants to the United States tend to have better health status than U.S.-born citizens (Stephen, Foote, Hendershot, & Schoenborn, 1994). These studies support the healthy migrant hypothesis. However, Abraido-Lanza et al. (1999) reasoned that if lower Hispanic mortality rates (compared with Whites) were merely a healthy migrant effect then there should be no differences in mortality between migrants from Latin America and those from other regions of the world, particularly Europe, since they were also affected by selective migration. Abraido-Lanza et al. found that European migrants did not have a mortality advantage relative to U.S.-born Whites similar to that of Hispanic migrants relative to U.S.-born Hispanics. Thus they concluded that the healthy migrant hypothesis was not a significant explanation for the Hispanic epidemiological paradox.

Risk Factors Hypothesis. The risk factors hypothesis states that the Hispanic mortality rate is greater than the White rate for some causes of death, yet greater than the White rate for others, because of the distribution of health risks and protective factors among Hispanics: in some ways Hispanics have a better health risk profile (such as a lower rate of smoking, a higher proportion of pregnant women seeking prenatal care, and a higher-fiber diet), but on the other hand Hispanics have higher rates of other health risk factors (such as lower rates of childhood immunizations, a higher prevalence of hypertension, and residence in areas with poorer-quality water and air). How these differences in health risks translate into differences in health outcomes is not known and has not been studied, at least not within the context of understanding the Hispanic epidemiological paradox; however, differences in risk factors could play a role in contributing to the lower incidence rates of certain diseases in Hispanics.

Summary

This chapter examined the health status of Hispanics/Latinos, a rapidly growing segment of the U.S. population. They are the largest non-White racial/ethnic group in the United States. Although persons of Mexican ancestry are the largest proportion of Hispanics/Latinos, there is a great deal of variation among the many subgroups that make up the Hispanic population. This variation can make it difficult to draw broad conclusions because in some cases the groups are so dissimilar that combining them obscures important information. However, some general comments can be made. In general, Hispanics/Latinos have a relatively good health profile given the group's overall socioeconomic status. In some cases, Hispanics have better health outcomes than White Americans. This is called the Hispanic epidemiological paradox. Hispanics as a group face barriers in accessing quality health care; they have a high rate of uninsured persons and must contend with language barriers as well.

For a case study, see Appendix A. See Appendix B for additional readings.

Key Words

Hispanic epidemiological paradox

Healthy migrant hypothesis

"Salmon bias" hypothesis

Data reliability hypothesis

Risk factors hypothesis

PART FIVE

CONCLUSIONS

CHAPTER FOURTEEN

ADDRESSING DISPARITIES IN HEALTH AND HEALTH CARE

Outline

Connecting Health Status and Health Care Disparities

I described the model of determinants of health in Chapter Seven. The model groups the causes of health status disparities into three broad categories: (1) socioenvironmental or contextual factors, (2) individual-level factors, and (3) biophysiological or genetic factors. The model of determinants of health is presented in Figure 14.1.

Socioenvironmental factors include factors external to the individual that impact health, such as environmental exposures, stress, poverty, poor-quality housing, or societal-level phenomena (such as a major economic downturn or war). Individual-level factors refer to characteristics of the person, including health behaviors,

FIGURE 14.1. DETERMINANTS OF HEALTH STATUS.

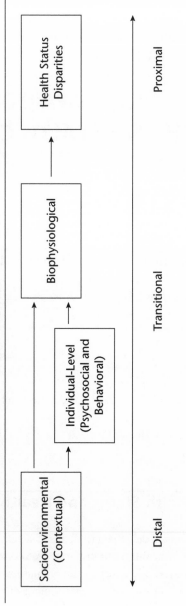

psychological factors, or the material resources or other assets owned by the person (such as their income, education, health insurance, and any other resource that can be employed to affect health). Biophysiological factors refer to the biological mechanisms that produce ill health.

The determinants of health model can be augmented to incorporate health care resources (see Figure 14.2). As was shown in Chapter Six, health care services can actually increase as well as decrease health status disparities. Disparities in health care access, utilization, or quality can lead to a widening of the racial/ethnic gap in health status. However, health care can also be an important part of the solution. Figure 14.2 shows that socioenvironmental and individual factors can have an important impact on access to and utilization and quality of health care received. Also note that the model demonstrates that although health care is one factor that determines health status, it is not the only factor. Some possible solutions to health status disparities can be health system-based solutions. However, there must be non–health care based solutions as well.

Addressing Health Status Disparities

England's King's Fund issued a 1995 report titled *Tackling Inequalities in Health: An Agenda for Action* (Benzeval et al., 1995). The report presented a four-level framework for addressing health inequalities:

1. Improving the physical environment
2. Addressing social and economic conditions
3. Improving access to appropriate and effective health and social services
4. Reducing barriers to adopting healthy lifestyles

The Bernzeval et al. model is consistent with the determinants of health model, as outlined in Figure 14.1. Levels 1 and 2 of the Bernzeval et al. model apply directly to the socioenvironmental category of the determinants of health model. Bernzeval et al. recognized that it would be difficult (and likely impossible) to address health inequalities as long as socioenvironmental inequalities persist.

As was outlined in Chapter Eight, there is substantial variation in socioeconomic status (SES) among the racial/ethnic groups. Although socioeconomic status does not fully account for racial/ethnic disparities in health status, SES is one of the determinants of the health status that contribute to health status disparities.

FIGURE 14.2.   HEALTH CARE DISPARITIES AND HEALTH DISPARITIES.

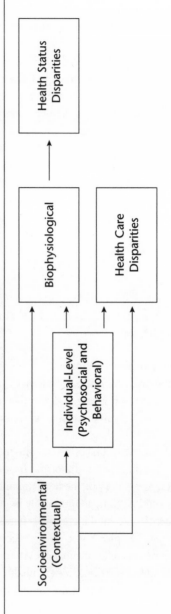

In the United States there have been some policies directed at addressing the distribution of wealth. And there have been some efforts to provide persons of low socioeconomic status with resources that help to counterbalance their low SES status (such as the earned income tax credit, the Section 8 housing program, food stamps, and Medicaid). Such programs are major components of the U.S. welfare state. However, they are not substantial enough to be a sufficient counterweight to the debilitating effects on health of low SES.

Level 3 of the model developed by Bernzeval et al. also conforms to the determinants of health model in its focus on the role of health care. Health care disparities are produced partly by socioeconomic factors, such as health insurance status or geographic location of health care facilities. Although health care facilities are typically available in urban areas, availability of health care services is a major limitation of the Indian Health Service and one of the primary health care challenges faced by American Indians (Korenbrot, Ehlers, & Crouch, 2003). Efforts to address this aspect of the health care disparities problem include the development of policies and programs that ensure universal access to health care. The United States remains the only industrialized country that does not ensure access to health for all citizens.

BOX 14.1.   EXAMPLES OF EFFORTS TO ADDRESS SOCIOECONOMIC DISPARITIES.

Section 8—housing choice vouchers allow very low-income families to choose and lease or rent safe, decent, and affordable privately owned housing.

The *Earned Income Tax Credit (EITC)* is a federal income tax credit for low-income workers who are eligible for and claim the credit. The credit reduces the amount of tax an individual owes and may be returned in the form of a refund.

The *Food Stamp Program* enables low-income families to buy nutritious food with coupons and Electronic Benefits Transfer (EBT) cards. Food-stamp recipients spend their benefits to buy eligible food in authorized retail food stores.

Medicaid is a program that pays for medical assistance for certain individuals and families with low incomes and resources. This program became law in 1965 and is jointly funded by the federal and state governments (including the District of Columbia and U.S. territories) to assist the states in providing medical long-term care assistance to people who meet the eligibility criteria. Medicaid is the largest source of funding for medical and health-related services for people with limited income.

Finally, Benzeval et al.'s (1995) Level 4 ("Reducing barriers to adopting healthy lifestyles") addresses health behavior—the individual-level factors of the determinants of health model. Health behavior is impacted by many things. Perceived health risk is one, but access to and availability of resources to support a healthy lifestyle play a role as well. It is more difficult to convince someone to develop an exercise program that includes aerobic activities, such as jogging or walking, if that person lives in a community with a high risk of becoming a victim of violent crime when venturing outdoors.

Humans are complex. Programs designed to modify health behavior have had mixed success. Often people have competing demands that relegate their own health status to a lower priority. However, although health behavior change is difficult, it is important to continue research to understand why racial/ethnic differences in health behaviors persist. Why do African Americans have lower smoking rates than Whites as teens, but a higher rate in adulthood? And once we know the answer, how can we use that knowledge to eliminate disparities in smoking-related deaths? Why do Hispanics/Latinos have a low rate of condom use? And can we use this knowledge to reduce the high rate of HIV transmission among Hispanics/Latinos? What strategies can be employed to reduce high rates of alcohol abuse among American Indians? The answers to these questions are important components to the elimination of health status disparities. However, our knowledge has not yet progressed to a point where consistently reliable interventions exist.

Addressing Health Care Disparities

Bernzeval's four-level framework is useful but has its limits. Although the Bernzeval model incorporates the role of health care into the framework, it only addresses health care access. It does not address health care services utilization, quality, cultural competency, or patient compliance. Cooper and Roter (2002) presented a framework that can be used to complement Bernzeval et al.'s model. The modified model is presented in Figure 14.3. The figure shows three levels of factors that affect patient outcomes. The first level presents three sources of barriers to obtaining care: personal/family, structural, and financial.

Barriers

Barriers are factors that can inhibit persons from accessing care. Barriers can also influence the individual's ability to engage the health care system in such a way as to ensure good quality care. For example, personal/family barriers can include language, which can impede access, make an individual less inclined to utilize health care

FIGURE 14.3. BARRIERS TO AND MEDIATORS OF EQUITABLE HEALTH CARE FOR RACIAL AND ETHNIC GROUPS.

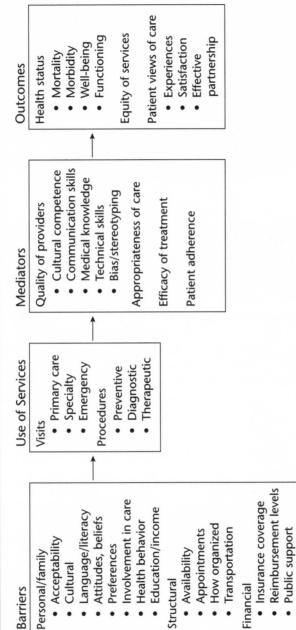

Barriers

Personal/family
- Acceptability
- Cultural
- Language/literacy
- Attitudes, beliefs
- Preferences
- Involvement in care
- Health behavior
- Education/income

Structural
- Availability
- Appointments
- How organized
- Transportation

Financial
- Insurance coverage
- Reimbursement levels
- Public support

Use of Services

Visits
- Primary care
- Specialty
- Emergency

Procedures
- Preventive
- Diagnostic
- Therapeutic

Mediators

Quality of providers
- Cultural competence
- Communication skills
- Medical knowledge
- Technical skills
- Bias/stereotyping

Appropriateness of care

Efficacy of treatment

Patient adherence

Outcomes

Health status
- Mortality
- Morbidity
- Well-being
- Functioning

Equity of services

Patient views of care
- Experiences
- Satisfaction
- Effective partnership

Source: Cooper and Roter, 2002.

BOX 14.2.   FIVE PRINCIPLES FOR ADDRESSING DISPARITIES.

Principle 1: Disparities must be recognized as a significant health care quality problem.

Principle 2: The collection of relevant and reliable data is needed to address disparities.

Principle 3: Health system performance measures should be stratified by socioeconomic position and race/ethnicity.

Principle 4: Populationwide performance measures should be adjusted for socioeconomic position and race/ethnicity.

Principle 5: Approaches to disparities should account for the relationship between socioeconomic position and race/ethnicity.

Source: Fiscella, Franks, Gold, and Clancy, 2000.

---

services even when they are available, or make it difficult to communicate effectively with the health care provider, thus increasing the risk of receiving lower-quality care.

Barriers can also be structural or financial. Structural barriers are those associated with the organization and distribution of health services, including geographic inaccessibility. Financial barriers relate to ability to pay for services. In the United States, lack of health insurance is a financial barrier that affects many people.

Racial/ethnic minorities suffer a disproportionate burden of barriers to obtaining care. Among the most prevalent barriers is lack of health insurance. Table 14.1 displays the racial/ethnic distribution of the uninsured. In 2001 fully 39.2 million Americans were uninsured. Of those, 46.1 percent were racial/ethnic minorities. Although Hispanics/Latinos comprised 12.5 percent of the total U.S. population, they were 26.3 percent of the uninsured. Thus they were overrepresented among the uninsured by a ratio of more than 2:1. Native Americans were nearly as overrepresented among the uninsured as Hispanics/Latinos. African Americans and Asians were not nearly as overrepresented as Native Americans and Hispanics/Latinos. However, every non-White racial/ethnic group was overrepresented among the uninsured. Clearly, the elimination of health insurance as a barrier to obtaining care is an important component to the elimination of health status disparities.

Use of Services

Each individual has a unique combination of personal, family, structural, and financial barriers. Some will have very few (or even none) of these barriers, others may have most (or even all) of them, and still others will have some barriers but not others. An

TABLE 14.1.   RACIAL/ETHNIC DISTRIBUTION AMONG THE UNINSURED, 2001.

Race/Ethnic Group	Percent of All Uninsured	Percent of U.S. Population	Ratio
White	53.9	75.1	0.72
Black	14.3	12.3	1.16
Hispanic/Latino	26.3	12.5	2.10
Asian (only)	3.7	3.6	1.0
Native American	1.8	0.9	2.0

BOX 14.3.   THREE LEVELS OF ACCESS TO CARE FOR VULNERABLE POPULATIONS.

Level 1: Access to the health care system (difficulty getting care, delay in care because of costs, and transportation problems)

Level 2: Structural barriers within the system (difficulty getting appointments and advice after hours and completing referrals to specialists)

Level 3: The ability of the provider to address patients' needs (awareness of patients' conditions and functional limitations, knowledge and clinical skills, cultural competence)

Source: Bierman, Magari, Jette, Splaine, and Wasson, 1998.

individual's unique combination of barriers, along with the degree to which the person perceives a need to use health services, will determine that individual's pattern of use of health services.

Mediators

The first two stages of the model address access to and utilization of health services. The third stage deals with quality of care. *Mediators* are characteristics of the doctor-patient encounter that enable good patient outcomes. Specifically, they include the degree to which the available health services offer good-quality providers (including being culturally competent, knowledgeable, and technically skillful) and provide appropriate care, whether or not the treatment regimen is effective, and whether the patient is adherent to the treatment regimen. Each of these areas is a potential point for intervention.

BOX 14.4. POINTS OF INTERVENTION FOR HEALTH DISPARITIES.

Socioenvironmental	Individual-Level	Health Care System
Community redevelopment	Reduce inactivity	Increase availability of health services
Job creation	Increase healthy eating	Provide universal access to health care and pharmaceuticals
Improved housing	Reduce/eliminate conception of ATOD	
Clean water	Increase health screenings	
Safe wastewater treatment	Improve education	Increase number of health care providers who are proficient in a second language
Elimination of exposures to environmental hazards	Improve health literacy	
	Improve English proficiency	
Reduced availability of alcohol, tobacco, and other drugs (ATOD)		
Increased availability of clean supermarkets		

Cultural Competency

Studies have demonstrated that minorities tend to be less satisfied with the health care they receive (Haviland, Morales, Reise, & Hays, 2003) and to feel that they have received care that is less "participatory" in terms of allowing for input and involvement of the patient (Doescher, Saver, Franks, & Fiscella, 2000; Cooper-Patrick et al., 2002). More highly participatory physicians tend to engender greater patient satisfaction (Kaplan, Greenfield, Gandek, Rogers, & Ware, 1996). Patient satisfaction is associated with important health/illness behaviors such as appointment keeping (Litt & Cuskey, 1984) and utilization of health services (Ivanov & Flynn, 1999; Carlson & Gabriel, 2001). Finally, previous studies have found that when patients are matched with their doctor by race/ethnicity, patients report that they are more satisfied with the care they received (LaVeist & Nuru-Jeter, 2002), that they have received more participatory care (Cooper et al., 2003), and that they are more likely to use needed health services (Saha et al.,

---

BOX 14.5.   WHAT IS CULTURAL COMPETENCY?

Lavizzo-Mourey and MacKenzie (1996) define *cultural competency* as "the demonstrated awareness and integration of three population-specific issues: health-related and cultural values, disease incidence and prevalence, and treatment efficacy." Anderson et al. (2003) described cultural competency this way: "a set of congruent behaviors, attitudes, and policies that come together in a system, agency, or among professionals and enable effective work in cross-cultural situations."

1999; LaVeist, Nuru-Jeter, & Jones, 2003). This is suggestive, although not direct evidence, that cultural competency is an important mediator of patient outcomes.

It has been projected that racial and ethnic minority populations in the United States will be an increasingly larger proportion of the U.S. population and eventually, by midcentury, will form the majority. As patients tend to prefer physicians of their own racial or ethnic group, the demand for minority physicians will likely increase in the coming decades. However, as Libby et al. (1997) have demonstrated, at the current rate of production the supply of minority physicians will fall short of future demand. These trends foreshadow a probable decreased likelihood of race concordance for African Americans and Hispanics in the future, a reduction of satisfaction among minority patients, and perhaps a decline in quality of care among minorities. These outcomes can be avoided by increasing minority physician production and placing greater emphasis on improving the ability of physicians to interact with patients who are racially, ethnically, or otherwise culturally different than they are.

Cultural competency seems to be an important key to addressing health disparities. Cultural competency can be taught. Evaluations of several programs designed to improve cultural competency in medical training programs have shown that such training programs can work (Crosson, Deng, Brazeau, Boyd, & Soto-Greene, 2004; Ferguson, Keller, Haley, & Quirk, 2003; Wachtler & Troein, 2003). But such training does not have to be limited to formal training settings.

The Office of Minority Health (OMH) of the Department of Health and Human Services (DHHS) has released fourteen standards on culturally and linguistically appropriate services (CLAS) in health care. The recommended standards cover three areas of competence requirements for health care for racial or ethnic minorities: (1) culturally competent care, (2) language access services, and (3) organizational support for cultural competence (OMH, 1999).

BOX 14.6.   STANDARDS FOR CULTURALLY AND LINGUISTI-CALLY APPROPRIATE HEALTH CARE SERVICES.

Culture and language have considerable impact on how patients access and respond to health care services. To ensure equal access to quality health care by diverse populations, health care organizations and providers should:

1. Promote and support the attitudes, behaviors, knowledge, and skills necessary for staff to work respectfully and effectively with patients and each other in a culturally diverse work environment.

2. Have a comprehensive management strategy to address culturally and linguistically appropriate services, including strategic goals, plans, policies, procedures, and designated staff responsible for implementation.

3. Utilize formal mechanisms for community and consumer involvement in the design and execution of service delivery, including planning, policy-making, operations, evaluation, training, and, as appropriate, treatment planning.

4. Develop and implement a strategy to recruit, retain, and promote qualified, diverse, and culturally competent administrative, clinical, and support staff that are trained and qualified to address the needs of the racial and ethnic communities being served.

5. Require and arrange for ongoing education and training for administrative, clinical, and support staff in culturally and linguistically competent service delivery.

6. Provide all clients with limited English proficiency (LEP) access to bilingual staff or interpretation services.

7. Provide oral and written notices, including translated signage at key points of contact, to clients in their primary language informing them of their right to receive no-cost interpreter services.

8. Translate and make available signage and commonly used written patient education material and other materials for members of the predominant language groups in service areas.

9. Ensure that interpreters and bilingual staff can demonstrate bilingual proficiency and receive training that includes the skills and ethics of interpreting and knowledge in both languages of the terms and concepts relevant to clinical or non-clinical encounters. Family or friends are not considered adequate substitutes because they usually lack these abilities.

10. Ensure that the clients' primary spoken language and self-identified race/ethnicity are included in the health care organization's management information system as well as any patient records used by provider staff.

11. Use a variety of methods to collect and utilize accurate demographic, cultural, epidemiological, and clinical outcome data for racial and ethnic

groups in the service area and become informed about the ethnic/cultural needs, resources, and assets of the surrounding community.

12. Undertake ongoing organizational self-assessments of cultural and linguistic competence and integrate measures of access, satisfactions, quality, and outcomes for CLAS into other organizational internal audits and performance improvement programs.

13. Develop structures and procedures to address cross-cultural ethical and legal conflicts in health care delivery and complaints or grievances by patients and staff about unfair, culturally insensitive or discriminatory treatment, or difficulty in accessing services or denial of services.

14. Prepare an annual progress report documenting the organizations' progress with implementing CLAS standards, including information on programs, staffing, and resources.

Source: Office of Minority Health, 1999.

Additional Keys to Success

There is a relatively small body of research literature describing interventions to address health status and health care disparities. The knowledge base is still evolving in this area, but I think it is important to end with a few final comments about some lessons that have been learned so far. And a few comments about things we don't yet know, but need to know.

Community-Based Participatory Research (CBPR)

Several studies have demonstrated that community representatives can be successfully integrated into research projects and interventions (Cornwall & Jewkes, 1995). Several studies have demonstrated the effectiveness of this approach in reducing health disparities (Stillman, Bone, Rand, Levine, & Becker, 1993; Voorhees et al., 1996). In the most successful partnerships, community leaders are involved in all aspects of the project, from agenda setting to program planning and development. They are considered team members, recognized for their expertise regarding the social, cultural, and other aspects of the community. They should have similar rights and expectations as other team members. They should be compensated for their time. And they should be included in the technical aspects of research design (Israel, Schulz, Parker, & Becker, 2001), including writing articles for publication. The CBPR approach helps to empower communities (Braun et al., 2003), providing community leaders with skills that will help to make the program sustainable (Metzler et al., 2003). The new skill sets also help community members to more independently and effectively take on other projects on other topics.

Cultural Tailoring

When possible, interventions should be tailored specifically to the target group's language and culture. This requires a strong understanding of the subtleties of the target's modes of communication. Tailored interventions have been successfully employed in terms of health education messages (Lauver, Settersten, Kane, & Henriques, 2003; Skinner, Strecher, & Hospers, 1994); however, there are not many well-controlled evaluations of this strategy in the research literature.

Community Health Workers

There is a large and consistent body of literature demonstrating the efficacy of community health workers in addressing health disparities (Gary et al., 2003, 2004; Corkery et al., 1997; Levine et al., 2003). Other studies have demonstrated their cost-effectiveness (Fedder, Chang, Curry, & Nichols, 2003).

By linking each of these strategies with the points of intervention for health disparities, we can produce a matrix that shows how each strategy can be best used. The matrix is provided in Table 14.2, which shows that community-based participatory research (CBPR) approaches are most successful in interventions targeted to socioenvironmental causes of health disparities. The CBPR approach is particularly effective in this realm because of its strong emphasis on fully engaging the community and harnessing the resources of the community for health improvement. Such a strategy may not be as effective when applied to interventions geared toward individual-level behavior change. CBPR could, however, be highly valuable in developing interventions for individual-level behavior change. CBPR seems least appropriate for interventions intended to change health systems. Such systems tend to be more top-down hierarchical organizations with professional managers.

Culturally tailored approaches seem highly likely to be effective in interventions targeted to the socioenvironmental and individual levels. This approach places emphasis on understanding the culture of the target community and tailoring a message to its specific needs and interests. One can envision a behavior change intervention targeted to heath care providers. Since this approach has not been as thoroughly tested as the CBPR or, especially, the community health worker models, my ratings in Table 14.2 should be viewed as speculative.

Finally, the community health worker model has been tested in many different settings and has power to be effective. It is perhaps least effective at influencing health

TABLE 14.2.   STRATEGIES AND POINTS OF INTERVENTION.

		Points of Intervention		
		Socioenvironmental	Individual	Health System
Strategy	Community-Based Participatory Research	Good	Fair	Poor
	Cultural Tailoring	Good	Good	Good
	Community Health Worker	Good	Good	Fair

system change, but within a health system that is seeking to make change, community health workers can be highly effective advocates for community interests.

Summary

This chapter outlined strategies for addressing health status and health care disparities. The chapter reintroduced the determinants of health model, with the addition of the role that health care disparities play in producing health status disparities. The model identifies three levels for the introduction of interventions: socioenvironmental, individual, and health care system. The chapter then discussed some existing strategies that attempt to intervene to reduce disparities at each of these levels. The chapter concluded with a discussion of three proven strategies that can be applied to the points of intervention. (See Appendix B for additional readings.)

Key Words

Cultural competence

Community-based participatory research (CBPR)

Community health workers

Cultural tailoring

Culturally and linguistically appropriate health care services (CLAS)

APPENDIX A

CASE STUDIES

Chapter Two Case Study

Since 1977, federal statistical agencies have used the four racial categories (American Indian or Alaska Native, Asian or Pacific Islander, Black, and White) and two ethnic categories (Hispanic origin and not of Hispanic origin) specified by the Office of Management and Budget (OMB) in Statistical Policy Directive 15. These are the minimum categories for reporting race and ethnicity. In 1994 OMB initiated a comprehensive review of the racial categories prescribed by Directive 15; as part of that review the Census Bureau conducted three sample surveys to test the results of variations in reporting race and ethnicity. This case presents the results of those samples.

The first test examines the effect of providing alternative variations of the questions on race and Hispanic origin. This survey, the National Content Survey (NCS), was conducted between March and June 1996. It focuses on the effects of the following three treatments tested in the NCS:

1. Adding a multiracial response category in the race question
2. Placing the Hispanic origin question immediately before the race question
3. Combining both of these changes

The results of adding a multiracial or biracial response category were as follows:

- About 1 percent of persons reported as multiracial in the variations of the race question that included a multiracial or biracial response category.
- The presence of a multiracial response category in the race question did not have statistically significant effects on the percentages of persons who reported as White, Black, American Indian, or Asian/Pacific Islander. This finding held regardless of the sequence of the race and Hispanic origin questions.
- Including a multiracial category in the race-followed-by-Hispanic-origin sequence reduced the percentage of persons reporting in the Other race category of the race question.

The results of varying the sequence of race and Hispanic origin questions were as follows:

- Placing the Hispanic origin question before the race question significantly reduced the number of people that did not respond to the Hispanic origin question
- Placing the Hispanic origin question before a race question that did not include a multiracial option had these effects:
    It reduced the percentage of persons reporting in the "other race" category of the race question
    It increased reporting by Hispanics in the White category of the race question

The results of allowing respondents to "mark one or more category" or to "mark all that apply" were as follows:

- The options for reporting more than one race did not affect the percentages reporting solely as White, Black, or American Indian. However, the percentages of persons selecting Alaska Native and Asian/Pacific Islander were affected by the way the questions were presented.
- When the race question and the Hispanic origin questions were combined into one question, a high percentage of responses included both Hispanic origin and one of the four major race categories currently allowed under Directive 15.

Source: U.S. Bureau of the Census, "Results of the 1996 Race and Ethnic Targeted Test," Population Division Working Paper No. 18, May 1997.

Discussion Questions

1. Given the many problems associated with creating a racial/ethnic classification scheme that accurately reflects the diversity of humans and the increasing diversity of the United States, should we simply stop collecting and reporting data by race?

2. Although eliminating the practice of collecting and reporting data by race is one option for a response to increasing diversity, another option would be to increase the number of categories used in the collection and reporting of data. Discuss the pros and cons of increasing the number of categories.

Chapter Six Case Study

Dr. Knox Todd and his colleagues (2002) conducted a study of African American and White patients who came to the emergency department with an isolated long-bone (leg) fracture. The study sought to determine whether there was a difference by race in the administration of analgesic (pain) medication. (This research team conducted a similar study among White and Hispanic/Latino patients from a different state.) This study found that White patients were 30 percent more likely to receive pain medication compared with African American patients with similar injuries (see Table A.1).

Discussion Question

1. What are some possible explanations for these findings?

Chapter Twelve Case Study

Mr. Yost is a sixty-three-year-old Korean American who has been in the United States for seven years. Dr. Yee is a thirty-one-year-old second-generation Chinese American family physician who has been seeing Mr. Yost for three years. They have a good

TABLE A.1. RACE DIFFERENCES IN USE OF ANALGESIC (PAIN) MEDICATION.

Analgesic Received?	Patient's Race	
	White	Black
Yes	67 (74%)	73 (57%)
No	23 (26%)	54 (43%)
Total	90	127

Source: Based on Todd, Deaton, D'Adamo, and Goe, 2002.

relationship, but early in their relationship Mr. Yost mentioned that he occasionally used "traditional" medications from Korea and India. Dr. Yee expressed his disapproval. Mr. Yost was somewhat surprised by Dr. Yee's reaction, given the doctor's Asian ancestry, but Mr. Yost liked the doctor so he decided he would continue to see him, but would never mention traditional medicine again.

Mr. Yost was feeling very ill. He suffered from general weakness, dizziness, nausea, and muscle pain. He came to see Dr. Yee. After a number of tests Dr. Yee had great difficulty finding a cause for Mr. Yost's illness. Dr. Yee began to suspect lead poisoning, but that is very rare among adults, unless exposed at work. Given Mr. Yost's job as an office worker, occupational lead exposure seemed unlikely. And Dr. Yee had not prescribed any drugs or other treatments that would elevate Mr. Yost's lead levels.

After blood tests, the doctor was able to determine that Mr. Yost was suffering from lead anemia (lead poisoning). But he could not figure out how this would have happened. What Mr. Yost never told Dr. Yee is that while on a recent trip to Korea, he visited a traditional Ayurvedic medical center where he obtained herbal medicines that he had been taking. Mr. Yee never connected his lead poisoning with the herbal medicines he took. After being treated for lead poisoning, Mr. Yost went back to taking the herbs.

Discussion Questions

1. Given that Mr. Yost didn't tell Dr. Yee about the herbal medicine, he will likely get lead poisoning again. What needs to happen to get Mr. Yost to give Dr. Yee the critical information he needs?
2. What role did Dr. Yee play in creating a scenario in which Mr. Yost will likely suffer lead poisoning for a second time?
3. Consider the various aspects of cultural conflict involved in this case.

   Eastern versus Western culture

   The culture of medicine versus the lay public

   Acculturated versus less acculturated APIs

Chapter Thirteen Case Study

Ana Gutierrez is a thirty-three-year-old woman who moved from Nicaragua to Maryland a few months ago. She is staying with her sister and her niece in a predominantly Spanish-speaking neighborhood, where her limited English has not been a problem.

Ana has been feeling ill, but has delayed a trip to the doctor because she was told to bring in an interpreter who is fluent in both Spanish and English. Ana doesn't know many people. The only person she could think to ask was her ten-year-old niece. She doesn't feel comfortable sharing personal medical information with a child and family member, but she feels she has no choice.

The doctor also feels uncomfortable with a child as the translator, but at the moment she is their only line of communication. He asks Ana's niece about Ana's medical history and asks her to describe what the problem is now. Ana doesn't want to share personal information with her niece, so she omits that she has recently had an abortion. Instead she tells her niece, "*He tenido un dolor muy fuerte en el estomago por varios dias.*" The niece translates this as "I have had a strong stomach pain for a few days." Because the doctor does not have complete information, he thinks that this may simply be a stomachache and that Ana may be exaggerating the pain, since there seems to be nothing wrong with her. He sends her home with a pain reliever.

Ana takes the medicine as instructed, but her pain continues to worsen. She is in so much pain by that night that she has to be rushed to the hospital. This time she is lucky enough to find a nurse who speaks Spanish and English. She tells the nurse that she had an abortion a few days ago, and because she was feeling ill, she went to a local healer in the area who gave her metamizole (a traditional medication banned in the United States but in common use in many parts of Latin America). The doctor is now able to adequately treat her. At the end of the visit he gives Ana some medication and tells her to take it three times a day, with food, for two weeks. He says if she does not, she may feel some stomach pains. He also informs her of some of the other side effects associated with this medicine: headaches and nausea.

The nurse translates the doctor's instructions as "*Tiene que tomar una pastilla despues de comer, tres veces al dia, puede ser que le de cefalea y nausea, eso es normal.*" (Take the medicine three times a day after each meal, and she may suffer from headaches and nausea, but that is normal.) The nurse has inadvertently shortened and slightly altered the message. She has also used a medical term (*cefalea*) to describe a headache instead of using the more commonly understood *dolor de cabeza*.

Discussion Questions

1. Should hospitals be required to hire interpreters as part of their staff?
2. Many studies have found that even professional translators make an alarming number of mistakes, many of which can adversely affect a patient. Why would someone who is "trained" make errors in translation? What are some solutions to this problem?
3. Should doctors be required to learn a second language as part of their medical training?

APPENDIX B

ADDITIONAL READINGS

Chapter One

Amaro, H., & Zambrana, R. E. (2000). Criollo, mestizo, mulato, LatiNegro, indigena, white, or black? The U.S. Hispanic/Latino population and multiple responses in the 2000 census. *American Journal of Public Health, 90*(11), 1724–1727.

Borak, J., Fiellin, M., & Chemerynski, S. (2004). Who is Hispanic? Implications for epidemiologic research in the United States. *Epidemiology, 15*(2), 240–244.

Comas-Diaz, L. (2001). Hispanics, Latinos, or Americanos: The evolution of identity. *Cultural Diversity and Ethnic Minority Psychology, 7*(2), 115–120.

Herman, M. (2004). Forced to choose: Some determinants of racial identification in multiracial adolescents. *Child Development, 75*(3), 730–748.

Karlsen, S. (2004). "Black like Beckham"? Moving beyond definitions of ethnicity based on skin colour and ancestry. *Ethnic Health, 9*(2), 107–137.

Massey, D. S., & Denton, N. A. (1994). *American apartheid: Segregation and the making of the underclass.* Cambridge, MA: Harvard University Press.

Chapter Two

Byrd, W. M., & Clayton, L. A. (2000). *An American health dilemma, volume one: A medical history of African Americans and the problem of race: Beginnings to 1900.* New York: Routledge.

Molnar, S. (2001). *Human variation, races, types, and ethnic groups* (5th ed.). Upper Saddle River, NJ: Prentice Hall.

Olson, S. (2003). *Mapping human history: Genes, race, and our common origins.* New York: Houghton Mifflin.

Chapter Three

Aratame, N., & Singelmann, J. (1998). Migration and race in the southern United States. *Research in Rural Sociology and Development, 7*(2), 113–130.

Burke, B. M. (1995). Mexican immigrants shape California's fertility future. *Population Today, 23*(9), 4–6.

Dunlevy, J. A. (1991). On the settlement patterns of recent Caribbean and Latin immigrants to the United States. *Growth and Change, 22*(1), 54–67.

Frey, W. H. (1998). Black migration to the South reaches record highs in 1990s. *Population Today, 26*(2), 1–3.

Hansen, N., & Cardenas, G. (1988). Immigrant and native ethnic enterprises in Mexican American neighborhoods: Differing perceptions of Mexican immigrant workers. *International Migration Review, 22*(2), 226–242.

Haverluk, T. (1997). The changing geography of U.S. Hispanics, 1850–1990. *Journal of Geography, 96*(3), 134–145.

Massey, D. S., & Denton, N. A. (1994). *American apartheid: Segregation and the making of the underclass.* Cambridge, MA: Harvard University Press.

Saenz, R. (1989). Selectivity of Mexican American intraregional migration in the Southwest. *Hispanic Journal of Behavioral Sciences, 11*(2), 148–155.

Sandefur, G. D., & Jeon, J. (1991). Migration, race and ethnicity, 1960–1980. *International Migration Review, 25*(2), 392–407.

Winsberg, M. D. (1986). Geographical polarization of whites and minorities in large U.S. cities, 1960–1980. *Population Today, 14*(3), 6–7.

Chapter Four

Hogue, C. J. R., Hargraves, M. A., & Collins, K. C. (2000). *Minority health in America: Findings and policy implications from the Commonwealth Fund Minority Health Survey.* Baltimore: Johns Hopkins University Press.

LaVeist, T. A. (2002). *Race, ethnicity, and health: A public health reader.* San Francisco: Jossey-Bass.

Shah, N. (2001). *Contagious divides: Epidemics and race in San Francisco's Chinatown.* Berkeley: University of California Press.

Chapter Five

Hollan, D. (2004). Self-systems, cultural idioms of distress, and the psycho-bodily consequences of childhood suffering. *Transcultural Psychiatry, 41*(1), 62–79.

Niehaus, D. J., Oosthuizen, P., Lochner, C., Emsley, R. A., Jordaan, E., Mbanga, N. I., et al. (2004). A culture-bound syndrome '*amafufunyana*' and a culture-specific event '*ukuthwasa*': Differentiated by a family history of schizophrenia and other psychiatric disorders. *Psychopathology, 37*(2), 59–63.

Pescosolido, B. A., Monahan, J., Link, B. G., Stueve, A., & Kikuzawa, S. (1999). The public's view of the competence, dangerousness, and need for legal coercion of persons with mental health problems. *American Journal of Public Health, 89*(9), 1339–1345.

Strakowski, S. M., Keck, P. E., Jr., Arnold, L. M., Collins, J., Wilson, R. M., Fleck, D. E., et al. (2003). Ethnicity and diagnosis in patients with affective disorders. *Journal of Clinical Psychiatry, 64*(7), 747–754.

Sumathipala, A., Siribaddana, S. H., & Bhugra, D. (2004). Culture-bound syndromes: The story of *dhat* syndrome. *British Journal of Psychiatry, 184*(2), 200–209.

Takeuchi, D. T., Mokuau, N., & Chun, C. A. (1992). Mental health services for Asian Americans and Pacific Islanders. *Journal of Mental Health Administration, 19*(3), 237–245.

U.S. Department of Health and Human Services. (1999). *Mental health: Culture, race, and ethnicity. A supplement to mental health: A report of the surgeon general.* Rockville, MD: Author.

Weissman, M. M., Bland, R. C., Canino, G. J., Faravelli, C., Greenwald, S., Hwu, H. G., et al. (1996). Cross-national epidemiology of major depression and bipolar disorder. *Journal of the American Medical Association, 276*(4), 293–299.

Chapter Six

Institute of Medicine. (2001). *Crossing the quality chasm: A new health system for the 21st century.* Washington, DC: National Academy Press.

Institute of Medicine. (2002). *Unequal treatment: Confronting racial and ethnic disparities of health care.* Washington, DC: National Academy Press.

Chapter Seven

LaVeist, T. A. (2002). *Race, ethnicity, and health: A public health reader.* San Francisco: Jossey-Bass.

Chapter Eight

Kawachi, I., & Berkman, L. F. (2003). *Neighborhoods and health.* New York: Oxford University Press.

Lichtenstein, P., Harris, J. R., Pedersen, N. L., & McClearn, G. E. (1993). Socioeconomic status and physical health: How are they related? An empirical study based on twins reared apart and twins reared together. *Social Science and Medicine, 36*(4), 441–450.

Marmot, M. G. (2004). *Status syndrome: How your social standing directly affects your health and life expectancy.* London: Bloomsbury.

Marmot, M. G., & Wilkinson, R. G. (1999). *Social determinants of health.* New York: Oxford University Press.

Chapter Nine

Block, G., Patterson, B. H., & Subar, A. F. (1992). Fruit, vegetables, and cancer prevention: A review of the epidemiologic evidence. *Nutrition and Cancer,18*(1), 1–29.

Kamimoto, L. A., Easton, A. N., Maurice, E., Husten, C. G., & Macera, C. A. (1998). Surveillance for five health risks among older adults—United States, 1993–1997. *Morbidity and Mortality Weekly Report, 48*(SS08), 89–130.

Pate, R. R., Pratt, M., Blair, S. N., Haskel, W. L., Macera, C. A., Bouchard, C., et al. (1995). Physical activity and public health: A recommendation from the Centers for Disease Control and Prevention and the American College of Sports Medicine. *Journal of the American Medical Association, 273*(5), 402–407.

U.S. Department of Health and Human Services (DHHS). (1996). *Physical activity and health: A report of the Surgeon General.* Atlanta: Author.

U.S. Department of Health and Human Services. (1998). *Tobacco use among U.S. racial/ethnic minority groups—African Americans, American Indians and Alaska Natives, Asian Americans and Pacific Islanders, and Hispanics: A report of the Surgeon General.* Atlanta: Author.

Chapter Ten

Byrd, W. M., & Clayton, L. A. (2000). *An American health dilemma: Vol. 1. A medical history of African Americans and the problem of race, beginnings to 1900.* New York: Routledge.

Byrd, W. M., & Clayton, L. A. (2002). *An American health dilemma: Race, medicine, and health care in the United States.* New York: Routledge.

Chapter Eleven

Galloway, J. M., Goldberg, B. W., & Alpert, J. S. (1999). *Primary care of Native American patients: Diagnosis, therapy, and epidemiology.* Boston: Butterworth-Heinemann.

Rhoades, E. R. (2000). *American Indian health: Innovations in health care, promotion, and policy.* Baltimore: Johns Hopkins University Press.

Chapter Twelve

Lin, K. M., & Cheung, F. (1999). Mental health issues for Asian Americans. *Psychiatric Services, 50*(6), 774–780.

Park, Y. J., Kim, H. S., Kang, H. C., & Kim, J. W. (2001). A survey of *hwa-byung* in middle-age Korean women. *Journal of Transcultural Nursing, 12*(2), 115–122.

Park, Y. J., Kim, H. S., Schwartz-Barcott, D., & Kim, J. W. (2002). The conceptual structure of *hwa-byung* in middle-aged Korean women. *Health Care for Women International, 23*(4), 389–397.

Workman, R. L. (2001). Tobacco use among Pacific Islanders: Risk-behavior surveys and data sets for the study of smoking behavior on Guam. *Asian American Pacific Islander Journal of Health, 9*(1), 15–24.

Chapter Thirteen

Aguirre-Molina, M., & Molina, C. W. (Eds.). (2003). *Latina health in the United States: A public health reader.* San Francisco: Jossey-Bass.

Aguirre-Molina, M., Molina, C. W., & Zambrana, R. E. (Eds.). (2001). *Health issues in the Latino community.* San Francisco: Jossey-Bass.

Chong, N. (2002). *The Latino patient: A cultural guide for health care providers.* Yarmouth, ME: Intercultural Press.

Chapter Fourteen

Beach, M. C., Cooper, L. A., Robinson, K. A., Price, E. G., Gary, T. L., Jenckes, M. W., et al. (2004). *Strategies for improving minority healthcare quality.* Rockville, MD: Agency for Healthcare Research and Quality.

Benzeval, M., Judge, K., & Whitehead, M. (1995). *Tackling inequalities in health.* London: King's Fund.

Cooper, L. A., Hill, M. N., & Powe, N. R. (2002). Designing and evaluating interventions to eliminate racial and ethnic disparities in health care. *Journal of General Internal Medicine, 17*(6), 477–486.

Green, C. R., Anderson, K. O., Baker, T. A., Campbell, L. C., Decker, S., Fillingim, R. B., et al. (2003). The unequal burden of pain: Confronting racial and ethnic disparities in pain. *Pain Medicine, 4*(3), 277–294.

REFERENCES

Abraido-Lanza, A. F., Dohrenwen, B. P., Ng-Mak, D. S., & Turner, J. B. (1999). The Latino mortality paradox: A test of the "salmon bias" and health migrant hypotheses. *American Journal of Public Health, 89*(10), 1543–1548.

Acevedo-Garcia, D. (2001). Zip code–level risk factors for tuberculosis: Neighborhood environment and residential segregation in New Jersey, 1985–1992. *American Journal of Public Health, 91*(5), 734–741.

Acevedo-Garcia, D. (2002). Residential segregation and the epidemiology of infectious diseases. In T. A. LaVeist (Ed.), *Race, ethnicity, and health: A public health reader.* San Francisco: Jossey-Bass.

Adams, H. E., & Cassidy, J. F. (1993). The classification of abnormal behavior. In P. B. Sutker & H. E. Adams (Eds.), *Comprehensive handbook of psychopathology* (2nd ed., pp. 3–25). New York: Plenum.

Albano, A. M., Chorpita, B. F., & Barlow, D. H. (1996). Childhood anxiety disorders. In E. J. Mash & R. A. Barkley (Eds.), *Child psychopathology* (pp. 196–241). New York: Guilford Press.

Ali, S., and Osberg, J. S. (1997). Differences in follow-up visits between African American and white Medicaid children hospitalized with asthma. *Journal of Health Care for the Poor and Underserved, 8*(1), 83–98.

Amaro, A., Vega, R. R., & Valencia, D. (2001). Gender, context, and HIV prevention among Latinos. In M. Aguirre-Molina, C. W. Molina, & R. Zambrana (Eds.), *Health issues in the Latino community.* San Francisco: Jossey-Bass.

American Psychiatric Association. (2000). *Diagnostic and statistical manual of mental disorders* (4th ed., rev.). Washington, DC: Author.

American Psychological Association. (1993). Guidelines for providers of psychological services to ethnic, linguistic, and culturally diverse populations. *American Psychologist, 48*(1), 45–48.

Amey, C. H., Albrecht, S. L., & Miller, M. K. (1996). Racial differences in adolescent drug use: The impact of religion. *Substance Use and Misuse, 31*(10), 1311–1332.

Amshel, C. E., & Caruso, D. M. (2000).Vietnamese "coining": A burn case report and literature review. *Journal of Burn Care and Rehabilitation, 21*(2), 112–114.

Andersen, R. M. (1995). Revisiting the behavioral model and access to medical care: Does it matter? *Journal of Health and Social Behavior, 36*(1), 1–10.

Anderson, L. M., Scrimshaw, S. C., Fullilove, M. T., Fielding, J. E., & Normand, J. (2003). Task Force on Community Preventive Services: Culturally competent healthcare systems: A systematic review. *American Journal of Preventive Medicine, 24*(Suppl. 3), 68–79.

Anderson, L. M., Wood, D. L., & Sherbourne, C. D. (1997). Maternal acculturation and childhood immunization levels among children in Latino families in Los Angeles. *American Journal of Public Health, 87*(12), 2018–2021.

Anderson, O. W. (1958). Infant mortality and social and cultural factors: Historical trends and current patterns. In E. G. Jaco (Ed.), *Patterns, physicians, and illness.* Glencoe, IL: Free Press.

Antai-Otong, D. (2002). Culturally sensitive treatment of African Americans with substance-related disorders. *Journal of Psychosocial Nursing and Mental Health Services, 40*(7), 14–21.

Anthony, J. C., & Echeagaray-Wagner, F. (2000). Epidemiologic analysis of alcohol and tobacco use. *Alcohol Health and Research World, 24*(4), 201.

Bachman, J. G., Wallace, J. M., Jr., O'Malley, P. M., Johnston, L. D., Kurth, C. L., & Neighbors, H. W. (1991). Racial/ethnic differences in smoking, drinking, and illicit drug use among American high school seniors, 1976–89. *American Journal of Public Health, 81*(3), 372–377.

Baker, D.W., Hayes, R., & Fortier, J. P. (1998). Interpreter use and satisfaction with interpersonal aspects of care for Spanish-speaking patients. *Medical Care, 36*(10), 1461–1470.

Balbach, E. D., Gasior, R. J., & Barbeau, E. M. (2003). R. J. Reynolds' targeting of African Americans, 1988–2000. *American Journal of Public Health, 93*(5), 822–827.

Balcazar, H., Castro, F. G., & Krull, J. L. (1995). Cancer risk reduction in Mexican American women: The role of acculturation, education, and health risk factors. *Health Education Quarterly, 22*(1), 61–84.

Bartels, S. J., Coakley, E., Oxman, T. E., Constantino, G., Oslin, D., Chen, H., et al. (2002). Suicidal and death ideation in older primary care patients with depression, anxiety, and at-risk alcohol use. *American Journal of Geriatric Psychiatry, 10*(4), 417–427.

Bassford, T. L. (1995). Health status of Hispanic elders. *Clinics in Geriatric Medicine, 11*(1), 25–38.

Bebbington, P., & Kuipers, L. (1994). The predictive utility of expressed emotion in schizophrenia: An aggregate analysis. *Psychological Medicine, 24*(3), 707–718.

Becker, E. L., & Landav, S. I. (1986). *International dictionary of medicine and biology.* New York: Oxford University Press.

Benzeval, M., Judge, K., & Whitehead, M. (1995), *Tackling inequalities in health.* London: King's Fund.

Bernasconi, R. (2001). Introduction. In R. Bernasconi (Ed.), *Concepts of race in the eighteenth century* (Vol. 1). Chicago: University of Chicago Press.

Berndt, E. R., Finkelstein, S. N., Greenberg, P. E., Howland, R. H., Keith, A., Rush, A. J., et al. (1998). Workplace performance effects from chronic depression and its treatment. *Journal of Health and Economics, 17*(5), 511–535.

Bertakis, K. D. (1981). Does race have an influence on patients' feelings toward physicians? *Journal of Family Practice, 13*(3), 383–387.

Besharov, D. J., & Gardiner, K. N. (1997). Trends in teen sexual behavior. *Child Youth Services Review, 19*(5–6), 341–367.

Bierman, A. S., Magari, E. S., Jette, A. M., Splaine, M., & Wasson, J. H. (1998). Assessing access as a first step toward improving the quality of care for very old adults. *Journal of Ambulatory Care Management, 21*(1), 17–26.

Blackburn, H., & Prineas, R. (1983). Diet and hypertension: Anthropology, epidemiology, and public health implications. *Progress in Biochemical Pharmacology, 19*(1), 31–79.

Blendon, R. J., Aiken, L. H., Freeman, H. E., & Corey, C. R. (1989). Access to medical care for black and white Americans: A matter of continuing concern. *Journal of the American Medical Association, 261*(2), 278–281.

Block, G., Patterson, B. H., & Subar, A. F. (1992). Fruit, vegetables, and cancer prevention: A review of the epidemiologic evidence. *Nutrition and Cancer, 18*(1), 1–29.

Blumenbach, J. F. (1797). *Institutions physiologiques.* Paris.

Bonkowsky, J. L., Frazer, J. K., Buchi, K. F., & Byington, C. L. (2002). Metamizole use by Latino immigrants: A common and potentially harmful home remedy. *Pediatrics, 109*(6), e98.

Borowsky, I. W., Resnick, M. D., Ireland, M., & Blum, R. W. (1999). Suicide attempts among American Indian and Alaska Native youth: Risk and protective factors. *Archives of Pediatric and Adolescent Medicine, 153*(6), 573–580.

Bosma, H., van de Mheen, H. D., Borsboom, G. J., & Mackenbach, J. P. (2001). Neighborhood socioeconomic status and all-cause mortality. *American Journal of Epidemiology, 153*(4), 363–371.

Bradshaw, B. S., & Frisbie, W. P. (1992). Morality of Mexican Americans and Mexican immigrants: Comparisons with Mexico. In J. R. Weeks & R. H. Chand (Eds.), *Demographic dynamics of the U.S.-Mexico border* (pp. 125–150). El Paso: Texas Western Press.

Braithwaite, R. L., & Arriola, R. J. (2003). Male prisoners and HIV prevention: A call for action ignored. *American Journal of Public Health, 93*(5), 759–763.

Braun, K. L., & Browne, C. (1998). Perceptions of dementia, caregiving, and help seeking among Asian and Pacific Islander Americans. *Health and Social Work, 23*(4), 262–274.

Braun, K. L., Ichiho, H. M., Kuhaulua, R. L., Aitaoto, N. T., Tsark, J. U., Spegal, R., et al. (2003, November). Empowerment through community building: Diabetes today in the Pacific. *Journal of Public Health Management and Practice* (Suppl.), S19–S25.

Braun, K. L., Mokuau, N., & Tsark, J. (1997). Cultural themes in health, illness, and rehabilitation among Native Hawaiians. *Topics in Geriatric Rehabilitation, 12*(3), 19–37.

Braun, K. L., & Nichols, R. (1996). Cultural issues in death and dying. *Hawaii Medical Journal, 55*(12), 260–264.

Braun, K. L., Yee, B. W., Browne, C. V., & Mokuau, N. (2004). Native Hawaiian and Pacific Islander elders. In K. E. Whitfield (Ed.), *Closing the gap: Improving the health of minority elders in the new millennium.* Waashington, DC: Gerontological Society of America.

Bridges, C. B., Winquist, A. G., Fukuda, K., Cox, N. J., Singleton, J. A., & Strikas, R. A. (2000). Prevention and control of influenza: Recommendations of the Advisory Committee on Immunization Practices (ACIP). *Morbidity and Mortality Weekly Report: Recommendations and Reports, 49*(1), 1–38.

Broman, C. L. (1996). Coping with personal problems. In H. W. Neighbors & J. S. Jackson (Eds.), *Mental health in black America* (pp. 117–129). Thousand Oaks, CA: Sage.

Broussard, B. A., Johnson, A., Himes, J. H., Story, M., Fichtner, R., Hauck, F., et al. (1991). Prevalence of obesity in American Indians and Alaska Natives. *American Journal of Clinical Nutrition, 53*(Suppl. 6), 1535S–1542S.

Brown, P. (1995). Race, class, and environmental health: A review and systematization of the literature. *Environmental Research, 69*(1), 15–30.

Brownson, R. C., & Bal, D. G. (1996). The future of cancer control research and translation. *Journal of Public Health Management Practice, 2*(2), 70–78.

Buchwald, D., Panwala, S., & Hooton, T. M. (1992). Use of traditional health practices by Southeast Asian refugees in a primary care clinic. *Western Journal of Medicine, 156*(5), 507–511.

Buckle, J. M., Horn, S. D., Oates, V. M., & Abbey, H. (1992). Severity of illness and resource use differences among White and Black hospitalized elderly. *Archives of Internal Medicine, 152*(8), 1596–1603.

Buffon, G. L. L. (1778). *Les époques de la nature.* Clermont-Ferrand, France.

Bullard, R. D. (2002). Solid waste sites and the black Houston community. In LaVeist, T. A. (Ed.), *Race, ethnicity, and health: A public health reader.* San Francisco: Jossey-Bass.

Butcher, J. N., Narikiyo, T., & Vitousek, K. B. (1993). Understanding abnormal behavior in cultural context. In P. B. Sutker & H. E. Adams (Eds.), *Comprehensive handbook of psychopathology* (2nd ed., pp. 83–105). New York: Plenum.

Caldas, S. J. (1994). Teen pregnancy: Why it remains a serious social, economic, and educational problem in the U.S. *Phi Delta Kappan, 75*(5), 402–406.

Campbell, D. W., Sharps, P. W., Gary, F. A., Campbell, J. C., & Lopez, L. M. (2002). Intimate partner violence in African American women. *Online Journal of Issues in Nursing, 7*(1), 5.

Campbell, R. L. (1981). *Campbell's psychiatric dictionary* (5th ed.). London: Oxford University Press.

Carlisle, D. M., Gardner, J. E., & Liu, H. (1998). The entry of underrepresented minority students into U.S. medical schools: An evaluation of recent trends. *American Journal of Public Health, 88*(9), 1314–1318.

Carlson, M. J., & Gabriel, R. M. (2001). Patient satisfaction, use of services, and one-year outcomes in publicly funded substance abuse treatment. *Psychiatric Services, 52*(9), 1230–1236.

Carrasquillo, O., Orav, E. J., Brennan, T. A., & Burstin, H. R. (1999). Impact of language barriers on patient satisfaction in an emergency department. *Journal of General Internal Medicine, 14*(2), 82–87.

Carrillo, J. E., Trevino, F. M., Betancourt, J. R., & Coustasse, A. (2001). Latino access to health care: The role of insurance, managed care, and institutional barriers. In M. Aguirre-Molina, C. Molina, & R. E. Zambrana (Eds.), *Health issues in the Latino community.* San Francisco: Jossey-Bass.

Catania, J. A., Kegeles, S. M., & Coates, T. J. (1990). Towards an understanding of risk behavior: An AIDS risk reduction model (ARRM). *Health Education Quarterly, 17*(1), 53–72.

Cavalli-Sforza, L. L., Menozzi, P., & Piazza, A. (1994). *The history and geography of human genes.* Princeton, NJ: Princeton University Press.

Centers for Disease Control and Prevention. (1998). Sexually transmitted disease surveillance, 1997. Atlanta: U.S. Department of Health and Human Services.

Centers for Disease Control and Prevention. (2000). HIV/AIDS among racial/ethnic minority men who have sex with men—United States, 1989–1998. *Morbidity and Mortality Weekly Report, 49*(1), 4–11.

Centers for Disease Control and Prevention. (2001). Pregnancy-related deaths among Hispanic, Asian/Pacific Islander, and American Indian/Alaska Native women—United States, 1991–1997. *Morbidity and Mortality Weekly Report, 50*(18), 361–364.

Centers for Disease Control and Prevention. (2002a). *Behavioral Risk Factor Surveillance System Survey data.* Atlanta: U.S. Department of Health and Human Services.

Centers for Disease Control and Prevention. (2002b). *HIV/AIDS surveillance report, 2002.* Atlanta: U.S. Department of Health and Human Services.

Centers for Disease Control and Prevention. (2002c). Traumatic brain injury among American Indians/Alaska Natives—United States, 1992–1996. *Morbidity and Mortality Weekly Report, 51*(14), 303–305.

Centers for Disease Control and Prevention. (2003). HIV/STD risks in young men who have sex with men who do not disclose their sexual orientation—six U.S. cities, 1994–2000. *Morbidity and Mortality Weekly Report, 52*(4), 81–100.

Centers for Disease Control and Prevention. (2004). Lead poisoning associated with Ayurvedic medications—five states, 2000–2003. *Morbidity and Mortality Weekly Report, 53*(26), 582–584.

Chao, A., & Tsay, P. (1998). A sample coverage approach to multiple-system estimation with application to census undercount. *Journal of the American Statistical Association, 93*(441), 283–293.

Chen, J., Rathore, S., Radford, M. J., Wang, Y., & Krumholz, H. M. (2002). Racial differences in the use of cardiac catheterization after acute myocardial infarction. In T. A. LaVeist (Ed.), *Race, ethnicity, and health: A public health reader* (pp. 644–656). San Francisco: Jossey-Bass.

Chi, I., Lubben, J. E., & Kitano, H. H. (1989). Differences in drinking behavior among three Asian-American groups. *Journal for the Study of Alcoholism, 50*(1), 15–23.

Chng, C. L., Wong, F. Y., Park, R. J., Edberg, M. C., & Lai, D. S. (2003). A model for understanding sexual health among Asian American/Pacific Islander men who have sex with men (MSM) in the United States. *AIDS Education and Prevention, 15*(1, Suppl. A), 21–38.

Choi, K. H., Catania, J. A., & Dolcini, M. M. (1994). Extramarital sex and HIV risk behavior among U.S. adults: Results from the National AIDS Behavioral Survey. *American Journal of Public Health, 84*(12), 2003–2007.

Clark, H. J., Lindner, G., Armistead, L., & Austin, B. J. (2003). Stigma, disclosure, and psychological functioning among HIV-infected and non-infected African American women. *Women's Health, 38*(4), 57–71.

Clark, R., Anderson, N. B., Clark, V. R., & Williams, D. R. (2002). Racism as a stressor for African Americans: A biopsychosocial model. In T. A. LaVeist (Ed.), *Race, ethnicity, and health: A public health reader* (pp. 319–339). San Francisco: Jossey-Bass.

Coe, K., Attakai, A., Papenfuss, M., Giuliano, A., Martin, L., & Nuvayestewa, L. (2004). Traditionalism and its relationship to disease risk and protective behaviors of women living on the Hopi reservation. *Health Care for Women International, 25*(5), 391–410.

Cohen, S., Frank, E., Doyle, W. J., Skoner, D. P., Rabin, B. S., & Gwaltney, J. M., Jr. (1998). Types of stressors that increase susceptibility to the common cold in healthy adults. *Journal of Health Psychology, 17*(3), 214–223.

Collins, C. A., & Williams, D. R. (2002). Racial residential segregation: A fundamental cause of racial disparities in health. In T. A. LaVeist (Ed.), *Race, ethnicity, and health: A public health reader* (pp. 369–389). San Francisco: Jossey-Bass.

Commission for Racial Justice, United Church of Christ. (1987). *Toxic wastes and race in the United States: A national report on the racial and socioeconomic characteristics of communities with hazardous waste sites.* New York: Public Data Access.

Conwell, Y., & Brent, D. (1995). Suicide and aging: Patterns of psychiatric diagnosis. *International Psychogeriatrics, 7*(2), 149–164.

Coonrod, D. V., Bay, R. C., & Balcazar, H. (2004). Ethnicity, acculturation, and obstetric outcomes: Different risk factor profiles in low- and high-acculturation Hispanics and in white non-Hispanics. *Journal of Reproductive Medicine, 49*(1), 17–22.

Cooper, L. A., Brown, C., Vu, H. T., Ford, D. E., & Powe, N. R. (2001). How important is intrinsic spirituality in depression care? A comparison of white and African American primary care patients. *Journal of General Internal Medicine, 16*(9), 634–638.

Cooper, L. A., & Roter, D. L. (2002). Patient-provider communication: The effect of race and ethnicity on process and outcomes of health care. In Institute of Medicine, *Unequal treatment: Confronting racial and ethnic disparities in health care* (pp. 336–380). Washington, DC: National Academies Press.

Cooper, L. A., Roter, D. L., Johnson, R. L., Ford, D. E., Steinwachs, D. M., & Powe, N. R. (2003). Patient-centered communication, ratings of care, and concordance of patient and physician race. *Annals of Internal Medicine, 139*(11), 907–915.

Cooper-Patrick, L., Gallo, J. J., Gonzales, J. J., Vu, H. T., Powe, N. R., Nelson, C., et al. (2002). Race, gender, and partnership in the patient-physician relationship. In T. A. LaVeist (Ed.), *Race, ethnicity, and health: A public health reader* (pp. 609–625). San Francisco: Jossey-Bass.

Corkery, E., Palmer, C., Foley, M. E., Schechter, C. B., Frisher, L., & Roman, S. H. (1997). Effect of a bicultural community health worker on completion of diabetes education in a Hispanic population. *Diabetes Care, 20*(3), 254–257.

Cornwall, A., & Jewkes, J. (1995). What is participatory action research? *Social Science and Medicine, 41*(12), 1667–1676.

Corrigan, P. W., & Penn, D. L. (1999). Lessons from social psychology on discrediting psychiatric stigma. *American Psychologist, 54,* 765–776.

Corti, M. C., Guralnik, J. M., Ferrucci, L., Izmirlian, G., Leveille, S. G., Pahor, M., et al. (1999). Evidence for a black-white crossover in all-cause and coronary heart disease mortality in an older population: The North Carolina EPESE. *American Journal of Public Health, 89*(3), 308–314.

Cossrow, N., & Falkner, B. (2004). Racial/ethnic issues in obesity and obesity-related comorbidities. *Journal of Clinical Endocrinal Metabolism, 89*(6), 2590–2594.

Coughlin, S. S., Uhler, R. J., Bobo, J. K., & Caplan, L. (2004). Breast cancer screening practices among women in the United States, 2000. *Cancer Causes and Control, 15*(2), 159–170.

Cowen, E. L. (1994). The enhancement of psychological wellness: Challenges and opportunities. *American Journal of Community Psychology, 22,* 149–179.

Crabbe, K. M. (1998). Etiology of depression among native Hawaiians. *Pacific Health Dialog, 5*(2), 341–345.

Crane, J. A. (1997). Patient comprehension of doctor-patient communication on discharge from emergency department. *Journal of Emergency Medicine, 15*(1), 1–7.

Crosson, J. C., Deng, W., Brazeau, C., Boyd, L., & Soto-Greene, M. (2004). Evaluating the effect of cultural competency training on medical student attitudes. *Family Medicine, 36*(3), 199–203.

Cruz, M. (1999). Alcohol and solvent abuse. In J. M. Galloway, B. W. Goldberg, & J. S. Alpert (Eds.), *Primary care of Native American patients: Diagnosis, therapy, and epidemiology* (pp. 263–268). Boston: Butterworth-Heinemann.

Curb, J. D., Aluli, N. E., Huang, B. J., Sharp, D. S., Rodriguez, B. L., Burchfield, C. M., et al. (1996). Hypertension in elderly Japanese Americans and adult native Hawaiians. *Public Health Reports, 111*(Suppl. 2), 53–55.

David, R. J., & Collins, J. W., Jr. (2002). Differing birthweight among infants of U.S. born blacks, African-born blacks, and U.S. born whites. In T. A. LaVeist (Ed.), *Race, ethnicity, and health: A public health reader* (pp. 252–264). San Francisco: Jossey-Bass.

Davis, D. J. (1999). Health care for Alaska Natives and Native Americans: Historical perspective. In J. M. Galloway, B. W. Goldberg, & J. S. Alpert (Eds.), *Primary care of Native American patients: Diagnosis, therapy, and epidemiology.* Boston: Butterworth-Heinmann.

Davis, F. G., Persky, V. W., Ferre, C. D., Howe, H. L., Barrett, R. E., & Haenszel, W. M. (1995). Cancer incidence of Hispanics and non-Hispanic whites in Cook County, Illinois. *Cancer, 75*(12), 2939–2945.

Davis, F. J. (1991). *Who is black? One nation's definition.* University Park: Pennsylvania State University Press.

Davis, S. F., Rosen, D. H., Steinberg, S., Wortley, P. M., Karon, J. M., & Gwinn, M. (1998). Trends in HIV prevalence among childbearing women in the United States, 1989–1994. *Journal of Acquired Immune Deficiency Syndrome, 19*(2), 158–164.

Dawson, D. A., Grant, B. F., Chou, S. P., & Pickering, R. P. (1995). Subgroup variation in U.S. drinking patterns: Results of the 1992 National Longitudinal Alcohol Epidemiologic Study. *Journal of Substance Abuse, 7*(3), 331–344.

Dean, M., Stephens, J. C., Winkler, C., Lomb, D. A., Ramsburg, M., Boaze, R., et al. (1994). Polymorphic admixture typing in human ethnic populations. *American Journal of Human Genetics, 55*(4), 788–808.

de Bruyn, T. (2002). HIV-related stigma and discrimination: The epidemic continues. *Canadian HIV/AIDS Policy Law Review, 7*(1), 8–14.

Dessio, W., Wade, C., Chao, M., Kronenberg, F., Cushman, L. E., & Kalmuss, D. (2004). Religion, spirituality, and healthcare choices of African American women: Results of a national survey. *Ethnicity and Disease, 14*(2), 189–197.

Diala, C., Muntaner, C., Walrath, C., Nickerson, K. J., LaVeist, T. A., & Leaf, P. J. (2000). Racial differences in attitudes toward professional mental health care and in the use of services. *American Journal of Orthopsychiatry, 70*(4), 455–464.

Diaz, T., Chu, S. Y., Buehler, J. W., Boyd, D., Checo, P. J., Conti, L., et al. (1994). Socioeconomic differences among people with AIDS: Results from a multistate surveillance project. *American Journal of Preventive Medicine, 10*(4), 217–222.

Doescher, M. P., Saver, B. G., Franks, P., & Fiscella, K. (2000). Racial and ethnic disparities in perceptions of physician style and trust. *Archives of Family Medicine, 9*(10), 1156–1163.

Dohrenwend, B. S., & Dohrenwend, B. P. (1984). Life stress and illness: Formulation of the issues. In B. S. Dohrenwend & B. P. Dohrenwend (Eds.), *Stressful life events and their contexts* (Vol. 2, pp. 1–27). New Brunswick, NJ: Rutgers University Press.

Dominitz, J. A., Samsa, G. P., Landsman, P., & Provenzale, D. (1998). Race, treatment, and survival among colorectal carcinoma patients in an equal-access medical system. *Cancer, 82*(12), 2312–2320.

Doty, M. M. (2003). *Insurance, access, and quality of care among Hispanic populations.* New York: Commonwealth Fund.

Dracup, K., & Moser, D. K. (1991). Treatment-seeking behavior among those with signs and symptoms of acute myocardial infarction. *Heart and Lung, 20*(5, Pt. 2), 570–575.

Dressler, W. W. (1991). Social class, skin color, and arterial blood pressure in two societies. *Ethnicity and Disease, 1*(1), 60–77.

Drewnowski, A., & Speter, S. E. (2004). Poverty and obesity: The role of energy density and energy costs. *American Journal of Clinical Nutrition, 79*(1), 6–16.

Duijkers, T. J., Drijver, M., Kromhout, D., & James, S. A. (1988). "John Henryism" and blood pressure in a Dutch population. *Psychosomatic Medicine, 50*(4), 353–359.

Duncan, O. D. (1961). A socioeconomic index for all occupations. In A. J. Reiss Jr. (Ed.), *Occupations and social status* (pp. 109–138). New York: Free Press.

Egede, L. E., & Bonadonna, R. J. (2003). Diabetes self-management in African Americans: An exploration of the role of fatalism. *Diabetes Education, 29*(1),105–115.

Egede, L. E., & Zheng, D. (2003). Racial/ethnic differences in influenza vaccination coverage in high-risk adults. *American Journal of Public Health, 93*(12), 2074–2078.

Eggers, P. W. (1995). Racial differences in access to kidney transplantation. *Health Care Financial Review, 17*(2), 89–103.

Ehresmann, K. R., White, K. E., Hedberg, C. W., Anderson, E., Korlath, J. A., Moore, K. A., et al. (1998). A statewide survey of immunization rates in Minnesota school age children: Implications for targeted assessment and prevention strategies. *Pediatric Infectious Disease Journal, 17*(8), 711–716.

Eisenbruch, M., & Handelman, L. (1990). Cultural consultation for cancer: Astrocytoma in a Cambodian adolescent. *Social Science and Medicine, 31*(12), 1295–1299.

Engels, F. (1999). *The condition of the working class in England.* London: Oxford University Press. (Originally published 1845)

Epstein, A. M., & Ayanian, J. Z. (2001). Racial disparities in medical care. *New England Journal of Medicine, 344*(19), 1471–1473.

Ertugrul, A., & Ulug, B. (2004). Perception of stigma among patients with schizophrenia. *Social Psychiatry and Psychiatric Epidemiology, 39*(1), 73–77.

Escarce, J. J., Epstein, K. R., Colby, D. C., & Schwartz, J. S. (1993). Racial differences in the elderly's use of medical procedures and diagnostic tests. *American Journal of Public Health, 83*(7), 948–954.

Escobar, J. I. (1987). Cross-cultural aspects of the somatization trait. *Hospital and Community Psychiatry, 38*(2), 174–180.

Faber, D. R., & Krieg, E. J. (2002). Unequal exposure to ecological hazards: Environmental injustices in the Commonwealth of Massachusetts. *Environmental Health Perspectives, 110*(Suppl. 2), 277–288.

Falcon, A., Aguirre-Molina, M., and Molina, C. W. (2001). Latino health policy: Beyond demographic determinism. In M. Aguirre-Molina, C. W. Molina, & R. E. Zambrana (Eds.), *Health issues in the Latino community* (pp. 3–22). San Francisco: Jossey-Bass.

Fang, J., Madhavan, S., Bosworth, W., & Alderman, M. H. (1998). Residential segregation and mortality in New York City. *Social Science and Medicine, 47*(4), 469–476.

Featherman, D. L., & Hauser, R. M. (1976). Prestige or socioeconomic scales in the study of occupational achievement? *Sociological Methods and Research, 4*(4), 403–422.

Fedder, D. O., Chang, R. J., Curry, S., & Nichols, G. (2003). The effectiveness of a community health worker outreach program on healthcare utilization of West Baltimore City Medicaid patients with diabetes, with or without hypertension. *Ethnicity and Disease, 13*(1), 22–27.

Ferguson, W. J., Keller, D. M., Haley, H. L., & Quirk, M. (2003). Developing culturally competent community faculty: A model program. *Academic Medicine, 78*(12), 1221–1228.

Fiscella, K., Franks, P., Gold, M. R., & Clancy, C. M. (2000). Inequality in quality: Addressing socioeconomic, racial, and ethnic disparities in health care. *Journal of the American Medical Association, 283*(19), 2579–2584.

Fitzgerald, E. F., Hwang, S. A., Langguth, K., Cayo, M., Yang, B. Z., Bush, B., et al. (2004). Fish consumption and other environmental exposures and their associations with serum PCB concentrations among Mohawk women at Akwesasne. *Environmental Research, 94*(2), 160–170.

Flaherty, J. A., & Meagher, R. (1980). Measuring racial bias in inpatient treatment. *American Journal of Psychiatry, 137*(6), 679–682.

Flaskerud, J. H., Uman, G., Lara, R., Romero, L., & Taka, K. (1996). Sexual practices, attitudes, and knowledge related to HIV transmission in low-income Los Angeles Hispanic women. *Journal of Sex Research, 33,* 343–353.

Fletcher, B. J. (1998). Spirituality, grieving, and mental well-being. In R. L. Jones (Ed.), *African American mental health* (pp. 135–149). Hampton, VA: Cobb & Henry.

Flores, G., Rabke-Verani, J., Pine, W., & Sabharwal, A. (2002). The importance of cultural and linguistic issues in the emergency care of children. *Pediatric Emergency Care, 8*(4), 271–284.

Flynn-Saldana, K. J., Kirsch, A., & Lister, M. E. (2003). Racial and ethnic disparities in childhood immunization coverage in North Carolina. *North Carolina Medical Journal, 64*(3), 106–110.

Folsom, A. R., Sprafka, J. M., Luepker, R. V., & Jacobs, D. R., Jr. (1988). Beliefs among Black and White adults about causes and prevention of cardiovascular disease: The Minnesota Heart Survey. *American Journal of Preventive Medicine, 4*(3), 121–127.

Ford, E., Newman, J., & Deosaransingh, K. (2000). Racial and ethnic differences in the use of cardiovascular procedures: Findings from the California Cooperative Cardiovascular Project. *American Journal of Public Health, 90*(7), 1128–1134.

Ford, E. S., & Cooper, R. S. (1995). Racial/ethnic differences in health care utilization of cardiovascular procedures: a review of the evidence. *Health Services Research, 30*(1, Pt. 2), 237–252.

Franzini, L., Ribble, J. C., & Keddie, A. M. (2002). Understanding the Hispanic paradox. In T. A. LaVeist (Ed.), *Race, ethnicity, and health: A public health reader* (pp. 280–310). San Francisco: Jossey-Bass.

Freedenthal, S., & Stiffman, A. R. (2004). Suicidal behavior in urban American Indian adolescents: A comparison with reservation youth in a southwestern state. *Suicide and Life Threatening Behavior, 34*(2), 160–171.

Frisbie, W. P., Cho, Y., & Hummer, R. A. (2002). Immigration and the health of Asian and Pacific Islander adults in the United States. In T. A. LaVeist (Ed.), *Race, ethnicity, and health: A public health reader* (pp. 231–251). San Francisco: Jossey-Bass.

Frohmberg, E., Goble, R., Sanchez, V., & Quigley, D. (2000). The assessment of radiation exposures in Native American communities from nuclear weapons testing in Nevada. *Risk Analysis, 20*(1), 101–111.

Fullilove, M. T. (1998). Abandoning "race" as a variable in public health research: An idea whose time has come. *American Journal of Public Health, 88*(9), 1297–1298.

Ganesan, K., Teklehaimanot, S., Akhtar, A. J., Wijegunaratne, J., Thadepalli, K., & Ganesan, N. (2003). Racial differences in preventive practices of African American and Hispanic women. *Journal of the American Geriatric Society, 51*(4), 515–518.

Garrett, M. D., & Menke, K. A. (2001). *Indians no more: Inconsistent classification of American Indians and Alaska Natives in Medicare.* Albuquerque, NM: National Indian Council on Aging.

Garte, S. (2002). The racial genetics paradox in biomedical research and public health. *Public Health Report, 117*(5), 421–425.

Gary, T. L., Batts-Turner, M., Bone, L. R., Yeh, H. C., Wang, N. Y., Hill-Briggs, F., et al. (2004). A randomized controlled trial of the effects of nurse case manager and community health worker team interventions in urban African-Americans with type 2 diabetes. *Controlled Clinical Trials, 25*(1), 53–66.

Gary, T. L., Bone, L. R., Hill, M. N., Levine, D. M., McGuire, M., Saudek, C., et al. (2003). Randomized controlled trial of the effects of nurse case manager and community health worker interventions on risk factors for diabetes-related complications in urban African Americans. *Preventive Medicine, 37*(1), 23–32.

Gazino, J. M., Manson, J. E., Buring, J. E., & Hennekens, C. H. (1992). Dietary antioxidants and cardiovascular disease. *Annals of the New York Academy of Science, 669,* 249–259.

Geronimus, A. T. (2002). Black-White differences in the relationship of maternal age to birthweight: A population-based test of the weathering hypothesis. In T. A. LaVeist (Ed.), *Race, ethnicity, and health: A public health reader* (pp. 213–230). San Francisco: Jossey-Bass.

Giacomini, M. K. (1996). Gender and ethnic differences in hospital-based procedure utilization in California. *Archives of Internal Medicine, 156*(11), 1217–1224.

Gleiberman, L., Harburg, E., Frone, M. R., Russell, M., & Cooper, M. L. (1993). Skin color, ancestry, and blood pressure among Whites in Erie County, New York. *Ethnicity and Disease, 3*(4), 378–386.

Goff, D. C., Ramsey, D. J., Labarthe, D. R., & Nichaman, M. Z. (1994). Greater case-fatality after myocardial infarction among Mexican Americans and women than among non-Hispanic Whites and men. *American Journal of Epidemiology, 139*(5), 474–483.

Gove, S. V. (1999). African American women's perceptions of weight: Paradigm shift for advanced practice. *Holistic Nurse Practitioner, 13*(4), 71–79.

Gregory, P. M., Rhoads, G. G., Wilson, A. C., O'Dowd, K. J., & Kostis, J. B. (1999). Impact of availability of hospital-based invasive cardiac services on racial differences in the use of these services. *American Heart Journal, 138*(3, Pt. 1), 507–517.

Grim, C. E., & Robinson, M. (2003). Salt, slavery, and survival: Hypertension in the African diaspora. *Epidemiology and Society, 14*(1), 120–122.

Guarnaccia, P. J., Canino, G., Rubio-Stipec, M., & Bravo, M. (1993). The prevalence of *ataques de nervios* in the Puerto Rico Disaster Study: The role of culture in psychiatric epidemiology. *Journal of Nervous and Mental Disorders, 181*(3), 157–165.

Hackbarth, D. P., Schnopp-Wyatt, D., Katz, D., Williams, J., Silvestri, B., & Pfleger, M. (2001). Collaborative research and action to control the geographic placement of outdoor advertising of alcohol and tobacco products in Chicago. *Public Health Report, 116*(6), 558–567.

Hackbarth, D. P., Silvestri, B., & Cosper, W. (1995). Tobacco and alcohol billboards in 50 Chicago neighborhoods: Market segmentation to sell dangerous products to the poor. *Journal of Public Health Policy, 16*(2), 213–230.

Hader, D., Smith, D., Moore, J., & Holmberg, S. (2001). HIV infection in women in the United States: Status at the millennium. *Journal of the American Medical Association, 285*(9), 1186–1192.

Hall, T. R., Hickey, M. E., & Young, T. B. (1992). Evidence for recent increases in obesity and non-insulin-dependent diabetes mellitus in a Navajo community. *American Journal of Human Biology, 4,* 547–553.

Halter, M. J. (2004). The stigma of seeking care and depression. *Archives of Psychiatric Nursing, 18*(5), 178–184.

Hammond, C., & Rudolph, K. D. (1996). Childhood depression. In E. J. Mash & R. A. Barkley (Eds.), *Child psychopathology* (pp. 153–195). New York: Guilford Press.

Han, P. K., Hagel, J., Welty, T. K., Ross, R., Leonardson, G., & Keckler, A. (1994). Cultural factors associated with health-risk behavior among the Cheyenne River Sioux. *American Indian/Alaska Native Mental Health Research, 5*(3), 15–29.

Harburg, E., Erfurt, J. C., Chape, C., Hauenstein, L. S., Schull, W. J., & Schork, M. A. (1973). Socioecological stressor areas and Black-White blood pressure: Detroit. *Journal of Chronic Diseases, 26*(9), 595–611.

Harden, M. J. (1999). *Voices of wisdom: Hawaiian elders speak.* Kula, HI: Aka Press.

Harris, D. R., Andrews, R., & Elixhauser, A. (1997). Racial and gender differences in use of procedures for Black and White hospitalized adults. *Ethnicity and Disease, 7*(2), 91–105.

Harrison, D. F., Wambach, K. G., Byers, J. B., Imershein, A. W., Levine, P., Maddox, K., et al. (1991). AIDS knowledge and risk behaviors among culturally diverse women. *AIDS Education and Prevention, 3*(2), 79–89.

Hart, K. D. (1997). Racial segregation and ambulatory care-sensitive admissions. *Health Affairs, 16*(1), 224–225.

Haselkorn, T., Stewart, S. L., & Horn-Ross, P. L. (2003). Why are thyroid cancer rates so high in Southeast Asian women living in the United States? The Bay Area Thyroid Cancer Study. *Cancer Epidemiology Biomarkers and Prevention, 12*(2), 144–150.

Hashibe, M., Gao, T., Li, G., Dalbagni, G., & Zhang, Z. F. (2003). Comparison of bladder cancer survival among Japanese, Chinese, Filipino, Hawaiian, and Caucasian populations in the United States. *Asian Pacific Journal of Cancer Prevention, 4*(3), 267–273.

Haviland, M. G., Morales, L. S., Reise, S. P., & Hays, R. D. (2003). Do health care ratings differ by race or ethnicity? *Joint Commission Journal on Quality and Safety, 29*(3), 134–145.

Hawaii Department of Health. (2004). *Hawaii cancer facts, 2003–2004: A sourcebook for planning and implementing programs for cancer prevention and control.* Honolulu: State of Hawaii Department of Health.

Hayes-Bautista, D. E., & Chapa, J. (2002). Latino terminology: Conceptual bases for standardized terminology. In T. A. LaVeist (Ed.), *Race, ethnicity, and health: A public health reader* (pp. 141–159). San Francisco: Jossey-Bass.

He, H., McCoy, H. V., Stevens, S. J., & Stark, M. J. (1998). Violence and HIV sexual risk behaviors among female sex partners of male drug users. *Women's Health, 27*(1–2), 161–175.

Henderson, S. O., Magana, R. N., Korn, C. S., Genna, T., & Bretsky, P. M. (2002). Delayed presentation for care during acute myocardial infarction in a Hispanic population of Los Angeles County. *Ethnicity and Disease, 12*(1), 38–44.

Herek, G. M., Capitanio, J. P., & Wildman, K. F. (2002). HIV-related stigma and knowledge in the United States: Prevalence and trends, 1991–1999. *American Journal of Public Health, 92*(3), 371–377.

Hoberman, H. (1992). Ethnic minority status and adolescent mental health services utilization. *Journal of Mental Health Administration, 19*(3), 246–263.

Hogue, C. J. R., & Hargraves, M. A. (2000). The Commonwealth Fund Minority Health Survey of 1994: An overview. In C. J. R. Hogue, M. A. Hargraves, & K. S. Collins (Eds.), *Minority health in America: Findings and policy implications from the Commonwealth Fund Minority Health Survey.* Baltimore: Johns Hopkins University Press.

House, J., & Williams, D. R. (2000). Understanding and reducing socioeconomic and racial/ethnic disparities in health. In B. D. Smedley & S. L. Syme (Eds.), *Promoting health: Intervention strategies from social and behavioral research* (pp. 81–124). Washington, DC: National Academies Press.

Howell, E. M., & Russette, L. (2004). An innovative blood lead screening program for Indian children. *Public Health Report, 119*(2), 141–143.

Hsu, F. L. K. (1971). Psychosocial homeostasis and *jen:* Conceptual tools for advancing psychological anthropology. *American Anthropologist, 73*(1), 23–44.

Hsu, L. K., & Folstein, M. F. (1997). Somatoform disorders in Caucasian and Chinese Americans. *Journal of Nervous and Mental Disorders, 185*(6), 382–387.

Hudson, T. J., Owen, R. R., Thrush, C. R., Han, X., Pyne, J. M., Thapa, P., et al. (2004). A pilot study of barriers to medication adherence in schizophrenia. *Journal of Clinical Psychiatry, 65*(2), 211–216.

Iannotta, J. G. (2002). *Emerging issues in Hispanic health.* Washington, DC: National Academies Press.

Institute of Medicine. (1994). *Reducing risks for mental disorders: Frontiers for preventive intervention research.* Washington, DC: National Academies Press.

Institute of Medicine. (2001). *Crossing the quality chasm: A new health system for the 21st century.* Washington, DC: National Academies Press.

Institute of Medicine. (2002).*Unequal treatment: Confronting racial and ethnic disparities of health care.* Washington, DC: National Academies Press.

Ishida, D. N., Toomata-Mayer, T. F., & Braginsky, N. S. (2001). Beliefs and attitudes of Samoan women toward early detection of breast cancer and mammography utilization. *Cancer, 91*(Suppl. 1), 262–266.

Israel, B. A., Schulz, A. J., Parker, E. A., & Becker, A. B. (2001). Community-campus partnerships for health. Community-based participatory research: policy recommendations for promoting a partnership approach in health research. *Education and Health, 14*(2), 182–197.

Ivanov, L. L., & Flynn, B. C. (1999). Utilization and satisfaction with prenatal care services. *Western Journal of Nursing Research, 21*(3), 372–386.

Jackson, S. A., Anderson, R. T., Johnson, N. J., & Sorlie, P. D. (2000). The relation of residential segregation to all-cause mortality: A study in Black and White. *American Journal of Public Health, 90*(4), 615–617.

Jacobs, E. A., Lauderdale, D. S., Meltzer, D., Shorey, J. M., Levinson, W., & Thisted, R. A. (2001). Impact of interpreter services on delivery of health care to limited-English-proficient patients. *Journal of General Internal Medicine, 16*(7), 468–474.

Jacobs, E. A., Shepard, D. S., Suaya, J. A., & Stone, E. L. (2004). Overcoming language barriers in health care: Costs and benefits of interpreter services. *American Journal of Public Health, 94*(5), 866–869.

James, S. A. (2002). John Henryism and the health of African Americans. In T. A. LaVeist (Ed.), *Race, ethnicity, and health: A public health reader* (pp. 350–368). San Francisco: Jossey-Bass.

James, S. A., Keenan, N. L., Strogatz, D. S., Browning, S. R., & Garrett, J. M. (1992). Socioeconomic status, John Henryism, and blood pressure in black adults: The Pitt County Study. *American Journal of Epidemiology, 135*(1), 59–67.

Jeffery, R. W., & French, S. A. (1996). Socioeconomic status and weight control practices among 20- to 45-year-old women. *American Journal of Public Health, 86*(7), 1005–1010.

Johnson, R. L., Saha, S., Arbelaez, J. J., Beach, C. M., & Cooper, L. A. (2004). Racial and ethnic differences in patient perceptions of bias and cultural competence in health care. *Journal of General Internal Medicine, 19*(2), 101–110.

Jones, C. P., LaVeist, T. A., & Lillie-Blanton, M. (1991). "Race" in the epidemiologic literature: An examination of the *American Journal of Epidemiology,* 1921–1990. *American Journal of Epidemiology, 134*(10), 1079–1084.

Jones, D. A., Ainsworth, B. E., Croft, J. B., Macera, C. A., Lloyd, E. E., & Yusuf, H. R. (1998). Moderate leisure-time physical activity: Who is meeting the public health recommendations? *Archives of Family Medicine, 7*(2), 285–289.

Jones-Webb, R., Snowden, L., Herd, D., Short, B., & Hannan, P. (1997). Alcohol-related problems among Black, Hispanic, and White men: The contribution of neighborhood poverty. *Journal of Studies on Alcohol, 58*(5), 539–545.

Jung, R. T. (1997). Obesity as a disease. *British Medical Bulletin, 53*(2), 307–321.

Kaholokula, J. K., Grandinetti, A., Crabbe, K. M., Chang, H. K., & Kenui, C. K. (1999). Depressive symptoms and cigarette smoking among Native Hawaiians. *Asia-Pacific Journal of Public Health, 11*(1), 60–64.

Kaplan, S. H., Greenfield, S., Gandek, B., Rogers, W. H., & Ware, J. E., Jr. (1996). Characteristics of physicians with participatory decision-making styles. *Annals of Internal Medicine, 124*(5), 497–504.

Kaufman, J. S., & Barkey, N. (1993). Hypertension in Africa: An overview of prevalence rates and causal risk factors. *Ethnicity and Disease,* 3(Suppl.), S83–101.

Kaufman, J. S., & Hall, S. A. (2003). The slavery hypertension hypothesis: Dissemination and appeal of a modern race theory. *Epidemiology, 14*(1), 111–118.

Kavanaugh, D. (1992). Recent developments in expressed emotion and schizophrenia. *British Journal of Psychiatry, 160,* 601–620.

Kawachi, I., & Berkman, L. F. (2003). *Neighborhoods and health.* New York: Oxford University Press.

Kawachi, I., Kennedy, B. P., & Wilkinson, R. G. (Eds.). (1999). *The society and population health reader: Income inequality and health.* New York: New Press.

Kennamer, J. D., Honnold, J., Bradford, J., & Hendricks, M. (2000). Differences in disclosure of sexuality among African American and White gay/bisexual men: Implications for HIV/AIDS prevention. *AIDS Education and Prevention, 12*(6), 519–531.

Kessler, R. C., McGonagle, K. A., Zhao, S., Nelson, C. B., Hughes, M., Eshleman, S., et al. (1994). Lifetime and 12-month prevalence of DSM-III-R psychiatric disorders in the United States: Results from the National Comorbidity Survey. *Archives of General Psychiatry, 51*(1), 8–19.

Kessler, R. C., Nelson, C. B., McGonagle, K. A., Liu, J., Swartz, M., & Blazer, D. G. (1996). Comorbidity of DSM-III-R major depressive disorder in the general population: Results from the U.S. National Comorbidity Survey. *British Journal of Psychiatry* (Suppl. 30), 17–30.

King, R. C., & Stansfield, W. D. (1990). *A dictionary of genetics.* New York: Oxford University Press.

Kirkman-Liff, B., & Mondragon, D. (1991). Language of interview: Relevance for research of southwest Hispanics. *American Journal of Public Health, 81*(11), 1399–1404.

Kirmayer, L. J., & Young, A. (1998). Culture and somatization: Clinical, epidemiological, and ethnographic perspectives. *Psychosomatic Medicine, 60*(4), 420–430.

Kiyohara, Y., Kubo, M., Kato, I., Tanizaki, Y., Tanaka, K., Okubo, K., et al. (2003). Ten-year prognosis of stroke and risk factors for death in a Japanese community: The Hisayama Study. *Stroke, 34*(10), 2343–2347.

Klag, M. J., Whelton, P. K., Coresh, J., Grim, C. E., & Kuller, L. H. (1991). The association of skin color with blood pressure in U.S. Blacks with low socioeconomic status. *Journal of the American Medical Association, 265*(5), 599–602.

Kleinman, A. (1977). Depression, somatization, and the "new cross-cultural psychiatry." *Social Science and Medicine, 11*(1), 3–10.

Klingler, D., Green-Weir, R., Nerenz, D., Havstad, S., Rosman, H. S., Cetner, L., et al. (2002). Perceptions of chest pain differ by race. *American Heart Journal, 144*(1), 51–59.

Klonoff, E. A., & Landrine, H. (2002). Is skin color a marker for racial discrimination? Explaining the skin color–hypertension relationship. In T. A. LaVeist (Ed.), *Race, ethnicity, and health: A public health reader* (pp. 340–349). San Francisco: Jossey-Bass.

Knapp, R. G., Keil, J. E., Sutherland, S. E., Rust, P. F., Hames, C., & Tyroler, H. A. (1995). Skin color and cancer mortality among Black men in the Charleston Heart Study. *Clinical Genetics, 47*(4), 200–206.

Komaromy, M., Grumbach, K., Drake, M., Vranizan, K., Lurie, N., Keane, D., et al. (1996). The role of black and Hispanic physicians in providing health care for underserved populations. *New England Journal of Medicine, 334*(20), 1305–1310.

Korenbrot, C. C., Ehlers, S., & Crouch, J. A. (2003). Disparities in hospitalizations of rural American Indians. *Medical Care, 41*(5), 626–636.

Kugler, J. P., Connell, F. A., & Henley, C. E. (1990). Lack of difference in neonatal mortality between blacks and whites served by the same medical care system. *Journal of Family Practice, 30*(3), 281–287.

Kumanyika, S. (2002). The minority factor in the obesity epidemic. *Ethnicity and Disease, 12*(3), 316–319.

Last, J. M. (1988). *A dictionary of epidemiology* (2nd ed.). New York: Oxford University Press.

Lauver, D. R., Settersten, L., Kane, J. H., & Henriques, J. B. (2003). Tailored messages, external barriers, and women's utilization of professional breast cancer screening over time. *Cancer, 97*(11), 2724–2735.

LaVeist, T. A. (1989). Linking residential segregation and the infant mortality race disparity. *Sociology and Social Research, 73*(1), 90–94.

LaVeist, T. A. (1993). Separation, poverty, and empowerment: Health consequences for African Americans. *Milbank Quarterly, 73*(1), 41–64.

LaVeist, T. A. (1994). Beyond dummy variables and sample selection: What health services researchers ought to know about race as a variable. *Health Services Research, 29*(1), 1–16.

LaVeist, T. A. (1995). Data sources for aging research on racial and ethnic groups. *Gerontologist, 35*(3), 328–339.

LaVeist, T. A., Nickerson, K., & Bowie, J. (2000). Attitudes about racism, medical mistrust, and satisfaction with care among African American and White cardiac patients. *Medical Care Research and Review, 57*(Suppl. 1), 146–161.

LaVeist, T. A., & Nuru-Jeter, A. (2002). Is doctor-patient race concordance associated with greater satisfaction with care? *Journal of Health and Social Behavior, 43*(3), 296–306.

LaVeist, T. A., Nuru-Jeter, A., & Jones, K. E. (2003). The association of doctor-patient race concordance with health services utilization. *Journal of Public Health Policy, 24*(3–4), 312–323.

LaVeist, T. A., & Wallace, J. (2000). Health risk and inequitable distribution of liquor stores in African American neighborhoods. *Social Science and Medicine, 51*(4), 613–617.

Lavizzo-Mourey, R., & Mackenzie, E. R. (1996). Cultural competence: Essential measurements of quality for managed care organizations. *Annals of Internal Medicine, 124*(10), 919–921.

Lee, E., & Mokuau, N. (2002). *Cultural diversity series: Meeting the mental health needs of Asian and Pacific Islander Americans.* Alexandria, VA: National Technical Assistance Center for State Mental Health Planning.

Lee, H., Bahler, R., Chung, C., Alonzo, A., & Zeller, R. A. (2000). Prehospital delay with myocardial infarction: The interactive effect of clinical symptoms and race. *Applied Nursing Research, 13*(3), 125–133.

Lee, R. E., & Cubbin, C. (2002). Neighborhood context and youth cardiovascular health behaviors. *American Journal of Public Health, 92*(3), 428–436.

Leff, J., & Vaughn, C. (1985). *Expressed emotion in families: Its significance for mental illness.* New York: Guilford Press.

Leigh, B., & Stall, R. (1993). Substance use and risky sexual behavior for exposure to HIV: Issues in methodology, interpretation, and prevention. *American Psychologist, 48*(10), 1035–1045.

Leigh, W. A., & Jimenez, M. A. (2002). *Women of color health data book.* Bethesda, MD: Office of Research on Women's Health, National Institutes of Health.

Levine, D. M., Bone, L. R., Hill, M. N., Stallings, R., Gelber, A. C., Barker, A., et al. (2003). The effectiveness of a community/academic health center partnership in decreasing the level of blood pressure in an urban African-American population. *Ethnicity and Disease, 13*(3), 354–361.

Liao, Y., Cooper, R. S., Cao, G., Durazo-Arvizu, R., Kaufman, J. S., Luke, A., et al. (1998). Mortality patterns among adult Hispanics: Finding from the NHIS, 1986 to 1990. *American Journal of Public Health, 88*(2), 227–232.

Libby, D. L., Zhou, Z., & Kindig, D. A. (1997). Will minority physician supply meet U.S. needs? *Health Affairs, 16*(4), 205–214.

Lichtenstein, P., Harris, J. R., Pedersen, N. L., & McClearn, G. E. (1993). Socioeconomic status and physical health: How are they related? An empirical study based on twins reared apart and twins reared together. *Social Science and Medicine, 36*(4), 441–450.

Lillie-Blanton, M., Schuster, C. R., & Anthony, J. C. (2002). Probing the meaning of racial/ethnic group comparisons in crack-cocaine smoking. In T. A. LaVeist (Ed.), *Race, ethnicity and health: A public health reader* (pp. 494–503). San Francisco: Jossey-Bass.

Lin, K. M. (1983). *Hwa-byung:* A Korean culture-bound syndrome? *American Journal of Psychiatry, 140*(1), 105–107.

Lin, N., & Ensel, W. M. (1989). Life stress and health: Stressors and resources. *American Sociological Review, 54*, 382–399.

Lin-Fu, J. S. (1988). Population characteristics and health care needs of Asian Pacific Americans. *Public Health Report, 103*(1),18–27.

Litt, I. F., & Cuskey, W. R. (1984). Satisfaction with health care: A predictor of adolescents' appointment keeping. *Journal of Adolescent Health Care, 5*(3), 196–200.

Liu, W. T. (1985). Asian/Pacific American elderly: Mortality differentials, health status, and use of health services. *Journal of Applied Gerontology, 4*(1), 35–64.

Long, J. C., Knowler, W. C., Hanson, R. L., Robin, R. W., Urbanek, M., Moore, E., et al. (1998). Evidence for genetic linkage to alcohol dependence on chromosomes 4 and 11 from an autosome-wide scan in an American Indian population. *American Journal of Medical Genetics, 81*(3), 216–221.

Lopez, S. R., Nelson, K. A., Polo, J. A., Jenkins, J., Karno, M., & Snyder, K. (1998, August). *Family warmth and the course of schizophrenia of Mexican Americans and Anglo Americans.* Paper presented at the International Congress of Applied Psychology, San Francisco.

Luke, D., Esmundo, E., & Bloom, Y. (2000). Smoke signs: Patterns of tobacco billboard advertising in a metropolitan region. *Tobacco Control, 9*(1), 16–23.

Lundberg, O. (1993). The impact of childhood living conditions on illness and mortality in adulthood. *Social Science and Medicine, 36*(8), 1047–1052.

Makimoto, K., Oda, H., & Higuchi, S. (2000). Is heavy alcohol consumption an attributable risk factor for cancer-related deaths among Japanese men? *Alcoholism, Clinical and Experimental Research, 24*(3), 382–385.

Mandelblatt, J. S., Yabroff, K. R., & Kerner, J. F. (1999). Equitable access to cancer services: A review of barriers to quality care. *Cancer, 86*(11), 2378–2390.

Mann, J. J., Oquendo, M., Underwood, M. D., & Arango, V. (1999). The neurobiology of suicide risk: A review for the clinician. *Journal of Clinical Psychiatry, 60*(Suppl. 2), 7–11.

Manson, S. M., Shore, J. H., & Bloom, J. D. (1985). The depressive experience in American Indian communities: A challenge for psychiatric theory and diagnosis. In A. Kleinman & B. Good (Eds.), *Culture and depression* (pp. 331–368). Berkeley: University of California Press.

Marin, B. V., Tschann, J. M., Gomez, C. A., & Kegeles, S. M. (1993). Acculturation and gender differences in sexual attitudes and behaviors: Hispanic vs. non-Hispanic White unmarried adults. *American Journal of Public Health, 83*(12), 1759–1761.

Marin, M. G., Johanson, W. G., Jr., & Salas-Lopez, D. (2002). Influenza vaccination among minority populations in the United States. *Preventive Medicine, 34*(2), 235–241.

Markides, K. S., & Coreil, J. (1986). The health of Hispanics in the southwestern United States: An epidemiologic paradox. *Public Health Report, 101*(3), 253–265.

Markides, K. S., & Machalek, R. (1984). Selective survival, aging, and society. *Archives of Gerontology and Geriatrics, 3*(3), 207–222.

Marmot, M. G., Adelstein, A. M., & Bulusu, L. (1984). Lessons from the study of immigrant mortality. *Lancet, 2,* 1455–1457.

Marsella, A. J., Oliveira, J. M., Plummer, C. M., & Crabbe, K. M. (1995). Native Hawaiian culture, mind, and well-being. In H. I. McCubbin, E. A. Thompson, A. I. Thompson, & J. E. Fromer (Eds.), *Resiliency in ethnic minority families* (pp. 93–113). Madison: Center for Excellence in Family Studies, University of Wisconsin.

Marsh, J. V., Brett, K. M., & Miller, L. C. (1999). Racial differences in hormone replacement therapy prescriptions. *Obstetrics and Gynecology, 93*(6), 999–1003.

Martin, L. M., Calle, E. E., Wingo, P. A., & Heath, C. W., Jr. (1996). Comparison of mammography and Pap test use from the 1987 and 1992 National Health Interview Surveys: Are we closing the gaps? *American Journal of Preventive Medicine, 12*(2), 82–90.

Mash, E. J., & Dozois, D. J. (1996). Childhood psychopathology: A developmental-systems perspective. In E. J. Mash & R. A. Barkley (Eds.), *Child psychopathology* (pp. 3–62). New York: Guilford Press.

Mayo, R. M., Ureda, J. R., & Parker, V. G. (2001). Importance of fatalism in understanding mammography screening in rural elderly women. *Journal of Women and Aging, 13*(1), 57–72.

McLaughlin, L., & Braun, K. (1998). Asian and Pacific Islander values: Considerations for health care decision making. *Health and Social Work, 23*(2), 116–126.

McMahon, L. F., Jr., Wolfe, R. A., Huang, S., Tedeschi, P., Manning, W., Jr., & Edlund, M. J. (1999). Racial and gender variation in use of diagnostic colonic procedures in the Michigan Medicare population. *Medical Care, 37*(7), 712–717.

Metzler, M. M., Higgins, D. L., Beeker, C. G., Freudenberg, N., Lantz, P. M., Senturia, K. D., et al. (2003). Addressing urban health in Detroit, New York City, and Seattle through community-based participatory research partnerships. *American Journal of Public Health, 93*(5), 803–811.

Miller, B. A., Kolonel, L. N., Berstein, L., Young, J. L., Swanson, G. M., West, D., et al. (Eds.). (1996). *Racial/ethnic patterns of cancer in the United States, 1988–1992.* Bethesda, MD: National Cancer Institute.

Miniño, A. M., Arias, E., Kochanek, K. D., Murphy, S. L., & Smith, B. L. (2002). Deaths: Final data for 2000. *National Vital Statistics Reports, 50*(15), 1–120.

Mishra, S. I., Luce-Aoelua, P. H., & Hubbell, F. A. (2000). Knowledge of and attitudes about cancer among American Samoans. *Cancer Detection, 24*(2), 186–195.

Mishra, S. I., Luce-Aoelua, P. H., & Wilkens, L. R. (1996). Cancer among indigenous populations: The experience of American Samoans. *Cancer, 78*(Suppl. 7), 1553–1557.

Mokuau, N., & Browne, C. (1994). Life themes of Native Hawaiian female elders: Resources for cultural preservation. *Social Work, 39*(1), 43–49.

Mokuau, N., Lukela, D., Obra, A., & Voeller, M. (1997). *Native Hawaiian spirituality: A perspective on connections.* Honolulu: University of Hawaii School of Social Work and Kamehameha Schools Bishop Estate Native Hawaiian Safe and Drug Free Schools and Communities Program.

Mokuau, N., Reid, N., & Napalapalai, N. (2002). *Ho'omana (spirituality): Views of native Hawaiian women.* Honolulu: University of Hawaii School of Social Work.

Mokuau, N., & Tauili'ili, P. (1998). Families with Native Hawaiian and Samoan roots. In E. W. Lynch & M. J. Hanson (Eds.), *Developing cross-cultural competence* (pp. 409–440). Baltimore: Brookes.

Montagu, A. (1942). *Man's most dangerous myth: The fallacy of race.* New York: World.

Montagu, A. (1964). The concept of race in the human species in the light of genetics. In A. Montagu (Ed.), *The concept of race.* New York: Free Press.

Morland, K., Poole, C., Roux, A. D., & Wing, S. (2002). Neighborhood characteristics associated with the location of food stores and service places. In T. A. LaVeist (Ed.), *Race, ethnicity, and health: A public health reader* (pp. 448–462). San Francisco: Jossey-Bass.

Morris, A. D. (1986). *Origins of the civil rights movements.* New York: Free Press.

Morrison, R. S., Wallenstein, S., Natale, D. K., Senzel, R. S., & Huang, L. L. (2002). "We don't carry that": Failure of pharmacies in predominantly non-White neighborhoods to stock opioid analgesics. In T. A. LaVeist (Ed.), *Race, ethnicity, and health: A public health reader* (pp. 463–472). San Francisco: Jossey-Bass.

Moscicki, E. K. (2001). Epidemiology of completed and attempted suicide: Toward a framework for prevention. *Clinical Neuroscience Research, 1,* 310–323.

Mosley, J. D., Appel, L. J., Ashour, Z., Coresh, J., Whelton, P. K., & Ibrahim, M. M. (2000). Relationship between skin color and blood pressure in Egyptian adults: Results from the National Hypertension Project. *Hypertension, 36*(2), 296–302.

Mountain, J. L., & Cavalli-Sforza, L. L. (1997). Multilocus genotypes, a tree of individuals, and human evolutionary history. *American Journal of Human Genetics, 61*(3), 705–718.

Moure-Eraso, R., & Friedman-Jimenez, G. (2001). Occupational health among Latino workers in the urban setting. In M. Aguirre-Molina, C. W. Molina, & R. E. Zambrana (Eds.), *Health issues in the Latino community* (pp. 327–358). San Francisco: Jossey-Bass.

Moure-Eraso, R., Wilcox, M., Punnett, L., Copeland, L., & Levenstein, C. (1994). Back to the future: Sweatshop conditions on the Mexico-U.S. border. I. Community health impact of *maquiladora* industrial activity. *American Journal of Industrial Medicine, 25*(3), 311–324.

Moure-Eraso, R., Wilcox, M., Punnett, L., MacDonald, L., & Levenstein, C. (1997). Back to the future: Sweatshop conditions on the Mexico-U.S. border. II. Occupational health impact of *maquiladora* industrial activity. *American Journal of Industrial Medicine, 31*(5), 587–599.

Moy, E., & Bartman, B. A. (1995). Physician race and care of minority and medically indigent patients. *Journal of the American Medical Association, 273*(19), 1515–1520.

Mui, A. C., & Burnette, D. (1994). Long-term care service use by frail elders: Is ethnicity a factor? *Gerontologist, 34*(2), 190–198.

Murray, C. J. L., & Lopez, A. D. (1996). The global burden of disease: A comprehensive assessment of mortality and disability from diseases, injuries, and risk factors in 1990 and projected to 2020. Cambridge, MA: Harvard School of Public Health.

Nakao, K., & Treas, J. (1994). Updating occupational prestige and socioeconomic sources: How the new measures measure up. In P. Marsden (Ed.), *Sociological methodology* (pp. 1–72). Washington, DC: American Sociological Association.

Nam, C. B., & Powers, M. G. (1983). *The socioeconomic approach to status measurement.* Houston, TX: Cap and Gown Press.

Napholz, L. (2000). Bicultural resynthesis: Tailoring an effectiveness trial for a group of urban American Indian women. *American Indian/Alaska Native Mental Health Research, 9*(3), 49–70.

Narikiyo, T. A., & Kameoka, V. A. (1992). Attributions of mental illness and judgments about help seeking among Japanese-American and White American students. *Journal of Counseling Psychology, 39,* 363–369.

National Center for Complementary and Alternative Medicine. (2004). *The use of complementary and alternative medicine in the United States.* Retrieved August 8, 2004, from http://nccam.nih.gov/news/camsurvey_fs1.htm.

National Center for Healt Statistics. (2003). *National Vital Statistics Reports, 52*(3), Sept. 18.

National Center for Health Statistics. (2003). *Health, United States, 2003.* Hyattsville, MD: Author, Centers for Disease Control and Prevention, U.S. Department of Health and Human Services.

National Institute on Alcohol Abuse and Alcoholism. (1995). *The physicians' guide to helping patients with alcohol problems.* Rockville, MD: National Institutes of Health.

National Institute on Drug Abuse. (1995). *Drug use among racial/ethnic minorities.* Rockville, MD: National Institutes of Health.

National Institutes of Health. (2002). *Women of color health data book.* Retrieved November 12, 2004, from http://www4.od.nih.gov/orwh/wocEnglish2002.pdf.

National Institutes of Health. (n.d.). *What are health disparities?* Retrieved November 12, 2004, from http://healthdisparities.nih.gov/whatare.html.

National Research Council. (1991). *Environmental epidemiology: Vol. 1. Public health and hazardous wastes.* Washington, DC: National Academies Press.

Neighbors, H. W., Musick, M. A., & Williams, D. R. (1998). The African American minister as a source of help for serious personal crises: Bridge or barrier to mental health care? *Health Education and Behavior, 25*(6), 759–777.

Newsholme, A. (1910). *39th annual report of the local government board* (CD5312). London.

Ng, C. H. (1997). The stigma of mental illness in Asian cultures. *Australian and New Zealand Journal of Psychiatry, 31*(3), 382–390.

Ngo-Metzger, Q., Massagli, M. P., Clarridge, B. R., Manocchia, M., Davis, R. B., Iezzoni, L. I., et al. (2003). Linguistic and cultural barriers to care. *Journal of General Internal Medicine, 18*(1), 44–52.

Nobles, M. (2000). History counts: A comparative analysis of racial/color categorization in U.S. and Brazilian censuses. *American Journal of Public Health, 90*(11), 1738–1745.

Novins, D. K., Beals, J., Moore, L. A., Spicer, P., Manson, S. M., & AI-SUPERPFP Team. (2004). Use of biomedical services and traditional healing options among American Indians: Sociodemographic correlates, spirituality, and ethnic identity. *Medical Care, 42*(7), 670–679.

Novins, D. K., Beals, J., Roberts, R. E., & Manson, S. M. (1999). Factors associated with suicide ideation among American Indian adolescents: Does culture matter? *Suicide and Life Threatening Behavior, 29*(4), 332–346.

Office of Minority Health. (1988). *Closing the gap: Heart disease, stroke, and minorities.* Washington, DC: U.S. Department of Health and Human Services.

Office of Minority Health. (1999). *Standards for culturally and linguistically appropriate health care services.* Retrieved August 10, 2004, from http://www.omhrc.gov/clas/ds.htm.

Pachter, L. M. (1994). Culture and clinical care: Folk illness beliefs and behaviors and their implications for health care delivery. *Journal of the American Medical Association, 271*(9), 690–694.

Padgett, D. A., & Glaser, R. (2003). How stress influences the immune response. *Trends in Immunology, 24*(8), 444–448.

Padgett, J., & Biro, F. M. (2003). Different shapes in different cultures: Body dissatisfaction, overweight, and obesity in African American and Caucasian females. *Journal of Pediatric and Adolescent Gynecology, 16*(6), 349–354.

Palafox, N., & Warren, A. (Eds.). (1980). *Cross-cultural caring: A handbook for health care professionals in Hawaii.* Honolulu: University of Hawaii School of Medicine.

Papa Ola Lokahi (Native Hawaiian Health Board). (1998). *Technical proposal for the Pacific Basin Regional Training Center.* Honolulu: Author.

Park, Y. J., Kim, H. S., Kang, H. C., & Kim, J. W. (2001). A survey of *hwa-byung* in middle-aged Korean women. *Journal of Transcultural Nursing, 12*(2), 115–122.

Pate, R. R., Pratt, M., Blair, S. N., Haskel, W. L., Macera, C. A., Bouchard, C., et al. (1995). Physical activity and public health: A recommendation from the Centers for Disease Control and Prevention and the American College of Sports Medicine. *Journal of the American Medical Association, 273*(5), 402–407.

Pearlman, D. N., Rakowski, W., Ehrich, B., & Clark, M. A. (1996). Breast cancer screening practices among Black, Hispanic, and White women: Reassessing differences. *American Journal of Preventive Medicine, 12*(5), 327–337.

Peete, C. T. (1999). The importance of place of residence in health outcomes research: How does living in an ethnic enclave affect low birth weight deliveries for Hispanic mothers? *Dissertation Abstracts International, 60,* 1777A.

Perez-Stable, E. J., Napoles-Springer, A., & Miramontes, J. M. (1997). The effects of ethnicity and language on medical outcomes of patients with hypertension or diabetes. *Medical Care, 35*(12), 1212–1219.

Pescosolido, B. A., Monahan, J., Link, B. G., Stueve, A., & Kikuzawa, S. (1999). The public's view of the competence, dangerousness, and need for legal coercion of persons with mental health problems. *American Journal of Public Health, 89*(9), 1339–1345.

Pinhey, T. K., Heathcote, G. M., & Rarick, J. (1994). The influence of obesity on the self-reported health status of Chamorros and other residents of Guam. *Asian American and Pacific Islander Journal of Health, 2*(3), 195–211.

Pinhey, T. K., Rubinstein, D. H., & Colfax, R. S. (1997). Overweight and happiness: The reflected self-appraisal hypothesis reconsidered. *Social Science Quarterly, 78,* 747–755.

Polednak, A. P. (1991). Black-White differences in infant mortality in 38 standard metropolitan statistical areas. *American Journal of Public Health, 81*(11), 1480–1482.

Portugal, A. M., & Claro, A. (1993). Virgin and martyr. *Conscience, 14*(1–2), 28–32.

Powell, K. E., Thompson, P. D., Caspersen, C. J., & Kendrick, J. S. (1987). Physical activity and the incidence of coronary heart disease. *Annual Review of Public Health, 8,* 253–287.

Pridemore, W. A. (2002). What we know about social structure and homicide: A review of the theoretical and empirical literature. *Violence and Victims, 17*(2), 127–156.

Pucci, L. G., Joseph, H. M., Jr., & Siegel, M. (1998). Outdoor tobacco advertising in six Boston neighborhoods: Evaluating youth exposure. *American Journal of Preventive Medicine, 15*(2), 155–159.

Quarles, B. (1987). *The Negro in the making of America.* New York: Collier.

Quigley, D., Handy, D., Goble, R., Sanchez, V., & George, P. (2000). Participatory research strategies in nuclear risk management for native communities. *Journal of Health Communication, 5*(4), 305–331.

Quinn, K. (2000). *Working with benefits: The health insurance crisis confronting Hispanic-Americans.* New York: Commonwealth Fund.

Raczynski, J. M., Taylor, H., Cutter, G., Hardin, M., Rappaport, N., & Oberman, A. (1994). Diagnoses, symptoms, and attribution of symptoms among Black and White inpatients admitted for coronary heart disease. *American Journal of Public Health, 84*(6), 951–956.

Rafanelli, C., Roncuzzi, R., Finos, L., Tossani, E., Tomba, E., Mangelli, L., et al. (2003). Psychological assessment in cardiac rehabilitation. *Psychotherapy and Psychosomatics, 72*(6), 343–349.

Ramirez, J. R., Crano, W. D., Quist, R., Burgoon, M., Alvaro, E. M., & Grandpre, J. (2004). Acculturation, familism, parental monitoring, and knowledge as predictors of marijuana and inhalant use in adolescents. *Psychology of Addictive Behaviors, 18*(1), 3–11.

Rawlings, J. S., & Weir, M. R. (1992). Race- and rank-specific infant mortality in a U.S. military population. *American Journal of Diseases of Children, 146*(3), 313–316.

Redfern, P. (2001). A Bayesian model for estimating census undercount, taking emigration data from foreign censuses. *International Statistical Review, 69*(2), 277–301.

Rezentes, W. C., III. (1996). *Ka lama kukui Hawaiian psychology: An introduction.* Honolulu: 'A'ali'i Books.

Risch, N., Burchard, E., Ziv, E., & Tang, H. (2002). Categorization of humans in biomedical research: Genes, race, and disease. *Genome Biology, 3*(7), comment 2007.

Riston, E. D. (1999). Alcohol, drugs, and stigma. *International Journal of Clinical Practice, 53*(7), 549–551.

Robert Wood Johnson Foundation. (2004). *Working toward dismantling the language barrier in health care.* Retrieved August 7, 2004, from http://www.rwjf.org/news/special/languageBarrier_2.jhtml.

Robinson, J. C. (1985). Racial inequality and the probability of occupation-related injury or illness. *Milbank Quarterly, 62*(4), 567–590.

Robinson, J. C. (1989). Exposure to occupational hazards among Hispanics, Blacks, and non-Hispanic Whites in California. *American Journal of Public Health, 79*(5), 629–630.

Romero, G. L., Wyatt, G. E., & Singer, M. (1998). HIV-related behaviors among recently immigrated and undocumented Latinas. *International Quarterly of Community Health Education, 18*(1), 89–105.

Romero-Daza, N., Weeks, M., & Singer, M. (1998). Much more than HIV! The reality of life on the streets for drug-using sex workers in inner-city Hartford. *International Quarterly of Community Health Education, 18*(1), 107–119.

Ross, C. E., & Mirowsky, J. (2001). Neighborhood disadvantage, disorder, and health. *Journal of Health and Social Behavior, 42*(3), 258–276.

Rutherford, M. S., & Roux, G. M. (2002). Health beliefs and practices in rural El Salvador: An ethnographic study. *Journal of Cultural Diversity, 9*(1), 3–11.

Ryan, C., Shaw, R., Pliam, M., Zapolanski, A. J., Murphy, M., Valle, H. V., et al. (2000). Coronary heart disease in Filipino and Filipino American patients: Prevalence of risk factors and outcomes of treatment. *Journal of Invasive Cardiology, 12*(3), 134–139.

Sacco, R. L., Boden-Albala, B., Gan, R., Chen, X., Kargman, D. E., Shea, S., et al. (1998). Stroke incidence among White, Black, and Hispanic residents of an urban community: The Northern Manhattan Stroke Study. *American Journal of Epidemiology, 147*(3), 259–268.

Saha, S., Komaromy, M., Koepsell, T. D., & Bindman, A. B. (1999). Patient-physician racial concordance and the perceived quality and use of health care. *Archives of Internal Medicine, 159*(9), 997–1004.

Saha, S., Taggart, S. H., Komaromy, M., & Bindman, A. B. (2000). Do patients choose physicians of their own race? *Health Affairs, 19*(1), 76–83.

Sameroff, A. J. (1993). Models of development and developmental risk. In C. H. Zeanah Jr. (Ed.), *Handbook of infant mental health* (pp. 3–13). New York: Guilford Press.

Sampson, R. J., & Laub, J. H. (1994). Urban poverty and the family context of delinquency: A new look at structure and process in a classic study. *Child Development, 65*(Spec. iss. 2), 523–540.

Schaefer, D. C., & Cheskin, L. J. (1998). Constipation in the elderly. *American Family Physician, 58*(4), 907–914.

Schaubroeck, J., Lam, S. S., & Xie, J. L. (2000). Collective efficacy versus self-efficacy in coping responses to stressors and control: A cross-cultural study. *Journal of Applied Psychology, 85*(4), 512–525.

Schoendorf, K., Hogue, C. J., Kleinman, J., & Rowley, D. L. (1992). Mortality among infants of Black as compared to White college graduates. *New England Journal of Medicine, 326*(23), 1522–1526.

Schulte, L. J., & Battle, J. (2003). The relative importance of ethnicity and religion in predicting attitudes towards gays and lesbians. *Journal of Homosexuality, 47*(2), 127–142.

Scribner, R., & Dwyer, J. H. (1989). Acculturation and low birth weight among Latinos in the Hispanic HANES. *American Journal of Public Health, 79*(9), 1263–1267.

Segen, J. C. (1992). *The dictionary of modern medicine.* Park Ridge, NJ: Parthenon.

Seifer, R., Sameroff, A. J., Baldwin, C. P., & Baldwin, A. (1992). Child and family factors that ameliorate risk between 4 and 13 years of age. *Journal of the American Academy of Child and Adolescent Psychiatry, 31*(5), 893–903.

Shaughnessy, L., Doshi, S. R., & Jones, S. E. (2004). Attempted suicide and associated health risk behaviors among Native American high school students. *Journal of School Health, 74*(5), 177–182.

Sheifer, S. E., Escarce, J. J., & Schulman, K. A. (2000). Race and sex differences in the management of coronary artery disease. *American Heart Journal, 139*(5), 848–857.

Shi, L. (1999). Experience of primary care by racial and ethnic groups in the United States. *Medical Care, 37*(10), 1068–1077.

Shyrock, H. S., Siegel, J. S., & Associates. (1976). *The methods and materials of demography* (cond. ed.). San Diego, CA: Academic Press.

Sikora, A. G., & Mulvihill, M. (2002). Trends in mortality due to legal intervention in the United States, 1979 through 1997. *American Journal of Public Health, 92*(5), 841–843.

Singh, G. K., & Yu, S. M. (2002). Adverse pregnancy outcomes: Differences between U.S.- and foreign-born women in major U.S. racial ethnic groups. In T. A. LaVeist (Ed.), *Race, ethnicity, and health: A public health reader* (pp. 265–279). San Francisco: Jossey-Bass.

Skinner, C. S., Strecher, V. J., & Hospers, H. (1994). Physicians' recommendations for mammography: Do tailored messages make a difference? *American Journal of Public Health, 84*(1), 43–49.

Smith, D. B. (1999). *Health care divided: Race and healing a nation.* Ann Arbor: University of Michigan Press.

Sobal, J., & Stunkard, A. J. (1989). Socioeconomic status and obesity: A review of the literature. *Psychological Bulletin, 105*(2), 260–275.

Soderfeldt, B., Soderfeldt, M., Ohlson, C. G., & Warg, L. E. (1996). Psychosomatic symptoms in human service work: A study on Swedish social workers and social insurance personnel. *Scandinavian Journal of Social Medicine, 24*(1), 43–49.

Sorlie, P. D., Backlund, E., Johnson, N. J., & Rogot, E. (1993). Mortality by Hispanic status in the United States. *Journal of the American Medical Association, 270*(20), 2464–2468.

Stark, A. J., Kane, R. L., Kane, R. A., & Finch, M. (1995). Effect on physical functioning of care in adult foster homes and nursing homes. *Gerontologist, 35*(5), 648–655.

Steinmetz, K. A., Potter, J. D., & Folsom, A. R. (1993). Vegetables, fruit, and lung cancer in the Iowa Women's Health Study. *Cancer Research, 53*(3), 536–543.

Stephen, E. H., Foote, K., Hendershot, G. E., & Schoenborn, C. A. (1994). *Health of the foreign-born population: United States, 1989–90.* Atlanta: Centers for Disease Control and Prevention.

Stillman, F. A., Bone, L. R., Rand, C., Levine, D. M., & Becker, D. M. (1993). Heart, body, and soul: A church-based smoking-cessation program for urban African Americans. *Preventive Medicine, 22*(3), 335–349.

Stinson, F. S., Grant, B. F., & Dufour, M. C. (2001). The critical dimension of ethnicity in liver cirrhosis mortality statistics. *Alcoholism: Clinical Experimental Research, 25*(8), 1181–1187.

Stoddard, J. L., Johnson, C. A., Boley-Cruz, T., & Sussman, S. (1997). Targeted tobacco markets: Outdoor advertising in Los Angeles minority neighborhoods. *American Journal of Public Health, 87*(7), 1232–1233.

Stolley, P. D. (1999). Race in epidemiology. *International Journal of Health Services, 29*(4), 905–909.

Stone, V. E., Mauch, M. Y., Steger, K., Janas, S. F., & Craven, D. E. (1997). Race, gender, drug use, and participation in AIDS clinical trials: Lessons from a municipal hospital cohort. *Journal of General Internal Medicine, 12*(3), 150–157.

Substance Abuse and Mental Health Services Administration. (2000). Retrieved February 22, 2005 from http://www.drugabusestatistics.samhsa.gov/nhsda.htm.

Substance Abuse and Mental Health Services Administration. (2001). Retrieved February 22, 2005 from http://www.drugabusestatistics.samhsa.gov/nhsda.htm.

Sue, S., & Morishima, J. K. (1982). *The mental health of Asian Americans.* San Francisco: Jossey-Bass.

Sue, S., Sue, D., Sue, L., & Takeuchi, D. (1995). Asian American psychopathology. *Cultural Diversity and Mental Health, 1*(1), 39–51.

Sufian, M., Friedman, S. R., Curtis, R., Neaigus, A., & Stepherson, B. (1991). Organizing as a new approach to AIDS risk reduction for intravenous drug users. *Journal of Addictive Diseases, 10*(4), 89–98.

Sumathipala, A., Siribaddana, S. H., & Bhughra, D. (2004). Culture-bound syndromes: The story of *dhat* syndrome. *British Journal of Psychiatry, 184,* 200–209.

Szwarcwald, C. L., Bastos, F. I., Barcellos, C., Pina, M. F., & Esteves, M. A. (2000). Health conditions and residential concentration of poverty: A study in Rio de Janeiro, Brazil. *Journal of Epidemiology and Community Health, 54*(7), 530–536.

Taira, D. A., Seto, T. B., & Marciel, C. (2001). Ethnic disparities in care following acute coronary syndromes among Asian Americans and Pacific Islanders during the initial hospitalization. *Cellular Molecular Biology, 47*(7), 1209–1215.

Takeuchi, D. T., Chung, R. C., & Shen, H. (1998). Health insurance coverage among Chinese Americans in Los Angeles County. *American Journal of Public Health, 88*(3), 451–453.

Tanjasiri, P., Wallace, S., & Shibata, K. (1995). Picture imperfect: Hidden problems among Asian and Pacific Islander elderly. *Gerontologist, 35*(6), 753–760.

Taylor, E. J. (1988). *Dorland's illustrated medical dictionary* (27th ed.). Philadelphia: Saunders.

Tharp, R. (1991). Cultural diversity and treatment of children. *Journal of Consulting and Clinical Psychology, 59*(6), 799–812.

Thompson, M. P., Kaslow, N. J., & Kingree, J. B. (2002). Risk factors for suicide attempts among African American women experiencing recent intimate partner violence. *Violence and Victims, 17*(3), 283–295.

Todd, K. H., Deaton, C., D'Adamo, A. P., & Goe, L. (2002). Ethnicity and analgesic practice. In T. A. LaVeist (Ed.), *Race, ethnicity and health: A public health reader* (pp. 507–515). San Francisco: Jossey-Bass.

Traustadottir, T., Bosch, P. R., & Matt, K. S. (2003). Gender differences in cardiovascular and hypothalamic-pituitary-adrenal axis responses to psychological stress in healthy older adult men and women. *Stress, 6*(2), 133–140.

Uba, L. (1992). Cultural barriers to health care for Southeast Asian refugees. *Public Health Report, 107*(5), 544–548.

U.S. Bureau of the Census. (1996). *Current population survey.* Washington, DC: Author.

U.S. Bureau of the Census. (2001). Population by race and Hispanic or Latino origin for the United States. Retrieved November 12, 2004, from http://www.census.gov/population/cen2000/phc-t1/tab01.pdf.

U.S. Commission on Civil Rights. (2004). *Broken promises: Evaluating the Native American health care system.* Washington, D.C.: Author.

U.S. Department of Health and Human Services. (1996). *Physical activity and health: A report of the surgeon general.* Atlanta: Author.

U.S. Department of Health and Human Services. (1998). *Tobacco use among U.S. racial/ethnic minority groups—African Americans, American Indians and Alaska Natives, Asian Americans and Pacific Islanders, and Hispanics: A report of the surgeon general.* Atlanta: Author.

U.S. Department of Health and Human Services. (1999). *Mental health: A report of the surgeon general.* Rockville, MD: Author.

U.S. Department of Health and Human Services. (2001). *Mental health: Culture, race, and ethnicity— a supplement to* Mental health: A report of the surgeon general. Rockville, MD: Author.

van Ryn, M., & Burke, J. (2002). The effect of patient race and socioeconomic status on physicians' perceptions of patients. In T. A. LaVeist (Ed.), *Race, ethnicity, and health: A public health reader* (pp. 547–575). San Francisco: Jossey-Bass.

van Sickle, D., Morgan, F., & Wright, A. L. (2003). Qualitative study of the use of traditional healing by asthmatic Navajo families. *American Indian and Alaska Native Mental Health Research, 11*(1), 1–18.

Vega, W. A., Kolody, B., Aguilar-Gaxiola, S., Alderete, E., Catalano, R., & Caraveo-Anduaga, J. (1998). Lifetime prevalence of DSM-III-R psychiatric disorders among urban and rural Mexican Americans in California. *Archives of General Psychiatry, 55*(9), 771–778.

Voorhees, C. C., Stillman, F. A., Swank, R. T., Heagerty, P. J., Levine, D. M., & Becker, D. M. (1996). Heart, body, and soul: Impact of church-based smoking cessation interventions on readiness to quit. *Preventive Medicine, 25*(3), 277–285.

Wachtler, C., & Troein, M. (2003). A hidden curriculum: Mapping cultural competency in a medical programme. *Medical Education, 37*(10), 861–868.

Wagner, E. H., LaCroix, A. Z., Buchner, D. M., & Larson, E. B. (1992). Effects of physical activity on health status in older adults: I. Observational studies. *Annual Review of Public Health, 13,* 451–468.

Wallace, J. M., Jr. (1999). Explaining race differences in adolescent and young adult drug use: The role of racialized social systems. *Drugs and Society, 14*(1–2), 21–36.

Wallace, J. M., Jr., Bachman, J. G., O'Malley, P. M., Johnston, L. D., Schulenberg, J. E., & Cooper, S. M. (2002). Tobacco, alcohol, and illicit drug use: Racial and ethnic differences among U.S. high school seniors, 1976–2000. *Public Health Report, 117*(Suppl. 1), S67–S75.

Wallace, S. P., Levy-Storms, L., Kington, R. S., & Andersen, R. M. (1998). The persistence of race and ethnicity in the use of long-term care. *Journals of Gerontology. Series B, Psychological Sciences and Social Sciences, 53*(2), S104–S112.

Weber, W. W. (1999). Populations and genetic polymorphisms. *Molecular Diagnosis, 4*(4), 299–307.

Weinrich, S. P., Weinrich, M. C., Keil, J. E., Gazes, P. C., & Potter, E. (1988). The John Henryism and Framingham type A scales: Measurement properties in elderly Blacks and Whites. *American Journal of Epidemiology, 128*(1), 165–178.

Weissman, M. M., Bland, R. C., Canino, G. J., Faravelli, C., Greenwald, S., Hwu, H. G., et al. (1996). Cross-national epidemiology of major depression and bipolar disorder. *Journal of the American Medical Association, 276*(4), 293–299.

Weissman, M. M., Bland, R. C., Canino, G. J., Faravelli, C., Greenwald, S., Hwu, H. G., et al. (1997). The cross-national epidemiology of panic disorder. *Archives of General Psychiatry, 54*(4), 305–309.

Weissman, M. M., Bland, R. C., Canino, G. J., Greenwald, S., Hwu, H. G., Joyce, P. R., et al. (1999). Prevalence of suicide ideation and suicide attempts in nine countries. *Psychological Medicine, 29*(1), 9–17.

Weissman, M. M., Bland, R. C., Canino, G. J., Greenwald, S., Hwu, H. G., Lee, C. K., et al. (1994). The cross-national epidemiology of obsessive compulsive disorder. *Journal of Clinical Psychiatry, 55*(Suppl.), 5–10.

Wen, M., Browning, C. R., & Cagney, K. A. (2003) Poverty, affluence, and income inequality: Neighborhood economic structure and its implications for health. *Social Science and Medicine, 57*(5), 843–860.

Wergowske, G., Blanchette, P. L., & Diaz, J. H. (1999). Aging and health among Pacific Islanders. *Clinical Geriatrics, 7*(7), 54–69.

Whittle, J., Good, J., Conigliaro, C. B., & Lofgren, R. P. (1993). Racial differences in the use of invasive cardiovascular procedures in the Department of Veterans Affairs medical system. *New England Journal of Medicine, 329*(9), 621–627.

Wildsmith, E. M. (2002). Testing the weathering hypothesis among Mexican-origin women. *Ethnicity and Disease, 12*(4), 470–479.

Williams, D. R. (1994). Race in health services research, 1966 to 1990. *Health Services Research, 29*(3), 261–274.

Williams, D. R., Neighbors, H. W., & Jackson, J. S. (2003). Racial/ethnic discrimination and health: Findings from community studies. *American Journal of Public Health, 93*(2), 200–208.

Wilson, M. G., May, D. S., & Kelly, J. J. (1994). Racial differences in the use of total knee arthroplasty for osteoarthritis among older Americans. *Ethnicity and Disease, 4*(1), 57–67.

Wilson, T. W., & Grim, C. E. (1991). Biohistory of slavery and blood pressure differences in blacks today: A hypothesis. *Hypertension,* 17(Suppl. 1), I122–I128.

Wolf, A. M., Spitz, A. H., Olson, G., Zavodska, A., & Algharaibeh, M. (2003). Characterization of the solid waste stream of the Tohono O'odham nation. *Journal of Environmental Health, 65*(8), 9–15, 25.

Wong, M. M., Klingle, R. S., & Price, R. K. (2004). Alcohol, tobacco, and other drug use among Asian American and Pacific Islander adolescents in California and Hawaii. *Addictive Behavior, 29*(1), 127–141.

Woolhandler, S., & Himmelstein, D. U. (1991). The deteriorating administrative efficiency of the U.S. health care system. *New England Journal of Medicine, 342*(18), 1253–1258.

World Health Organization. (1946). *Constitution of the World Health Organization.* Retrieved February 17, 2005 from http://w3.whosea.org/aboutsearo/pdf/const.pdf.

World Health Organization. (2000). Obesity: Preventing and managing the global epidemic. Geneva: Author.

Yamashiro, G., & Matsuoka, J. K. (1997). Help-seeking among Asian and Pacific Americans: A multiperspective analysis. *Social Work, 42*(2), 176–186.

Yankauer, A. (1950). The relationship of fetal and infant mortality to residential segregation. *American Sociological Review, 15*(5), 644–648.

Yi, J. K. (1995). Acculturation, access to care, and use of preventive health services by Vietnamese women. *Asian American and Pacific Islander Journal of Health, 3*(1), 30–41.

Yoon, Y. H., Yi, H., Grant, B. F., Stinson, F. S., & Dufour, M. C. (2003). Liver cirrhosis mortality in the United States, 1970–2000. Bethesda, MD: National Institute on Alcohol Abuse and Alcoholism.

Yusuf, H. R., Croft, J. B., Giles, W. H., Anda, R. F., Casper, M. L., Caspersen, C. J., et al. (1996). Leisure-time physical activity among older adults, United States, 1990. *Archives of Internal Medicine, 156*(12), 1321–1326.

Zhang, A. Y., Snowden, L. R., & Sue, S. (1998). Differences between Asian and White Americans' help-seeking and utilization patterns in the Los Angeles area. *Journal of Community Psychology, 26*(4), 317–326.

Zuckerman, S., Haley, J., Roubideaux, Y., & Lillie-Blanton, M. (2004). Health service access, use, and insurance coverage among American Indians/Alaska Natives and Whites: What role does the Indian Health Service play? *American Journal of Public Health, 94*(1), 53–59.

NAME INDEX

A

Abbey, H., 121
Abraido-Lanza, A. F., 277
Acevedo-Garcia, D., 137
Adelstein, A. M., 278
Aguirre-Molina, M., 261
Albano, A. M., 87, 91
Albrecht, S. L., 191
Alderman, M. H., 137
Algharaibeh, M., 234
Ali, S., 121, 212
Alonzo, A., 198
Amey, C. H., 191
Amshel, C. E., 257
Andersen, R. M., 112, 121, 127
Anderson, L. M., 121, 274
Anderson, N. B., 150
Anderson, O. W., 158
Anderson, R. T., 137
Andrews, R., 121
Antai-Otong, D., 200
Anthony, J. C., 141, 191
Arango, V., 89
Arbelaez, D. S., 254
Arias, E., 89
Armistead, L., 200

Arriola, R. J., 216
Austin, B. J., 200
Ayanian, J. Z., 106

B

Backlund, E., 277
Backman, J. G., 191
Bahler, R., 198
Baker, D. W., 271
Bal, D. G., 181
Balbach, E. D., 141
Balcazar, H., 274
Balcaze, H., 274
Baldwin, A., 102
Baldwin, C. P., 102
Barbeau, E. M., 141
Barcellos, C., 174
Barkey, N., 155
Barlow, D. H., 87
Bartels, S. J., 251
Bartman, B. A., 123
Bastos, F. I., 174
Battle, J., 216
Bay, R. C., 274
Beach, C. M., 254
Beals, J., 236, 240

Bebbington, P., 103
Becker, A. B., 295
Becker, D. M., 295
Becker, E. L., 21
Berkman, L. F., 214, 234
Bernier, F., 16
Bernzeval, M., 285
Bertakis, K. D., 123
Betancourt, J. R., 270
Bindman, A. B., 123, 124, 213
Biro, F. M., 219
Blackburn, H., 154
Blanchette, P. L., 248
Blendon, R. J., 212
Block, G., 184
Bloom, J. D., 100
Blum, R. W., 240
Blumenbach, J. F., 16, 17
Bobo, J. K., 196
Boley-Cruz, T., 141
Bonadonna, R. J., 199
Bone, L. R., 295
Bonkowsky, J. L., 275
Borowsky, I. W., 240
Borsboom, G. J., 174
Bosch, P. R., 151
Bosma, H., 174

SUBJECT INDEX

A

Aboriginal social pathology theory, 240

Accidents (unintentional injuries): AIANs (American Indians/Alaska Natives) and, 237–238*fig*; alcohol and motor vehicle, 239*t*; labor law violations and, 272

Acculturation: APIs (Asian/Pacific Islanders) health status and, 258; Hispanics/Latinos health status and, 274–275. *See also* Cultural differences

Acculturation/immigration theory of health disparities, 147–149

Acute condition, 72*b*, 210*b*

AD (Alzheimer's disease), 96

ADHD (attention-deficit/hyperactivity disorder), 93–95

ADLs (activities of daily living): comparative morbidity and, 78–80; defining, 79*b*

Advisory Committee on Immunization Practices (CDC), 196

Affective functioning, 84*b*

African American culture: *John Henryism* hypothesis and, 124, 144–147*b*; male-to-male sex taboo of, 216

African Americans: alcohol consumption among, 192*fig*; Black medical schools and, 3, 4*b*; changing status (1619-2004) of, 2*fig*; death rates/causes of death among, 206–211*t*, 216–218; health care access/utilization by, 211–213; living near toxic waste sites, 140–141; low birth weight by mother's age, 144*fig*; low SES as major health risk of, 213–222*fig*; maternal and child health of, 220*t*–221; mortality crossover and, 68–72; perceived health care discrimination by, 117, 118*t*; preventive service utilization by, 196*t*–197*fig*; slave experience of, 1; slavery hypertension hypothesis on, 153, 154–155; smoking behavior by, 221–222*fig*; Tuskegee Syphilis Study and, 3, 4*b*; utilization of

mental health services by, 103–104; wealth among total U.S. population and, 169*t*

Age adjustment (age-standardization), 57*b*

Age adjustment mortality rates: AIAN (American Indians/Alaska Natives), 226*t*–227, 238*fig*, 246*t*; alcohol-related liver cirrhosis, 193*fig*; APIs (Asian/Pacific Islanders), 245–246*t*; comparing African Americans to other groups, 206–207*t*; Hispanics/Latinos (2001), 264*t*; historical trends in, 55–57*fig*; of HIV/AIDS by race/ethnicity, 215*fig*; homicide by race/ethnicity, 217*fig*; income inequality (1999) vs., 176*fig*; by race/ethnicity (1940-2000), 57*fig*; by race/ethnicity (1999), 47*b*; by race/ethnicity (2001), 59*fig*; by sex, 56*fig*. *See also* Mortality rates

AIAN (American Indian/Alaska Native). *See* Alaska Natives; American Indians